Atlas of Immunohistology

ATLAS OF IMMUNOHISTOLOGY

Raymond R. Tubbs, DO

Gordon N. Gephardt, MD

Robert E. Petras, MD

Department of Pathology
The Cleveland Clinic Foundation
Cleveland, Ohio

AMERICAN SOCIETY OF CLINICAL PATHOLOGISTS PRESS
CHICAGO

NOTICE

Trade names for equipment and supplies described herein are included as suggestions only. In no way does their inclusion constitute an endorsement or preference by the American Society of Clinical Pathologists. The ASCP did not test the equipment, supplies, or procedures and, therefore, urges all readers to read and follow all manufacturers' instructions and package insert warnings concerning the proper and safe use of products.

COVER

Hodgkin's disease. As illustrated here, when immunostained for S-100 protein, some cases show positive staining in the Reed-Sternberg cells and mononuclear variants (ABC-PO with AEC in a paraffin section of tissue fixed in Bouin's solution, hematoxylin counterstain). *Chapter 5, Figure 5–54.*

LIBRARY OF CONGRESS CATALOGING-IN-PUBLICATION DATA

Tubbs, Raymond R., 1946–
Atlas of immunohistology.

Bibliography; p.
Includes index.
1. Immunohistochemistry—Atlases. I. Gephardt, Gordon N. II. Petras, Robert E. III. Title.
[DNLM: 1. Histocytochemistry—atlases. 2. Immunologic Technics—atlases. QS 17 T884a]
RB46.5.T83 1986 616.07′5 85-18499
ISBN 0–89189–205–2
ISBN 0–89189–206–0 (bk. & slides)

89 88 87 86 6 5 4 3 2 1

Contents

APPENDIX

Figures

2 Immunohistologic Methods 8

3 Specimen Processing and Quality Assurance 25

4 Endocrine Pathology 33

5 Lymphoproliferative Disorders 45

Tables

Preface

Immunohistochemistry is rapidly growing as an important diagnostic tool in surgical pathology. This new staining technique will have a profound impact on the practice of diagnostic pathology because it enables more accurate diagnoses based on the antigenic properties of the lesions as well as their morphology. We hope that practitioners of both clinical and surgical pathology will benefit from the information contained in this volume.

This manual and atlas is designed to serve as an interpretive and methodologic source. The text describes the principles and applications of immunohistochemistry with special attention to potential methodologic problems and the interpretive errors that can result from such problems. The figures, which appear at the end of the chapters, illustrate the principles and provide examples of typical immunohistologic findings in the diseases and antigens considered in the chapter. The legends provide guidelines for interpretation. An optional slide set, consisting of 101 color transparencies selected from the figures in the text, is available. Cross-references to these slides appear in the legends and in the "Guide to Optional Slide Set."

Detailed protocols for performing the stains are provided in the appendixes. The approximate working dilutions and reagent sources are also provided. We have specified the commercial sources in many instances, not as an endorsement of the specific product but rather to facilitate the implementation of the immunohistochemical protocols in the laboratory.

The bibliography, at the end of the book, consists of selected references for the topics covered in each chapter.

We have not tried to provide a compendium of literature on immunohistochemistry. Other texts and review articles accomplish this task well. Rather, our main objective is to provide a source of usable, well-illustrated material to emphasize a practical methodologic and interpretive approach to immunohistochemistry. Also, we have chosen to limit the scope of the atlas to light microscopic applications; immunoelectron microscopy is not discussed.

We appreciate the patience exercised by our wives, Mary Ellen, Suzanne, and Susan, and by our children during the preparation of this manuscript. The critical reviews by William R. Hart, MD, Howard S. Levin, MD, and James Whitehead, PhD, are acknowledged and their helpful suggestions appreciated. We appreciate the support of our colleagues in laboratory medicine at the Cleveland Clinic and their integration of immunohistochemical techniques into diagnostic pathology. We also appreciate the electron micrographs kindly provided by James T. McMahon, PhD—he provided all the electron micrographs in this atlas; the hepatocellular carcinomas immunostained for carcinoembryonic antigen, by Thomas Bauer, MD, PhD; the immmunostained leukemia cytocentrifuge preparations, by Richard A. Savage, MD, and Andrew Fishleder, MD; and the immunostained cytology preparations, by the late Steven Becker, MD. Finally, we wish to acknowledge the excellent medical illustration skills of Jeffrey J. Loerch, who prepared the diagrams of methods (Chapters 2 and 3); the expert professional secretarial skills of Ms Sandy Hemphill in the word processing of the manuscript; the valuable advice given by Mr Rad Clark on the photomicrographs; the excellent immunohistochemical preparations generated by histotechnologists supervised by Mrs Linda Vargo; and the specimen preparation and processing by technologists under the direction of Mrs Susan Petras, Mrs Gwendolyn Cianflocco, Mrs Susan Arcuri, and Ms Kathy Herris, supervisor.

1 Principles and Practice

Immunohistologic methods were introduced in 1941 by Coons, after he successfully labeled antibodies with fluorescent material. Immunofluorescence soon became an indispensable diagnostic tool for the evaluation of numerous autoimmune diseases mediated by immune complexes or autoantibody deposition. As experience with immunofluorescence was acquired, it became clear that the special instrumentation required for immunofluorescence and the impermanence of preparations limited its usefulness.

Subsequently, immunohistologic systems using enzyme labels were developed. These systems permitted the localization of tissue antigens in permanent preparations and concomitant morphologic evaluation by light microscopy. Enzyme immunomicroscopy became practical after antibodies were successfully conjugated with enzymes and unlabeled antibody methods were developed. An extensive body of literature now documents the usefulness of enzyme-labeled antibody, unlabeled antibody (antienzyme), and biotin-avidin methods in the identification of tissue antigens by the formation of permanent colored reaction products in histologic sections, giving superb morphologic detail.

Although immunohistology is an important technique in diagnosis, its use must be kept in proper perspective. The results of all immunomicroscopic methods should be viewed as adjunctive and supportive in formulating a pathologic diagnosis. These methods should not be used as the primary mode of diagnosis for any illness because they are not freestanding, independent, primary methods of diagnosis. Immunomicroscopic methods provide but one piece of the several pieces of information to be integrated in formulating the final diagnosis. The amount of corroborative evidence they produce may be of relatively minor importance, or it may be a major factor in determining the final integrated pathologic classification for a given disease state. Histopathologic interpretation tempered and refined by experience and consultation remains the cornerstone of pathologic diagnosis.

Specificity screening with frozen tissue and fixed, paraffin-embedded tissue has been done at the Cleveland Clinic Foundation Department of Pathology for some of the antigen systems illustrated in this atlas. The screen that we have developed for frozen tissue sections consists of approximately 75 normal and neoplastic tissues to evaluate antigens not detectable in paraffin-embedded fixed tissues. To evaluate antigens preserved in paraffin tissue sections, a series of approximately 150 normal and neoplastic tissues were optimally fixed in Bouin's solution for specificity screening. Each tissue was optimally fixed by immersion of very thin segments of tissue in ample volumes of fixative for only two hours. The antibodies tested against the frozen and paraffin tissue specificity screens were evaluated by the avidin-biotinylated peroxidase complex (ABC-PO) technique.

The detailed protocols provided in this manual assume the use of the immersion ABC-PO procedure for the biotinylated secondary or tertiary ABC-PO steps. Development of the ABC-PO immersion procedure was necessary to accommodate the large number of immunostained preparations done daily at our institution. For laboratories with fewer applications, the ABC-PO immersion procedure may not be cost-effective, and a simple flat-slide incubation for all of the procedure steps may be desired. In this case, the volumes of secondary antibody and ABC-PO reagent will need to be reduced proportionately.

The immersion procedure is possible because of the sensitivity of the ABC-PO procedure: very low concentrations of biotinylated secondary antibody and ABC-PO reagent can be used in large volumes of buffer. Furthermore, the solutions can be stored and reused if positive and negative controls are monitored daily. For some antigens (eg, T4 on lymphocytes) or for tissues replete with endogenous biotin, staining may best be done with a flat-slide incubation, using the indirect procedure.

For pathologists who wish to begin doing immunohistochemistry, we suggest that prostate-specific antigen or prostatic acid phosphatase detected by the rabbit IgG ABC-PO method be used (Appendix C-8). Prostate tissue is readily available to optimize fixation, processing, dilutions, and staining, and the immunostaining patterns of antigen distribution are well defined.

2 Immunohistologic Methods

This chapter will focus on the reagents and methods employed in immunohistochemistry. First, the different immunohistologic methods will be discussed, with emphasis on enzyme immunohistochemistry and its specific techniques. Then systems using peroxidase as a label and the tissue biochemistry and practical use of chromogens for peroxidase will be discussed. Finally, specific techniques, including biotin-avidin techniques, will be presented and illustrated.

In immunohistochemistry, the reaction of the primary antibody may be with an immunoglobulin, a polypeptide hormone, or an antigen of other chemical composition. Reactions occurring between primary and secondary and between secondary and tertiary reagents are immunoglobulin–anti-immunoglobulin reactions. The amino terminal (Fab) portion of the immunoglobulin, composed of the variable regions of the heavy and light chains, is the antigen combining site.

Immunofluorescence

Immunofluorescence is a time-honored immunohistologic method employing a variety of labels, including fluorescein, rhodamine, Texas red, and other compounds. The advantages include the relative ease of use of the reagents and the fact that only washing steps are needed after antibody labeling, not the addition of more reagents as is required for development of an enzyme reaction product in other techniques. The disadvantages include the need for a special immunofluorescence microscope, the autofluorescence of some biologic tissues, the quenching of fluorescence and lack of permanency in most systems, and the poor correlation of immunofluorescence with morphologic features visible by light microscopy.

Immunogold/Silver Colloid Procedures

Procedures with immunogold/silver colloid are most useful in immunoelectron microscopy, in which the gold particle can be seen to directly overlie the morphologic organelle or other feature of interest. With relatively large amounts of labeled gold at an antigen site, a red or blue color can be visualized by conventional light microscopy. Also, reduced gold can be used to precipitate metallic silver from salts such as silver lactate.

To achieve the sensitivity of unlabeled or avidin-biotinylated peroxidase methods, overnight incubation in gold-labeled antibodies is necessary. Silver precipitation methods should be done in total darkness.

Enzyme Immunohistochemistry

In enzyme immunohistochemistry, an enzyme-substrate-chromogen reaction that yields colored reaction products is used to mark the location of extracellular or cellular antigens. The disadvantages include the use of potentially hazardous chromogens in some systems and false-positive reactions due to endogenous enzyme activity. The advantages include wide flexibility of localization techniques having varying sensitivity and specificity, permanency of reaction products, ability to counterstain or multilabel immunostained slides for light microscopic correlation (**FIGURES 2–1** through **2–13**), and no need for special equipment beyond that usually available in the histology laboratory.

Although other enzyme labels have theoretical advantages over peroxidase (**FIGURES 2–9** through **2–13**), most enzyme immunohistochemical systems used still employ peroxidase. Glucose oxidase is not present in human tissue as an endogenous enzyme and thus has a theoretical advantage. However, we have found the kinetics of the enzyme-substrate-chromogen reaction to be inferior to those of peroxidase and its substrates. We have found peroxidase to be the most useful and reliable enzyme label for immunohistochemistry. Furthermore, endogenous peroxidase activity can be blocked by the use of methanolic hydrogen peroxide. Actually, endogenous enzyme is a problem only in peripheral blood and bone marrow contaminated with polymorphonuclear leukocytes that have endogenous myeloperoxidase activity (lymph node usually has no or negligible endogenous peroxidase). Even this problem can be circumvented to some degree with hydrogen peroxide/acetone preincubation, but some antigens do not survive exposure to this kind of pretreatment. Thus, for certain specimens, such as peripheral blood, the use of an enzyme label other than peroxidase, such as alkaline phosphatase or glucose oxidase, may be helpful.

The characteristics of the available chromogens for peroxidase are outlined in Table 2–1. Tetramethylbenzidine (TMB) and benzidine yield blue reaction products. Both of these reagents are insoluble in organic solvents and can be dehydrated in alcohols and xylene as permanent preparations. The chromogens *o*-phenylenediamine (OPD), *m*-phenylenediamine (MPD), and Hanker-Yates reagent (*p*-phenylenediamine and pyrocatechol) can similarly be dehydrated but differ in the relative sensitivity and tinctorial properties of the reaction product. TMB, OPD, and MPD yield suboptimal tissue precipitation and are more useful for enzyme immunoassay than for enzyme immunohistochemistry. Diaminobenzidine (DAB) is similarly insoluble in organic solvents and yields a brown reaction product.

In our experience, aminoethylcarbazole (AEC) has been the most "sensitive" of all the peroxidase chromogens. AEC yields a red reaction product that, when counterstained with hematoxylin, is an easy preparation to interpret analogous to a hematoxylin and eosin stain; but the reaction product is soluble in organic solvents. Thus, AEC-developed preparations must be mounted in Aquamount or similar water-based media; but when the coverslip edges are sealed with nail polish or a similar preparation, slides are semipermanent. Preparations made in this way have been viewed by our group for up to four years following preparation, with no loss in intensity of staining and no observed diffusion of the AEC reaction product in the tissue. AEC reaction products are especially advantageous in tissue with abundant hemo-

TABLE 2–1. Peroxidase Chromogens

Chromogen	Color of Reaction Product	Solubility in Organic Solvents	Carcinogenicity
Benzidine	Blue	No	Yes
TMB[a]	Blue	No	Uncertain
DAB	Brown	No	Uncertain
DAB + $NiCl_2$	Blue-black	No	Uncertain
MPD[a]	Brown	No	Uncertain
OPD[a]	Brown	No	Uncertain
AEC	Red	Yes	Uncertain
4CN	Blue	Yes	Uncertain; toxic
HYR	Brown-black	No	No
HYR + $NiCl_2$	Blue-black	No	No

ABBREVIATIONS: AEC = 3-amino-9-ethylcarbazole, 4CN = 4-chloro-1-naphthol, DAB = 3,3′-diaminobenzidine, HYR = Hanker-Yates reagent (*p*-phenylenediamine and pyrocatechol), MPD = *m*-phenylenediamine, OPD = *o*-phenylenediamine, TMB = tetramethylbenzidine.

[a]These chromogens are more useful in enzyme immunoassay. Suboptimal precipitation at tissue sites limits their usefulness in immunohistochemistry.

siderin or melanin, which remain brown and contrast well with the specific red AEC reaction product (**FIGURES 2–7** and **2–8**).

The documented risk of carcinogenicity with benzidine and federal restrictions regarding its use have essentially precluded its use in diagnostic laboratories. Conflicting evidence exists in the literature for DAB, and further studies of carcinogenicity are needed for TMB, DAB, and AEC.

Immunohistochemical Techniques

The available techniques for immunohistochemistry are diagrammed in **FIGURES 2–14** through **2–22**. In immunohistochemical techniques, the primary antibody (rabbit anti-human Ig) binds to the tissue antigen (human Ig) through the Fab portion of the primary antibody (**FIGURE 2–14**). The location of the tissue antigen is determined by a colored reaction product produced by the oxidized chromogen when hydrogen peroxide is reduced in the presence of the enzyme peroxidase. (The peroxidase is usually extracted from horseradish.)

In the direct technique, the primary antibody is linked covalently to the enzyme peroxidase (**FIGURE 2–15**). When the antibody reacts with the antigen, the peroxidase-labeled primary antibody remains localized at the antigen locus in the tissue.

The indirect immunoperoxidase procedure employs a secondary antibody (goat anti-rabbit IgG) that has been conjugated with the enzyme peroxidase (**FIGURE 2–16**). The secondary antibody binds to the primary antibody (rabbit anti-human IgG).

The labeled antigen technique is a modified indirect immunoperoxidase procedure (**FIGURE 2–17**). The primary antibody, rabbit anti-human IgG, binds to its tissue antigen. Then the peroxidase-conjugated human IgG is added to the section and binds to the primary antibody. The reaction product is developed at sites of peroxidase-conjugated antigen (human IgG).

The unlabeled or peroxidase-antiperoxidase (PAP) technique is illustrated in **FIGURE 2–18**. The primary antibody (rabbit anti-human Ig) binds to the tissue antigen through the Fab portion of the primary antibody. The secondary reagent is goat anti-rabbit IgG, and the tertiary reagent is the PAP complex, which consists of a soluble preformed complex of peroxidase and rabbit antiperoxidase, a rabbit IgG molecule. The secondary reagent (goat anti-rabbit IgG) forms a molecular bridge between the rabbit Ig primary antibody and the rabbit IgG in the tertiary reagent (PAP complex).

Because protein A binds IgG from different species, it can be used to link PAP complexes to primary antibodies of a different species. Thus, in the protein A modification of the unlabeled PAP technique, the secondary reagent is protein A, which binds the Fc portions of IgG from several species. In the setting illustrated in **FIGURE 2–19**, protein A forms a molecular bridge between the Fc portions of the rabbit IgG molecules present in the tertiary (rabbit anti-peroxidase) and the primary (rabbit anti-human IgG) reagents. Antibodies directed against human insulin at one time were most widely available as guinea pig primary antibodies rather than rabbit antibodies. In this setting, protein A can be used to link the Fc portion of guinea pig IgG to the PAP complex to localize insulin in human tissue. However, this localization may now be accomplished more efficiently with a biotinylated secondary antibody.

A variety of biotin-avidin immunohistochemical procedures have been developed. Each procedure exploits the extraordinary avidity of avidin, an egg white protein (molecular weight 68,000), for biotin, a cofactor necessary for human intermediary metabolism. Avidin has four potential receptor sites for biotin, and the complex formed between the two molecules is extremely stable (the dissociation constant is 1×10^{-15} M). Of the many combinations of biotin and avidin that can be used, three are now commonly employed in immunohistochemistry: the indirect biotin-avidin technique (**FIGURE 2–20**), the avidin-biotinylated peroxidase complex (ABC-PO) technique (**FIGURE 2–21**), and the biotinylated primary antibody modification of the ABC-PO technique (**FIGURE 2–22**).

The indirect biotin-avidin technique uses a biotinylated goat anti-rabbit IgG (**FIGURE 2–20**). This biotinylated antibody can be used at half the concentration of the bridge secondary antibodies used in the unlabeled PAP technique, since the biotin is already linked to the anti-rabbit IgG. The biotin moieties bind essentially irreversibly to the avidin-peroxidase, and the anti-rabbit IgG binds to the rabbit IgG primary antibody (anti-human IgG). The enzyme peroxidase is localized to the antigen focus by virtue of its conjugation with avidin.

Of the three biotin-avidin techniques, we have found the ABC-PO technique to be the most satisfactory (**FIGURE 2–21**). (Originally all avidin-biotinylated complex techniques used peroxidase, and the abbreviation ABC sufficed. Now there are a variety of enzymes other than peroxidase that are used; therefore, an additional designation is necessary to specify which enzyme is being used.) If biotinylated primary antibodies are available, the simpler, modified ABC-PO technique may also be used (**FIGURE 2–22**).

The ABC-PO technique depends on the formation of a complex array by cross-linkage between soluble preformed complexes of avidin-DH and biotinylated peroxidase. There are no accessible biotins on the avidin-biotin complex, only biotin-binding sites. For a given antigen locus, a relatively large number of enzyme molecules are localized as compared with the other available methods. A secondary biotin-labeled reagent, affinity-purified goat anti-rabbit IgG, forms a molecular bridge between the preformed avidin-biotin complex and the rabbit IgG in the primary rabbit anti-human IgG antibody.

In our experience, the sensitivity of the ABC method exceeds that of the unlabeled PAP method. For example, with the PAP technique, systems for detecting polypeptide hormones such as gastrin previously required overnight incubation with primary antibodies. Now, the ABC method produces superior staining after 30-minute incubations with the same primary antibodies.

The ABC-PO procedure can be modified as diagrammed in **FIGURE 2–22**. The primary antibody can be directly biotinylated and the secondary reagent omitted. Biotin moieties in the primary antibody bind to the avidin in the avidin-biotin complex, and the biotinylated primary antibody binds to its corresponding antigen directly in the tissue. In this manner, biotinylated primary antibody is directly linked to the soluble avidin-biotin complex. This formulation avoids potential cross-reactivities between the biotinylated secondary antibodies (such as biotinylated anti-rabbit IgG) and antigens in the tissues (such as human IgG). Such possible cross-reactivities are unlikely when affinity-purified reagents are used, but in the sensitivity range of the ABC technique they are not entirely theoretical. Also, elimination of the additional step reduces the time required to perform the test. Biotinylated probes can also be used in this system to identify viruses by detection of in situ hybridization (see Chapter 12), but denaturation of DNA by heat, formamide, or other methods is a prerequisite.

The extraordinary sensitivity of the ABC-PO procedure permits the use of a rapid modification. Since reagent incubations are reduced from approximately 1.5 hours to 15 minutes, the technique becomes much less labor-intensive and perhaps more cost-effective. The macromolecular complex composed of tertiary avidin-biotinylated peroxidase, biotinylated secondary antibody, and primary antibody, are all formed in fluid phase while the tissue is being prepared for application of antibodies. For frozen tissue, such alacrity is helpful in further preservation of structural detail. The primary antibodies must be used at a much higher concentration, but the volumes of reagent are so small that generally only 5 μL of stock need be used for incubation. Thus, the end result is that the same amount of primary antibody is used with either the rapid or the conventional ABC-PO technique. It cannot be assumed that all antigens are equally evaluable with the rapid modification; each system must be evaluated independently.

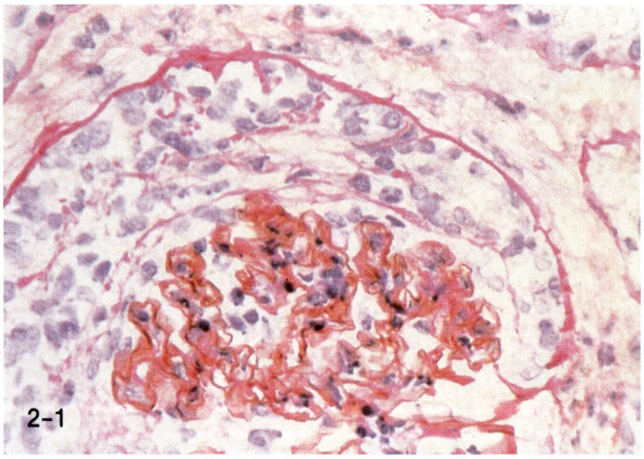

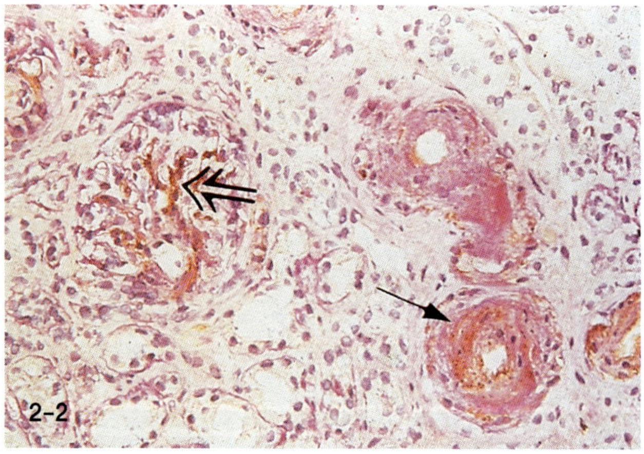

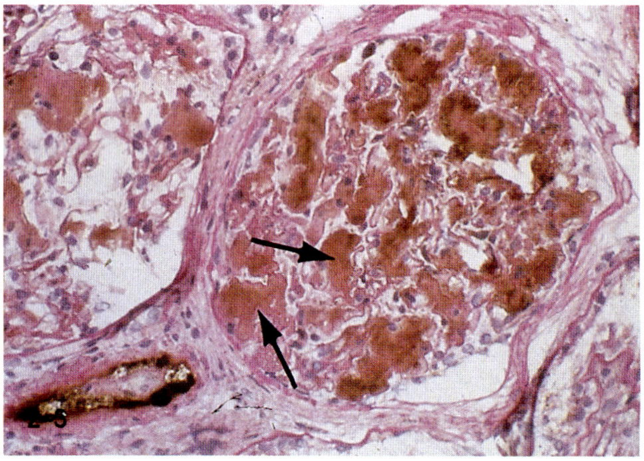

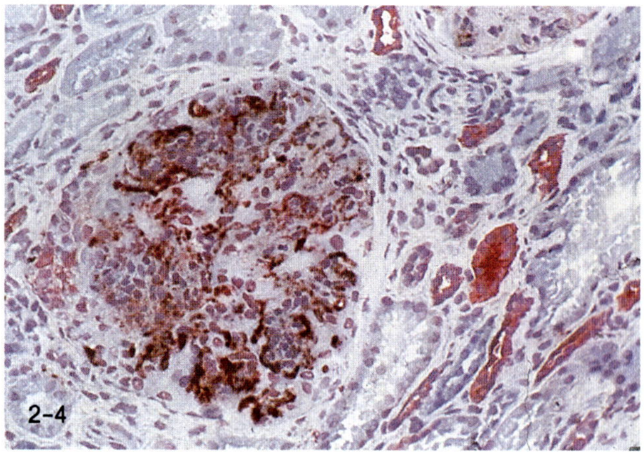

FIGURE 2–1. Anti–glomerular basement membrane disease. Diffuse generalized deposits of IgG (brown) in the glomerular basement membrane can be simultaneously correlated with a cellular extracapillary crescent occupying the urinary space (IMPAS with DAB, hematoxylin counterstain). *Slide 1.*

FIGURE 2–2. Henoch-Schönlein purpura. Vascular (arrow) and mesangial (double arrow) granular deposits of C3 (IMPAS with DAB, hematoxylin counterstain).

FIGURE 2–3. Renal amyloidosis. Homogeneous deposits of IgA (arrows) are visible (IMPAS with HYR, hematoxylin counterstain).

FIGURE 2–4. Systemic lupus erythematosus nephritis with cellular crescents. Generalized deposits of C3 (HYR, brown) in a glomerulus and a tubular epithelial cell containing cytokeratins (AEC, red) are visible. The glomerular crescent is negative for AE1/3 (for C3: direct IMP with HYR; for AE1/3: ABC-PO with AEC, hematoxylin counterstain). *Slide 2.*

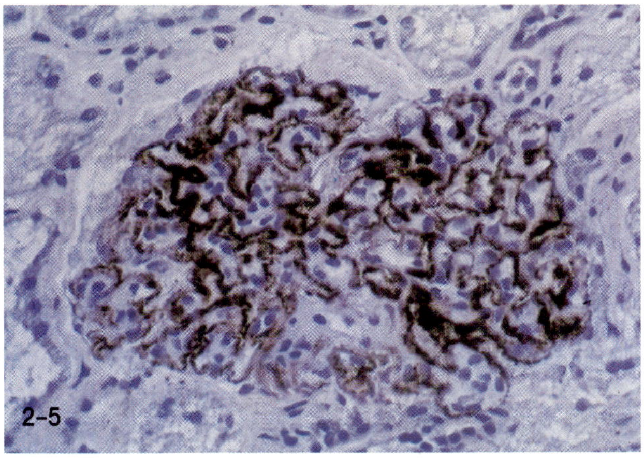

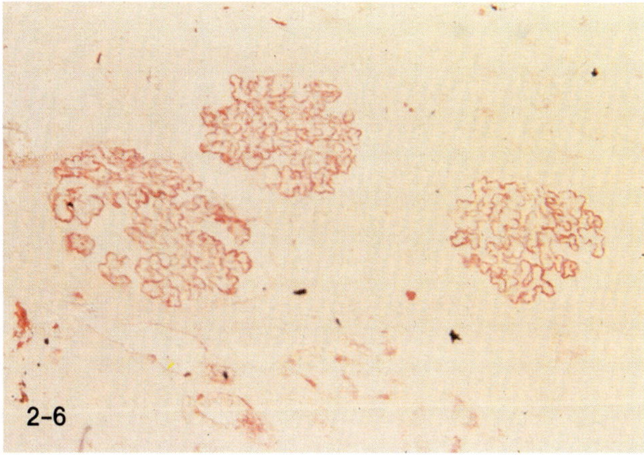

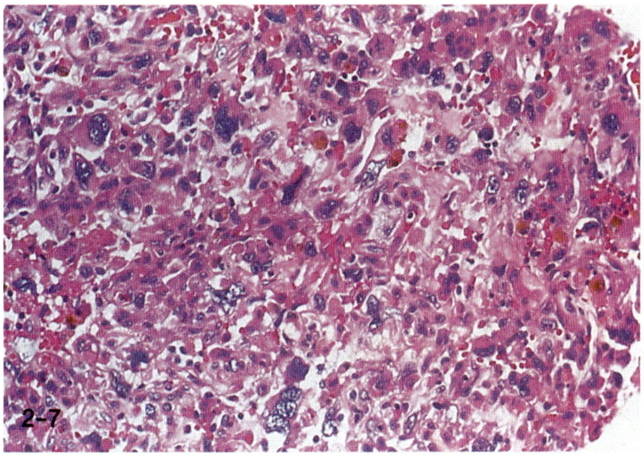

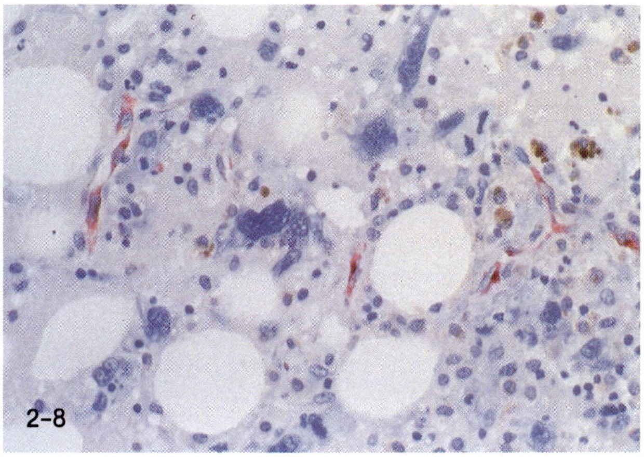

FIGURE 2–5. Membranous glomerulopathy, one variant of lupus nephritis. Generalized granular deposits of IgM (brown) are visible in the glomerular basement membrane (direct IMP with HYR, hematoxylin counterstain).

FIGURE 2–6. Membranous glomerulopathy. Diffuse generalized granular deposits of IgG in the peripheral capillary basement membrane are visible (direct IMP with AEC, no counterstain).

FIGURE 2–7. Sarcoma of salivary gland. Figures 2–7 and 2–8 are from the same case. Recent and remote hemorrhage with hemosiderin deposition (brown) are evident in this figure (H & E).

FIGURE 2–8. Same case as 2–7. The brown hemosiderin deposits, which could possibly be confused with some peroxidase chromogen reaction products, are clearly differentiated from the red reaction product of AEC with factor VIII (rabbit ABC-PO with AEC, hematoxylin counterstain).

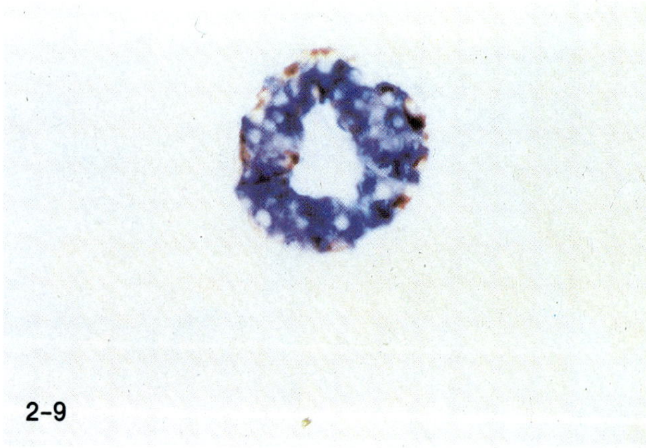

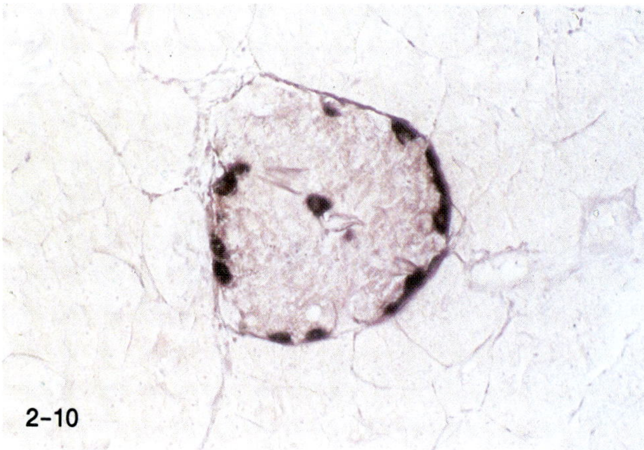

FIGURE 2–9. Pancreatic islet cells with double label. Glucagon (brown) was detected using ABC-PO with HYR. Insulin (blue) was detected using ABC-AP with fast blue (no counterstain).

FIGURE 2–10. Pancreatic islet cells immunostained for glucagon (brown; ABC-GO, no counterstain).

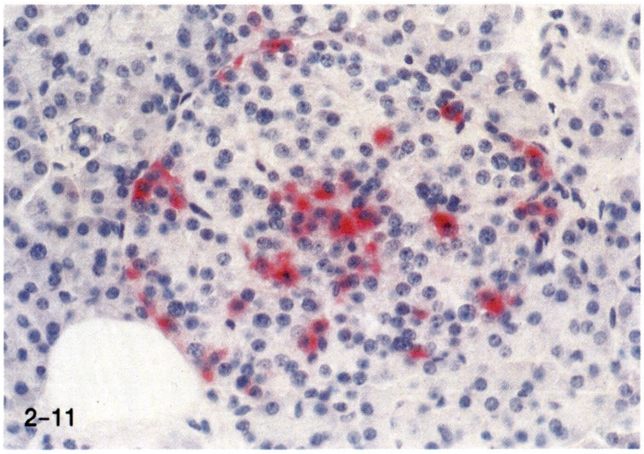

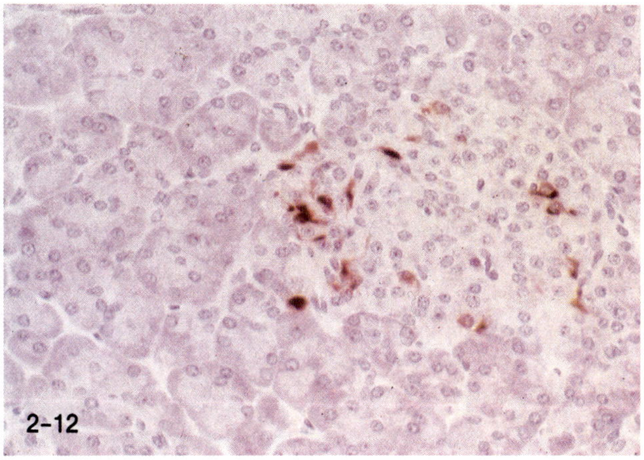

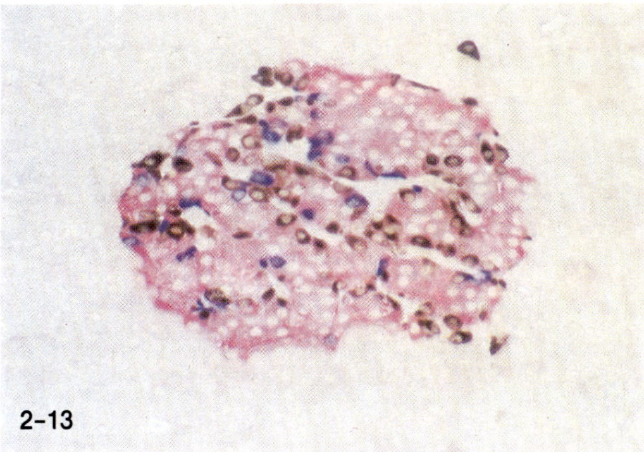

FIGURE 2–11. Pancreatic islet cells immunostained for somatostatin (red; ABC-AP with fast red, hematoxylin counterstain).

FIGURE 2–12. Pancreatic islet cells immunostained for somatostatin (brown; ABC-PO with HYR, hematoxylin counterstain).

FIGURE 2–13. Pancreatic islet cells with triple-label. Glucagon (brown; ABC-PO with DAB), somatostatin (blue; ABC-AP with fast blue), and insulin (red; ABC-AP with fast red) are simultaneously visible (no counterstain). *Slide 3.*

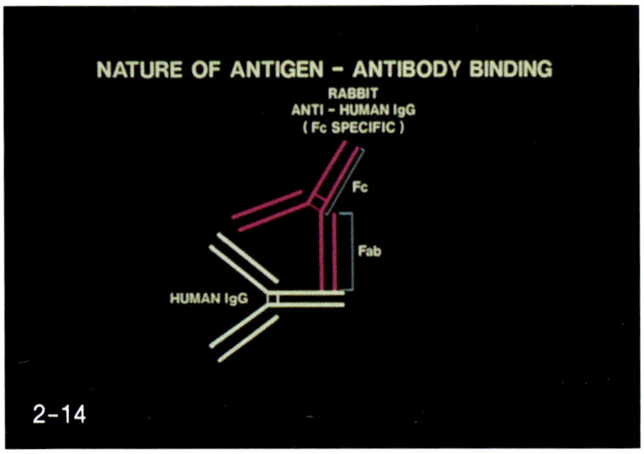

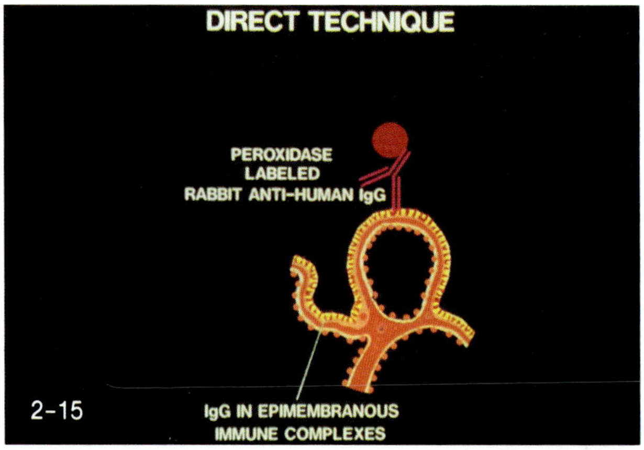

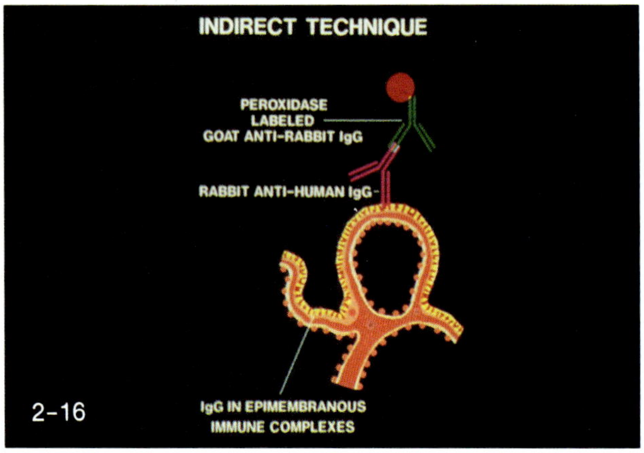

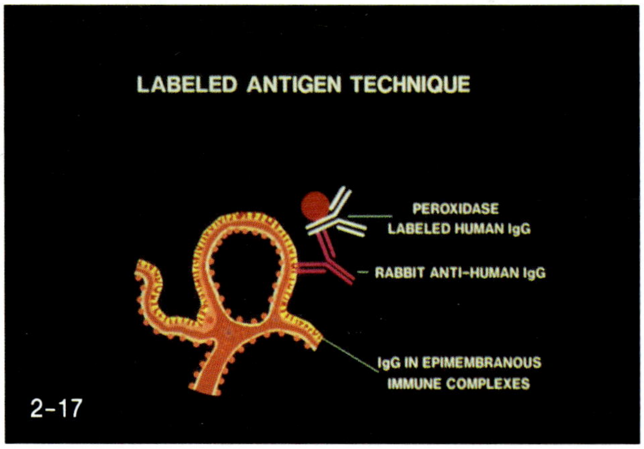

FIGURE 2–14. Nature of antigen-antibody binding. The Fab portion of the antibody in this instance binds to the Fc portion of its IgG immunoglobulin antigen.

FIGURE 2–15. Direct immunoperoxidase technique (direct IMP).

FIGURE 2–16. Indirect immunoperoxidase technique. *Slide 4.*

FIGURE 2–17. Labeled antigen technique.

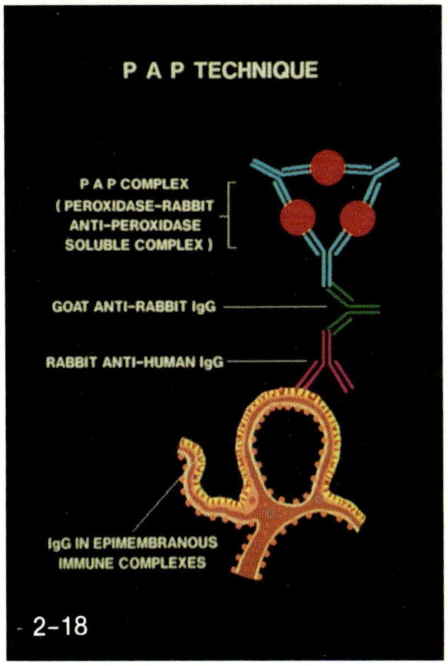

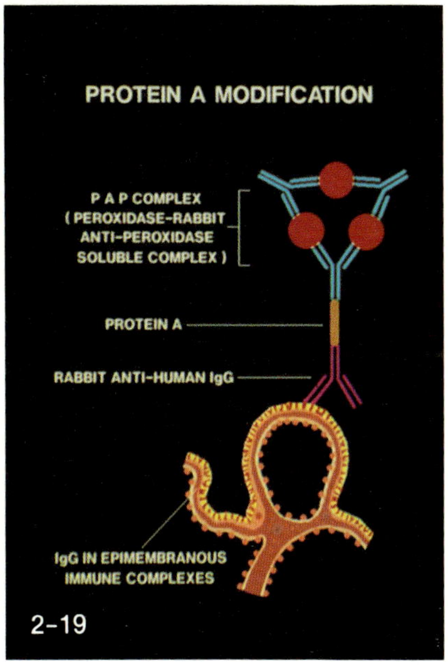

FIGURE 2–18. Unlabeled peroxidase-antiperoxidase (PAP) technique. *Slide 5.*
FIGURE 2–19. Protein A modification of the unlabeled PAP technique.

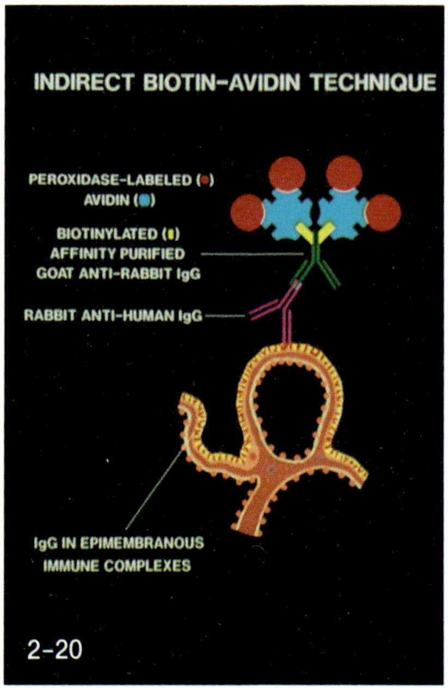

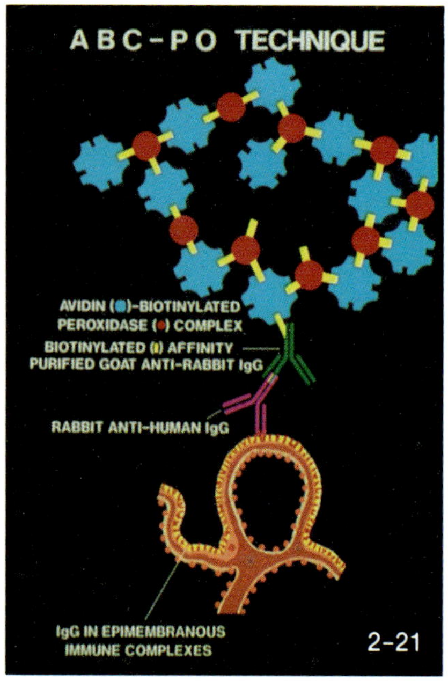

FIGURE 2–20. Indirect biotin-avidin immunoperoxidase technique.
FIGURE 2–21. Avidin-biotinylated peroxidase complex (ABC-PO) immunoperoxidase technique. *Slide 6.*

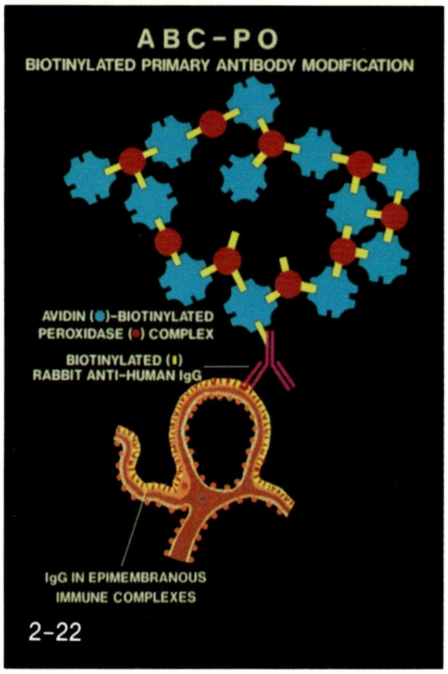

FIGURE 2–22. Biotinylated primary antibody modification of ABC-PO immunoperoxidase technique.

3 Specimen Processing and Quality Assurance

Originally, immunofluorescence techniques were developed for frozen tissue sections and individual cell suspensions, and immunoperoxidase techniques were developed for paraffin-embedded material. However, it has subsequently become clear that both types of antigen detection systems are readily applicable to all kinds of specimens. Thus, frozen sections of specimens from kidneys, lymph nodes, and solid tumors, originally prepared for immunofluorescence techniques, can readily be used in immunoperoxidase techniques. Similarly, immunofluorescence can also be used to study antigens in paraffin sections. The ability to detect a given antigen satisfactorily depends not so much on the immunomicroscopic method used as on factors related to tissue processing and quality of reagents, such as molar ratios of antibody to label, avidity of antibody for the tissue antigens, quality control of the buffer, and the degree of optimization of methods, particularly with regard to dilutions of multiple reagents in complex procedures.

It is difficult to generalize about optimal tissue processing for all antigens. Each immunohistologic system should be optimized independently. First, determine whether frozen tissue sections or fresh cell suspensions are essential for accurate detection of the antigen in question. Parallel comparative studies of frozen sections and fixed paraffin sections must be done to determine whether fixation and dehydration or other processing steps irreversibly alter the antigen. Second, if fixation renders antigen detection suboptimal, determine whether enzyme pretreatment with trypsin or pronase will unmask the desired antigen in paraffin sections and whether the resulting morphologic detail and overall quality of the preparation are superior to that which can be realized in frozen tissue sections. Third, if paraffin sections are to be used, determine optimal fixation conditions. Some antigens, such as polypeptide hormones, are best preserved in Bouin's solution. Others, such as blood group–associated antigens, are better preserved in absolute alcohol. For some antigens, paraffin sections (no matter which fixative is used) may be inferior to frozen tissue sections, eg, surface/cytoplasmic immunoglobulins in lymphoproliferative disease. Test conditions must be independently evaluated for each antigen.

Table 3–1 summarizes our experience with regard to optimal tissue processing and fixation conditions for the antigen systems detailed.

Anomalous Immunostaining

ENDOGENOUS ENZYMES

The ideal enzyme label for immunohistochemistry uses a nonmammalian enzyme, thus avoiding spurious color reaction products due to the action of endogenous enzymes such as myeloperoxidase, hemoglobin pseudoperoxidase, and leukocyte alkaline phosphatase. Unfortunately, enzymes that fulfill this criterion, such as glucose oxidase, lack optimal chromogen-substrate kinetics. Until bacterial or other enzymes that are not expressed endogenously in humans are identified, or until assay conditions for other enzymes are improved, the pathologist must avoid this problem by blocking endogenous peroxidase activity or by developing techniques to localize relatively large amounts of glucose oxidase at antigen foci. Preliminary results with the avidin-biotinylated alkaline phosphatase (ABC-AP) method offer some promise (see Appendix C-10).

For endogenous peroxidases and pseudoperoxidases, preincubation of paraffin sections in 0.5% hydrogen peroxide in methanol is usually satisfactory for inactivation; however, frozen tissue sections may be destroyed by methanol and the necessary concentrations of hydrogen peroxide. Some antigens survive pretreatment with 1% hydrogen peroxide in acetone. The mechanism by which endogenous enzyme activity is blocked is not clear. Enzymes are not supposed to be consumed during a chemical reaction; therefore, the disruption of activity may in fact be due to structural damage of the molecule by methanol or acetone during the interaction with substrate, or due to other forms of inhibition related to the relatively high concentration of substrate being used, or due to the accumulation of a toxic product.

Endogenous alkaline phosphatase may be inhibited with 1 mM of levamisole. This substance will inhibit the activity of all alkaline phosphatase isoenzymes except the intestinal form.

Finally, if it is not possible to obliterate endogenous enzyme staining, the appropriate negative controls may be used for comparison in conjunction with the specifically stained preparations. The negative control permits the delineation of endogenous enzyme activity, which can then be acknowledged during interpretation of the immunostained section.

ENDOGENOUS BIOTIN

Biotin is a necessary cofactor for intermediary metabolism and may accumulate in body tissues, particularly those of the liver and kidney. The binding qualities of endogenous biotin are not apparent in paraffin sections of fixed material but can be a problem in interpreting frozen tissue sections. Endogenous biotin, when exposed to avidin-labeled reagents, including ABC-PO complexes, will bind the avidin-containing compounds, producing spurious staining patterns when the color reaction product is developed (**FIGURE 3–1**). Endogenous biotin can be blocked by the avidin-biotin flush technique developed by Wood and Warnke (Appendix C–1). When sequentially exposed to an excess of avidin and biotin, tissue sites with endogenous biotin are effectively masked, and the usual immunostaining procedure can then be done. The flush technique is diagrammed in **FIGURE 3–2**.

NONSPECIFIC ANTIBODY BINDING

Any reagent used for immunohistochemistry has the potential for nonspecific binding to various tissue components. Generally, this problem occurs at higher concentrations of reagent protein. For example, in the unlabeled peroxidase-antiperoxidase (PAP) technique, the most significant problem occurs with binding of the secondary reagent, since it must be used at approximately twice the concentration of the other antibodies used in the sequence of the technique. However, nonspecific binding of the primary antibody is even more serious. Controls must be used carefully to identify such nonspecific binding problems and eliminate them if possible.

Tables 3–2 and 3–3 summarize the ideal negative and positive controls for immunohistology. The tissue control slide, which uses tissues known to contain the antigen in question, confirms the reactivity of the system. The negative control sections detect potential nonspecific

TABLE 3–1. Optimal Tissue Processing for Antigens

Antigen	Antibody		Preferred Technique	Frozen Sections	Fixatives for Paraffin Sections			
	Polyclonal (species)	Monoclonal (mouse)			Hollande's/ Bouin's	Formalin	Absolute Ethanol	B-5
Polypeptide hormones								
Insulin	Guinea pig	NA	ABC-PO	A	P	A	A	NA
Glucagon	Rabbit	NA	ABC-PO	A	P	A	A	NA
Somatostatin	Rabbit	NA	ABC-PO	A	P	A	A	NA
Gastrin	Rabbit	NA	ABC-PO	A	P	A	A	NA
Growth hormone	Rabbit	NA	ABC-PO	A	A	P	A	NA
Prolactin	Rabbit	NA	ABC-PO	A	A	P	A	NA
ACTH	Rabbit	NA	ABC-PO	A	A	P	A	NA
LH	Rabbit	NA	ABC-PO	A	A	P	A	NA
FSH	Rabbit	NA	ABC-PO	A	A	P	A	NA
TSH	Rabbit	NA	ABC-PO	A	A	P	A	NA
Thyroglobulin	Rabbit	NA	ABC-PO	A	P	A	A	NA
Thyroxine	Rabbit	NA	ABC-PO	A	P	A	A	NA
Calcitonin	Rabbit	NA	ABC-PO	A	P	A	A	NA
Immunoglobulins								
Extracellular immune complexes	Goat or rabbit	NA	Direct	P	NA	A[a]	NA	NA
Cell membrane–associated (lymphocytes)	Goat	NA	Direct	P	NA	NA	NA	NA
Cytoplasmic immunoglobulin (plasma cells)	Goat or rabbit	NA	ABC-PO	A	P	A	A	A
Oncodevelopmental antigens and cytoskeletal filaments								
Keratins	Rabbit	P	ABC-PO	P	A	A[a]	A	NA
Carcinoembryonic antigen	Rabbit	NA	ABC-PO	A	P	A	A	A
α-fetoprotein	Rabbit	NA	ABC-PO	A	P	A	NA	NA

Hematopoietic differentiation antigens								
T3, T11, T4, T6, T8, T9, T10, T12, Leu-1 through 15, B1, B2, HLA-DR, J5	NA	P	ABC-PO or indirect	P	NA	NA	NA	NA
Leu-M1, Dako CLA	NA	P	ABC-PO or indirect	P	A	A	NA	A
LN 1, 2, 3	NA	P	ABC-PO or indirect	A	A	NA	NA	P
Tissue-associated antigens								
Prostatic acid phosphatase	Rabbit	NA	ABC-PO	NA	A	P	NA	NA
Prostate-specific antigen	Rabbit	NA	ABC-PO	NA	A	A	A	P
Uro-2, 3, 4	NA	P	ABC-PO or indirect	P	NA	NA	NA	NA
MEL-1, 5	NA	P	ABC-PO or indirect	P	NA	NA	NA	NA
Melanoma-associated antigen	NA	P	ABC-PO or indirect	P	NA	NA	NA	NA
OC129, Ca 19-9	NA	P	ABC-PO or indirect	P	NA	NA	NA	NA
Organisms								
HBsAg	Goat	NA	ABC-PO	A	P	A	NA	NA
HBcAg	Rabbit	NA	ABC-PO	A	P	A	NA	NA
Biotinylated DNA probes	NA	NA	Biot-ABC	P	NA	A[a]	NA	NA
Epithelial membrane antigen	NA	P	ABC-PO or indirect	P	A	A	NA	NA
Mesenchymal antigens								
VIII R:Ag	Rabbit or mouse	NA	ABC-PO	P	A	A	NA	P
Myoglobin	Rabbit	NA	ABC-PO	A	P	A	NA	NA
Myosin	NA	P	ABC-PO or indirect	P	NA	NA	NA	NA
Desmin	NA	P	ABC-PO or indirect	P	NA	NA	NA	NA
Vimentin	NA	P	ABC-PO or indirect	P	NA	NA	NA	NA

ABBREVIATIONS: A = adequate results can be achieved under these conditions, but other factors such as background staining or intensity of specific staining may be suboptimal; ABC-PO = avidin-biotinylated peroxidase complex technique; ACTH = adrenocorticotropic hormone; Biot-ABC = biotinylated primary modification of ABC-PO technique; Dako CLA = Dako common leukocyte antigen; FSH = follicle-stimulating hormone; HBcAg = hepatitis-B core antigen; HBsAg = hepatitis-B surface antigen; LH = luteinizing hormone; NA = not applicable; P = preferred (best or only choice in our experience); VIII R:Ag = factor VIII–related antigen; TSH = thyroid-stimulating hormone.

NOTE: This table summarizes the most commonly employed antigens for immunohistochemistry; other less commonly employed antigens are not included.

[a]Following trypsin or pronase treatment.

TABLE 3–2. Working Controls: Tissue Control Slide (Pancreas Control)

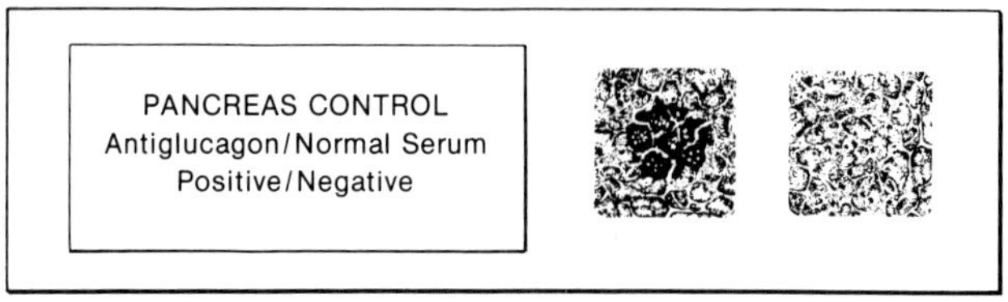

LEFT SIDE—Positive control	RIGHT SIDE—Negative control
Treated with antibody to the antigen in question	Treated with the IgG fraction of preimmune rabbit serum
Tissue Known to contain antigen in question, in this case, normal pancreas from control block	Tissue Known to contain antigen in question, in this case, normal pancreas from control block
Reagent Sequence Rabbit antiglucagon, 1:1,000 (primary antibody) Biotinylated anti-rabbit IgG, 1:400 ABC-PO AEC Hematoxylin	Reagent Sequence Preimmune rabbit IgG, 1:1,000 Biotinylated anti-rabbit IgG, 1:400 ABC-PO AEC Hematoxylin
Interpretation Ideally, should stain positively, which confirms that the system will identify glucagon.	Interpretation Ideally, should be negative (show no staining). If stains positively, indicates abnormal or undesirable reaction due to any of the following: • nonspecific binding of primary reagents, in this case, rabbit IgG • nonspecific binding of biotinylated secondary antibody • endogenous biotin bound by ABC-PO • endogenous peroxidase reaction with AEC. Other undesirable positive staining could indicate tissue characteristics, such as the presence of hemosiderin and necrosis.

ABBREVIATIONS: ABC-PO = avidin-biotinylated peroxidase complex, AEC = aminoethylcarbazole.

NOTE: This table also appears as Slide 8 in the optional slide set.

binding of primary antibody, secondary antibody, tertiary complex (ABC-PO), and endogenous enzyme activity. A negative control is done for both the unknown patient test case and for the positive control tissue. For the negative control section, the IgG fraction of normal serum from which the primary antibody was derived is used. Preferably, the IgG fraction of nonimmune normal serum is diluted to the same immunoglobulin concentration as the specific

TABLE 3–3. Working Controls: Test Slide from Patient's Tissue

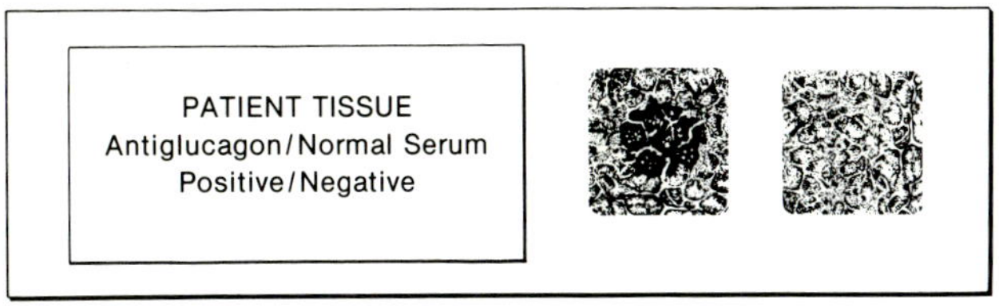

LEFT SIDE—Test tissue	RIGHT SIDE—Negative control
Treated with antibody to the antigen in question	Treated with the IgG fraction of preimmune rabbit serum
Tissue	**Tissue**
Abnormal tissue from the patient under study	Abnormal tissue from the patient under study
Reagent Sequence	**Reagent Sequence**
Rabbit antiglucagon, 1:1,000 (primary antibody) Biotinylated anti-rabbit IgG, 1:400 ABC-PO AEC Hematoxylin	Preimmune rabbit IgG, 1:1,000 Biotinylated anti-rabbit IgG, 1:400 ABC-PO AEC Hematoxylin
Interpretation	**Interpretation**
If the abnormal tissue contains glucagon, a positive reaction occurs.	Ideally, should be negative (show no staining). If stains positively, indicates abnormal or undesirable reaction due to any of the following: • nonspecific binding of primary reagents, in this case, rabbit IgG • nonspecific binding of biotinylated secondary antibody • endogenous biotin bound by ABC-PO • endogenous peroxidase reaction with AEC. Other undesirable positive staining could indicate tissue characteristics, such as the presence of hemosiderin and necrosis.

ABBREVIATIONS: ABC-PO = avidin-biotinylated peroxidase complex, AEC = aminoethylcarbazole.

NOTE: This table also appears as Slide 9 in the optional slide set.

primary antibody. Ideally, this normal IgG fraction is derived from preimmune serum from the individual animal or pool of animals that was the source of the reagent before immunization. The final concentration of the nonimmune immunoglobulin should equal that of the primary antibody. All of the reagents subsequently applied to the tissue section are identical to those used after the specific primary antibody has been added to the corresponding section. This sequence will also provide a control for nonspecific binding of the secondary antibody and of the tertiary complex and for endogenous enzyme activity.

For each antigen, the following controls should be employed (Tables 3–2 and 3–3):

Positive Control. The control block contains representative amounts and distribution of the desired antigen. The same staining pattern should occur in the control block in each run.

Negative Control. One negative control is a section of tissue from the tissue control block incubated with the IgG fraction of preimmune serum from the same species from which the primary antibody comes, eg, immunoglobulin fraction of preimmune rabbit serum (Table 3–2, right). Nonspecific binding of rabbit IgG to components of the tissue can be identified reliably if the dilutions of the preimmune rabbit IgG are equivalent to the dilution of the rabbit primary antibody. Another negative control is preimmune IgG applied to the specimen from the patient under study (Table 3–3, right).

Both of the negative controls are designed to detect nonspecific binding of components of rabbit IgG to the tissue. This kind of nonspecific reaction may not be diffuse and may be so selective as to simulate specific staining (**FIGURES 3–1** through **3–5**). The negative controls also identify nonspecific binding of secondary and tertiary reagents and endogenous peroxidase activity. Ideally, there should be no nonspecific staining, and both negative control sections should show no staining.

A positive stain in the negative control may indicate a problem at several levels in the sequence of the reaction, and requires that other corrective steps be taken. Nonspecific binding of secondary reagents can be prevented by preincubation of tissue sections in nonimmune serum of the same species from which the secondary antibody was derived. For example, in the rabbit PAP technique, preincubation in normal goat serum before addition of rabbit primary antibody will help prevent nonspecific binding of the goat anti-rabbit secondary antibody. Hyperimmune serum provides more efficient blocking (see Hume and Gordon). If preimmune serum becomes bound at dilutions equivalent to primary antibody dilutions, little can be done except to increase the dilutions of the primary antibody. For some antibodies with low avidity, this may not be possible, and the system may be deemed entirely unreliable.

When frozen tissue sections or cytocentrifuged preparations of cell suspensions are used, binding of antibody may occur via the Fc receptor for IgG that is expressed on a variety of cell populations. Fc receptors are not restricted to hematopoietic cells but may be expressed by carcinomas and other tissues as well. It may be possible to circumvent this type of binding problem by using $F(ab')_2$ fragments of antibodies. Binding to Fc receptors in large part depends on the immunoglobulin concentration, and in our experience monoclonal antibodies rarely if ever bind by this mechanism.

FIGURES 3–3 through **3–5** illustrate that these considerations are of more than theoretical interest. These illustrations show the effect of overfixation with Bouin's solution in evaluating tissues for polypeptide antigens. The specimen evaluated was a segment of normal pancreas removed with a pancreatic cyst. The material was processed immediately after receipt from the surgical suite. Thin segments, 1 to 2 mm thick, of grossly normal-appearing pancreas from the same area of this tissue specimen were compared. Separate blocks were fixed for 0.5, 1, 2, 4, 18, and 72 hours, and then immunostained with rabbit antiglucagon by the ABC-PO technique. The negative control consisted of appropriately diluted preimmune rabbit serum. Positive reactions in an appropriate distribution in pancreatic islets and absent staining in negative control sections were obtained with rabbit antiglucagon and rabbit preimmune serum in tissues fixed for 0.5 to 4 hours (**FIGURES 3–3**

and 3–4). However, in specimens fixed for periods longer than 4 hours, the nonimmune rabbit serum produced immunostained islets in an apparently selective fashion, superficially resembling the distribution of beta cells (**FIGURE 3–5**).

A variety of techniques are available to assure the quality of primary antibody reagents with regard to specificity. These include time-honored procedures such as competitive-binding radioimmunoassay, immunoelectrophoresis, and enzyme-linked immunoabsorbent assay. However, in our experience these quality control procedures, though important, are still insufficient for immunohistochemistry. Specifically, reagents that demonstrate excellent specificity by methods such as immunoelectrophoresis and whose antibody activity can be abolished by preabsorption with antigen may nevertheless work very poorly in tissue because of other factors, such as the molar conjugation ratio of enzyme to antibody protein.

OTHER ANOMALOUS REACTIONS

Unanticipated positive cross-reactivities may sometimes be observed in immunohistology. For example Leu-7 (**FIGURE 3–6**), a mouse monoclonal antibody that recognizes the large granular lymphocytes, which are, in part, responsible for natural killer cell activity, also reacts intensely with the Schwann cells of peripheral nerve tissue (**FIGURE 3–7**); and T8, a mouse monoclonal antibody that reacts with subsets of T-cells, also binds to splenic sinusoidal endothelium. Such specific and real cross-reactivities probably reflect shared epitopes between apparently unrelated tissues.

Tissue Specificity Screening

In any given tissue section, many antigens may be represented in the exposed tissue. The presence or absence of reactivity with a given antibody may profile antibody selectivity for a large number of antigens in a single tissue section. Furthermore, it has been our experience that reagents demonstrating certain specificities in a fluid phase, such as radioimmunoassay or immunoelectrophoresis, may not react as anticipated in the tissue sections. These anomalous reactivities may appear either as suboptimal intensity due to suboptimal ratios of labels to antibody protein or as unexpected cross-reactivities.

To take anomalous reactivities into account and to become familiar with the spectrum of reactivities for each antigen, the pathologist should develop tissue specificity screens before applying immunohistochemical procedures in the laboratory. These screens should include a frozen tissue screen and a fixed paraffin-embedded tissue screen. If most of the immunostaining is to be done prospectively, with the type and quality of fixation controlled, it is best to choose a screen with appropriate fixatives. Thus, most of the paraffin-embedded material will be fixed in Bouin's or Hollande's solution. The screen should be chosen from a variety of normal and neoplastic tissues, and a large number of blocks will not be needed if they are chosen and processed carefully. The reactivities of the antibodies should be recorded. Appropriate blocks should then be chosen as control blocks and used "in-run" each time the immunohistochemical stain is done thereafter.

Guidelines for Resolving Immunostaining Problems

Like other test systems in the laboratory, immunohistochemical systems may break down. However, with suitable positive and negative controls, anomalous immunostaining can be detected. Although some problems cannot be resolved, many can be rectified by means of a systematic approach.

ANOMALOUS POSITIVE STAINING

Anomalous positive staining is said to occur when negative control sections are positive. The determination is made by evaluating both the control tissue and tissue from the patient being evaluated (Tables 3–2 and 3–3). First, determine whether the system conditions, especially fixation conditions, have been optimized (Table 3–1). If fixation is not the obvious source of error, the procedure should then be repeated to exclude a simple technical error, for example, primary antibody may have been applied to the negative control section or primary antibody may have flowed onto the negative control section during incubation. Dilutions of the serum applied to the negative control should also be checked: the immunoglobulin concentration of the preimmune or nonimmune serum applied to the negative control should approximate the dilution of the primary antibody. The immunoglobulin concentration should be equivalent, especially if the apparent crude dilutions for the serum are equivalent without accounting for the antibody concentration per se.

If anomalous positive staining still persists, the dilutions of the primary antibody and preimmune system should be checked against another block to be sure that they have been optimized. Generally, the highest dilutions of a primary antibody that give satisfactory staining of known positive controls are preferred. It may be necessary to block nonspecific binding sites with hyperimmune serum (see Hume and Gordon). Finally, it should be determined whether endogenous biotin is contributing to anomalous positive staining. If this is the case, a flush technique or a system not using biotin-avidin should be employed.

In most cases, this systematic approach will resolve questions of anomalous positive staining. However, when tissue factors that cannot be identified make it impossible to evaluate the tissue, another block, which may be better fixed, can be chosen. If the persistent problem is either endogenous enzyme activity in a very small population of cells that can be accounted for, or is easily recognized endogenous enzyme activity in one piece of tissue in a block containing several segments of tissue, it may still be possible to interpret the stains.

One should always exercise the option of using another block of tissue if it is available. If another block is not available and anomalous results cannot be resolved, it is best simply not to interpret the preparation to avoid acquiring misleading information.

ANOMALOUS NEGATIVE RESULTS

A second major problem that may occur is the absence of specific staining in the sample being evaluated or lack of anticipated or specific staining in the positive control. To resolve this problem, first check for technical error, such as omission of an antibody step in the sequence, dilution of antibody in distilled water, omission of the antibody from the section, omission of the substrate in the chromogen-substrate step of the sequence, or use of organic solvents to dehydrate aminoethylcarbazole and similar chromogens. Also, review the fixation and processing conditions in the system (Table 3–1) to ensure that optimal conditions have been used. In addition, review the dehydrating and clearing steps in relationship to the chromogen used, fungal or bacterial contamination of reagents, and inappropriate dilutions or calculation errors in making dilutions. Rarely, a paradoxical inhibition of specific staining analogous to the prozone effect can be seen at very high concentrations of antibody.

The necessity of determining optimal immunohistochemical systems for individual applications cannot be overemphasized. **FIGURES 3–8** through **3–11** illustrate the effect of different fixatives on the detection of prostate-specific antigen. No single fixative or processing method can be recommended as perfect for every immunohistochemical system. Each must be evaluated individually for determination of optimum conditions.

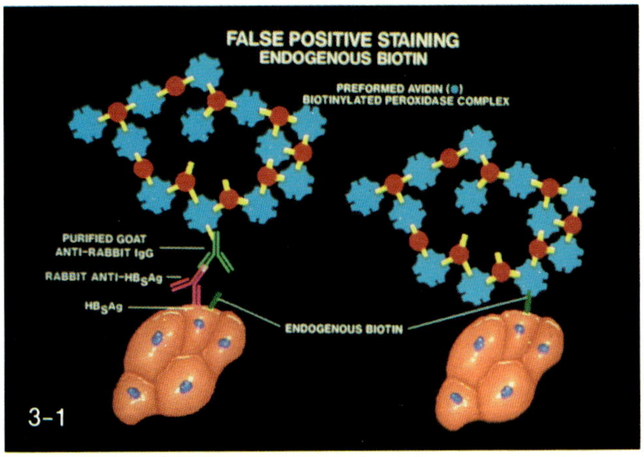

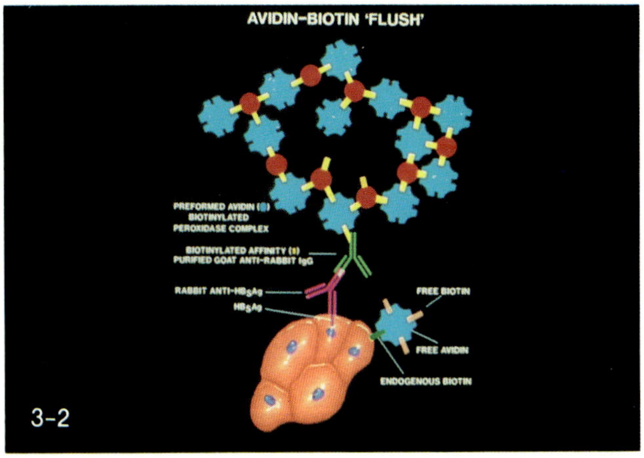

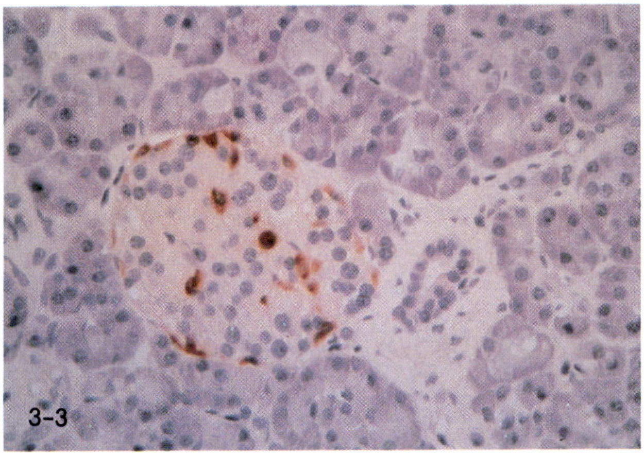

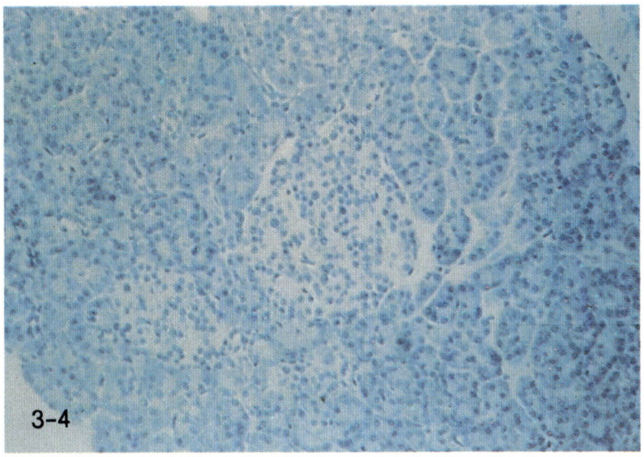

FIGURE 3–1. False-positive staining due to endogenous biotin. A positive reaction in the hepatocytes may represent binding of the avidin-biotin complex (ABC) to endogenous biotin, rather than a specific reaction with HBsAg.

FIGURE 3–2. Avidin-biotin flush technique. This flush technique is used to mask endogenous biotin. The tissue section is first exposed to excess avidin and then to biotin, a process that renders the endogenous biotin unavailable for binding to the ABC. *Slide 7.*

FIGURE 3–3. Normal pancreatic tissue. Figures 3–3 and 3–4 are from the same paraffin block. This tissue was fixed for 2 hours in Bouin's solution and stained for glucagon (red) with rabbit anti-glucagon, the primary antibody (ABC-PO with AEC, hematoxylin counterstain). See Table 3–2.

FIGURE 3–4. Tissue from same paraffin block as in Figure 3–3. In this slide, the IgG fraction of nonimmune rabbit serum was used instead of primary antibody. No positive staining is present. This sample acts as the negative glucagon control (ABC-PO with AEC, hematoxylin counterstain). See Table 3–2.

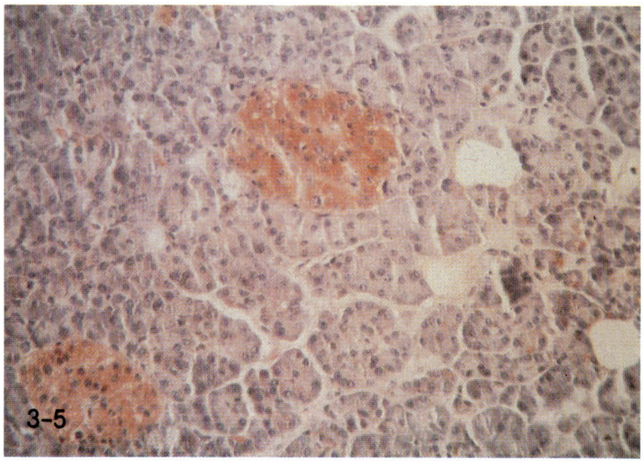

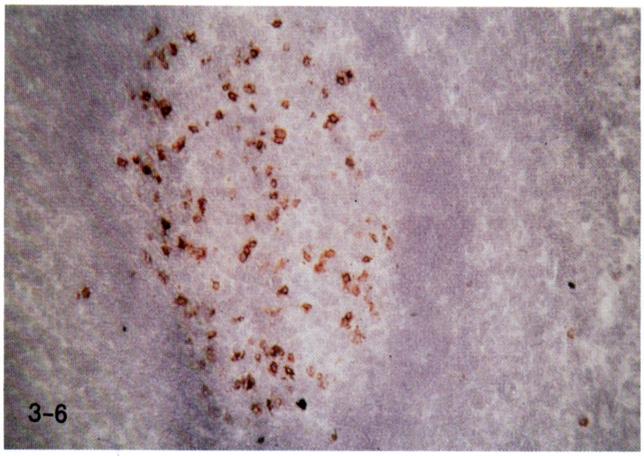

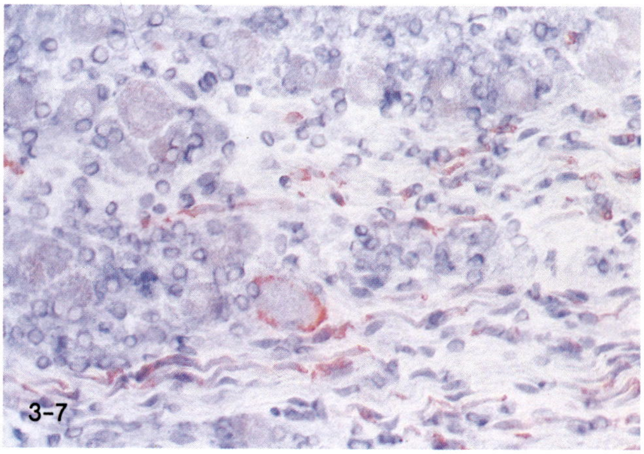

FIGURE 3–5. Normal pancreatic tissue, but fixed overnight in Bouin's solution. This slide shows anomalous binding of nonimmune normal rabbit IgG to overfixed tissue. The IgG fraction of nonimmune rabbit serum was used instead of primary antibody. The normal rabbit IgG binds selectively to islet cells (red), creating superficial resemblance to beta cell distribution (ABC-PO with AEC, hematoxylin counterstain).

FIGURE 3–6. Normal tonsil stained with Leu-7 monoclonal antibody. Some cells in the germinal center are stained (ABC-PO with AEC, hematoxylin counterstain).

FIGURE 3–7. Normal Schwann cells of peripheral nerve also stain positively (red) when Leu-7 monoclonal antibody is used (ABC-PO with AEC, hematoxylin counterstain).

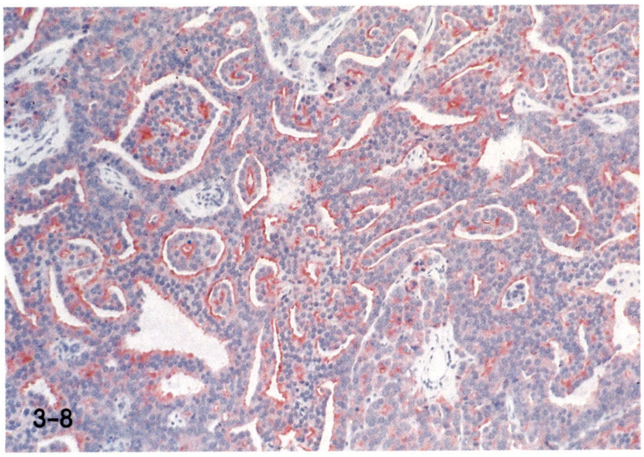

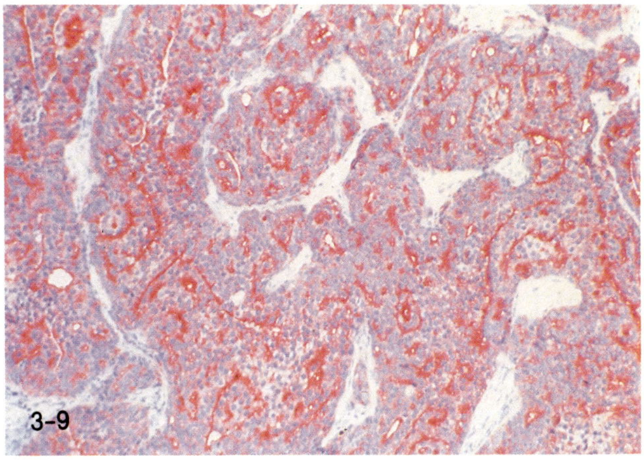

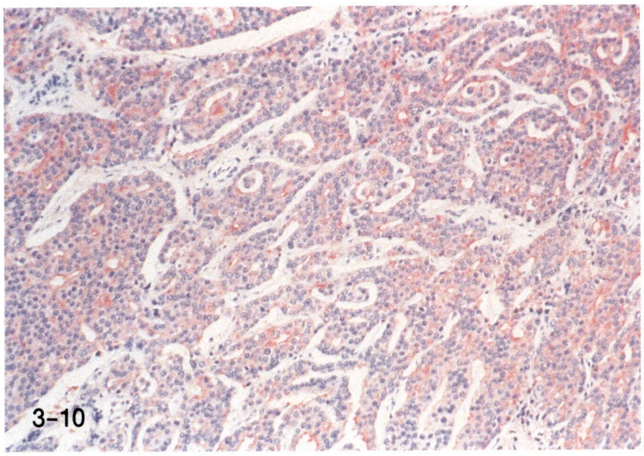

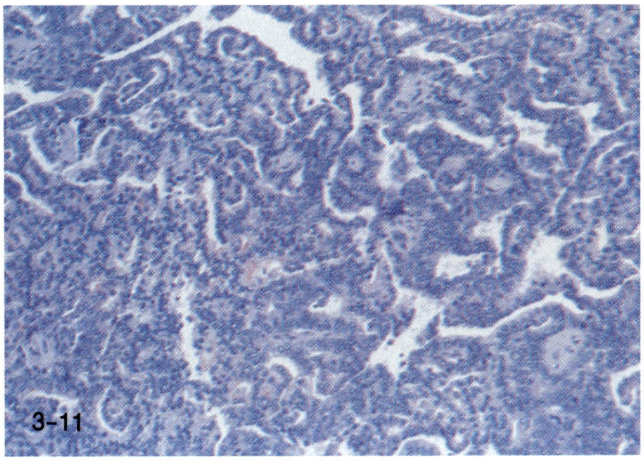

FIGURE 3–8. Effect of fixatives on detection of prostate-specific antigen. In Figures 3–8 through 3–11, paraffin sections of adenocarcinoma of prostate gland, fixed in different solutions, were stained with the same concentration of primary antibody (rabbit anti-prostate-specific antigen). This section was fixed with B-5 (ABC-PO with AEC, hematoxylin counterstain).

FIGURE 3–9. Prostate carcinoma. This section was fixed with formalin (ABC-PO with AEC, hematoxylin counterstain).

FIGURE 3–10. Prostate carcinoma. This section was fixed with absolute ethanol (ABC-PO with AEC, hematoxylin counterstain).

FIGURE 3–11. Prostate carcinoma. This section was fixed with Bouin's solution (ABC-PO with AEC, hematoxylin counterstain).

4 Endocrine Pathology

Immunohistochemical techniques in endocrine pathology have been primarily used in the evaluation of endocrine neoplasia. In this regard, immunohistochemical applications fall into four major categories: (1) classification of neoplasia, (2) clinicopathologic correlation, (3) direction of follow-up serum hormonal assays, and (4) prognosis.

The Pancreas

NORMAL IMMUNOHISTOLOGY

A knowledge of normal pancreatic immunohistology is essential for the interpretation and selection of control blocks. Beta cells containing immunoreactive insulin make up 60% to 80% of normal islets and tend to occupy a central position in the islet (**FIGURES 4–1** and **4–2**). The glucagon-secreting alpha cells (**FIGURES 4–2** and **4–3**) and delta cells containing immunoreactive somatostatin (**FIGURE 4–4**) are present in lesser numbers than are beta cells and are preferentially clustered toward the periphery of the islets. PP-cells secrete pancreatic polypeptide (PP) and make up only 0.5% to 1% of total islet cells. These cells are irregularly dispersed, demonstrating increased concentrations in the area of the pancreas developed embryologically from the ventral bud. Therefore, the usual blocks selected for immunohistochemistry from the pancreatic body or tail are unsuitable as PP-cell controls. G-cells containing gastrin are nonexistent in the normal adult pancreas. Also whether or not D1-cells containing vasoactive intestinal polypeptide (VIP) are present in pancreas is controversial. Therefore, we use gastric antrum and duodenum as positive controls for these antigens (**FIGURE 4–5**).

Over the years, a number of histochemical stains have been used to demonstrate the various islet cells in tissue sections. Experience has shown that the sensitivity and specificity of these stains are invariably inferior to those of immunohistochemistry.

ISLET CELL TUMORS

Pancreatic islet cell tumors are relatively uncommon, and only about 20% of them elaborate sufficient levels of hormone to induce a recognized clinical syndrome. Radioimmunoassay or immunohistochemical techniques will demonstrate hormone production in virtually all cases. Table 4–1 lists the hormones and other antigens that have been found in islet cell tumors either alone or in combination. Most of the antibodies

TABLE 4–1. Hormones and Other Antigens Identified in Islet Cell Tumors

Insulin
Glucagon
Somatostatin
Gastric inhibitory polypeptide (GIP)
Proinsulin
Secretin
Gastrin
Adrenocorticotropic hormone (ACTH)
Vasoactive intestinal polypeptide (VIP)
Melanin-stimulating hormone (MSH)
Pancreatic polypeptide (PP)
Calcitonin
Parathormone
Serotonin
5-Hydroxyindoleacetic acid (HIAA)
Dopamine
Human chorionic gonadotropin (HCG)
β-HCG
Prostatic acid phosphatase
α-1-Antitrypsin

TABLE 4–2. Malignancy Rate Based on Hormones Secreted by Islet Cell Tumors

Primary Immunocyto-chemical Hormone Secreted by Tumor	No. of Cases	Malignancies No. (%)
Pancreatic polypeptide	10	0
Insulin	27	4 (15)
Glucagon	13	8 (62)
Gastrin	24	16 (67)
Vasoactive intestinal polypeptide	21	16 (76)
None detected	30	15 (50)

SOURCE: Heitz P, Kasper M, Polak J, et al: Pancreatic endocrine tumors: Immunocytochemical analysis of 125 tumors. *Hum Pathol* 1982;13:263–271. Adapted with permission.

NOTE: Some tumors contained several hormones.

directed against these antigens can be obtained commercially. Our experience as well as that of others has shown that many islet cell tumors are multihormonal; therefore, classification is based on the predominant hormone present.

We are careful to note the presence of minor hormonal constituents. This information helps direct the selection of serum hormonal determinations in clinical follow-up. Metastases or recurrence, especially after chemotherapy, may demonstrate the minor hormonal components only. Also, on occasion, demonstration of the minor hormonal component is important to the individual clinical situation and may save the patient unnecessary additional surgeries; **FIGURES 4–6** through **4–8** illustrate such a case. The typical islet cell tumor illustrated in **FIGURE 4–6** was removed from a 62-year-old man who had elevated serum levels of VIP and calcitonin. Immunohistochemistry performed on the resected specimen demonstrated both VIP and calcitonin (**FIGURES 4–7** and **4–8**). The demonstration of calcitonin in this case helped save this patient an unnecessary neck exploration to look for a medullary thyroid carcinoma. The postoperative serum calcitonin and VIP levels returned to normal.

Table 4–2 illustrates a classification of islet cell tumors based on tissue immunohistochemistry. This classification seems to serve in predicting the likelihood of metastasis; however, for individual cases, there are no reliable criteria for predicting malignancy.

In the future, immunohistochemistry may be helpful in predicting malignancy in pancreatic endocrine tumors. There is evidence that production of several hormones (especially hormones considered ectopic to the pancreas) and expression of certain oncodevelopmental antigens (especially human chorionic gonadotropin) may be markers of malignant potential. More work in this area needs to be done.

The immunohistology of a typical insulinoma is illustrated in **FIGURE 4–9**. It is often helpful to select blocks for immunohistochemistry from the interface of tumor and normal pancreas because the residual normal islets will serve as a useful internal control.

Gastrinomas **(FIGURE 4–10)** are second in frequency to insulinomas. Pancreatic islet cell hyperplasia often seen in gastrinoma is considered an effect of high gastrin levels and not a cause. If no tumor can be found in the pancreas at laparotomy in patients with the Zollinger-Ellison syndrome, the surgical pathologist must urge the surgeon to continue looking for a gastrinoma because approximately 20% are extrapancreatic, occurring in the duodenal wall, stomach, biliary tree, splenic hilum, or ovary.

Electron microscopy has been used in evaluating these tumors. Characteristic morphology of neuroendocrine granules allows the identification of normal islet cells and the classification of some tumors. In practice, however, we have found that electron microscopy tends to be time-consuming and is subject to significant sampling errors, especially in multihormonal tumors. Also, ultrastructural morphologies of neoplastic granules overlap, making evaluation difficult. In general, we find immunohistochemistry easier and more reliable.

In summary, immunohistochemistry is the most reliable method for classifying pancreatic endocrine tumors. The recently published classification scheme based on tissue immunohistochemistry (Table 4–2) appears to have prognostic significance. Demonstration of minor hormones is important in follow-up and in clinicopathologic correlation. Finally, demonstration of multiple hormones, especially hormones considered ectopic to the pancreas or certain oncodevelopmental antigens such as human chorionic gonadotropin, may eventually prove to be specific markers for malignancy.

The Anterior Pituitary

NORMAL IMMUNOHISTOLOGY

Normal human pituitary glands obtained at autopsy serve adequately as controls for immunohistochemistry. Antibodies directed against growth hormone (GH), follicle-stimulating hormone (FSH), prolactin, luteinizing hormone (LH), thyroid-stimulating hormone (TSH), and adrenocorticotropic hormone (ACTH) are commercially available. A representative positive normal control for ACTH is illustrated in **FIGURE 4–11**.

PITUITARY ADENOMAS

As with pancreatic endocrine neoplasia, routine light microscopic examination of pituitary adenomas cannot predict hormonal activity or behavior. Historical classification of pituitary adenomas based on tinctorial appearance (acidophilic adenoma, basophilic adenoma, and chromophobe adenoma) and other classification schemes have been shown to be insufficient to cover the complex clinicopathologic aspects of these tumors.

The application of immunohistochemistry to the study of pituitary adenomas appears to be limited to classification and clinicopathologic correlation only. Paraffin-embedded tissue, preferably fixed in formalin, is optimal for these evaluations. The immunologic demonstration of hormones in tissue sections correlates well with both clinical manifestations and serum hormonal elevations but seems to be of little prognostic significance. **FIGURE 4–12** illustrates a growth hormone–producing pituitary adenoma in a patient with acromegaly. This tumor, like many pituitary adenomas, demonstrated one hormone only. However, multihormonal adenomas are not infrequent, and distinguishing between adenoma and hyperplasia may at times be difficult. The diffuse staining illustrated in **FIGURE 4–12** is a common pattern, but perinuclear staining has also been reported. Neither the absolute number of positive cells nor the pattern of staining (diffuse versus perinuclear) correlates with severity of clinical symptoms or degree of serum hormonal elevation.

Electron microscopy is a useful tool in studying pituitary adenomas. Although cell identification based solely on electron microscopy is difficult, electron microscopy may disclose the presence of neuroendocrine granules in tumors that have been negative by immunohistochemical techniques. Perhaps the hormone levels in these tumors are too low to be detected by immunologic stains or perhaps the anterior pituitary contains as yet unidentified hormones.

Immunohistochemistry is a useful tool for classification and clinicopathologic correlation in pituitary adenomas. However, we do not advocate its routine use unless clinical correlation is desired.

The Thyroid

NORMAL IMMUNOHISTOLOGY

Knowledge of normal thyroid immunohistology is important for interpretation and selection of control blocks. **FIGURE 4–13** illustrates a normal thyroglobulin control. Either incidental thyroidectomy (as part of a neck dissection) or nodular goiter can be used as a positive control. Not all follicular epithelial cells nor all colloid will stain positively or with the same intensity. This is particularly true when nodular goiter is used as a control. A calcitonin control illustrates the intrafollicular location of C-cells (**FIGURE 4–14**), which should not be misinterpreted as unwanted cross-reactivity. Many normal thyroid sections will be devoid of C-cells and unsuitable for positive C-cell controls. Therefore, we suggest using either a medullary thyroid carcinoma (**FIGURE 4–15**) or thyroid tissue demonstrating C-cell hyperplasia (**FIGURE 4–16**) as control blocks.

FOLLICULAR, PAPILLARY, AND MEDULLARY CARCINOMA

FIGURES 4–17 through **4–24** illustrate the utility of thyroglobulin and calcitonin immunohistology in differential diagnosis. Although thyroid origin can often be suggested on the basis of routine light microscopy, as in the metastatic papillary carcinoma illustrated in **FIGURE 4–17**, thyroid origin can be proved definitively by demonstrating immunoreactive thyroglobulin (**FIGURE 4–18**). Virtually all papillary and follicular thyroid neoplasias demonstrate positive immunoreactivity for thyroglobulin. Medullary carcinomas and metastatic carcinomas involving the thyroid are invariably negative, and anaplastic carcinomas show immunoreactive thyroglobulin in the more differentiated portions only. **FIGURES 4–19** and **4–20** illustrate a metastatic carcinoma involving the liver. This patient had a history of medullary thyroid carcinoma and had undergone a thyroidectomy and resections of multiple local recurrences. The histologic findings in **FIGURE 4–19** are somewhat unusual for medullary thyroid carcinoma, and stains for amyloid were negative. However, positive immunostaining for calcitonin established this lesion as metastatic medullary thyroid carcinoma (**FIGURE 4–20**).

Immunohistochemistry is now the only reliable method for demonstrating C-cell hyperplasia. Medullary thyroid carcinomas associated with familial syndromes are associated with C-cell hyperplasia in the surrounding thyroid. Thus, identification of C-cell hyperplasia justifies the screening of family members by serum calcitonin determinations. Normal thyroid usually contains four to ten C-cells per low-power field, some in clusters of two or three. However, in C-cell hyperplasia, many more C-cells are seen, and they are often clustered in groups of 10 to 20, with occasional nodule formation.

In summary, routine immunohistochemical techniques are not necessary for diagnosis in most forms of thyroid neoplasia; but on occasion immunologic demonstration of thyroglobulin and calcitonin can be invaluable in differential diagnosis, especially in metastases. In addition, immunohistochemistry is the only reliable method for demonstrating C-cell hyperplasia.

The Adrenal Gland

Uses of immunohistochemistry in the study of neoplasia of the adrenal gland have been limited to isolated case reports of clinicopathologic correlation. Immunoreactive aldosterone can be identified in cortical adenomas, and hormones such as ACTH (**FIGURE 4–21**), VIP, and somatostatin have been reported in pheochromocytoma.

Other Neuroendocrine Tumors

Occasionally, neuroendocrine tumors arise in other peripheral locations. Carcinoid tumors, for example, may arise in teratomas (**FIGURE 4–22**) and may contain polypeptide hormones (**FIGURES 4–23** and **4–24**), which can be immunostained.

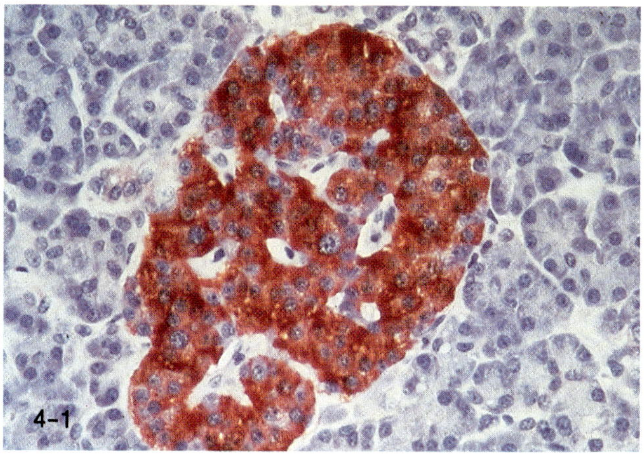

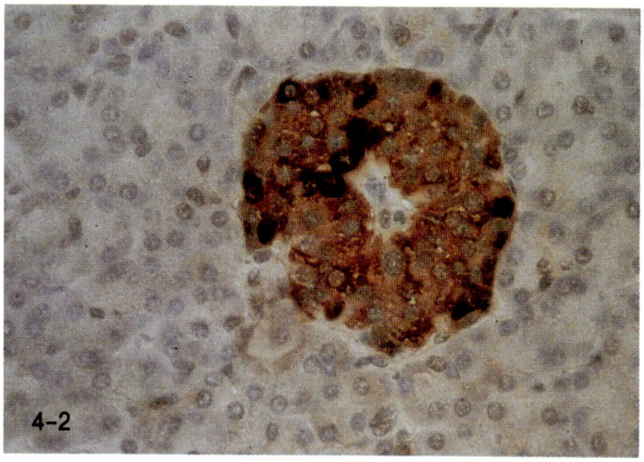

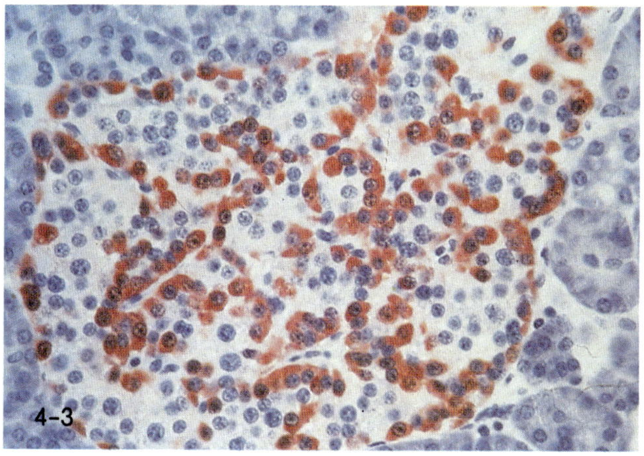

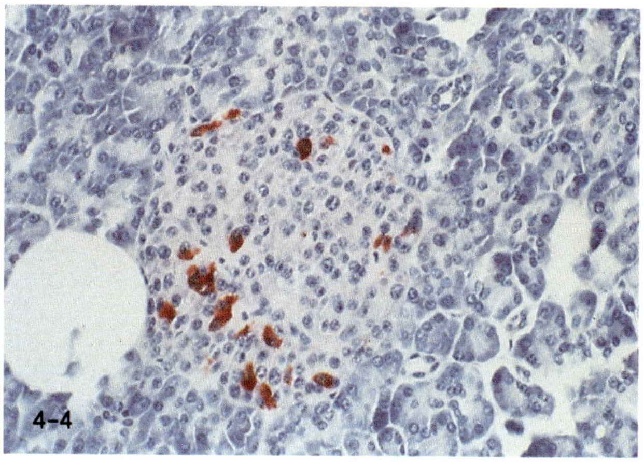

FIGURE 4–1. Pancreatic islet cells show immunoreactive insulin (red) in the beta cells (ABC-PO with AEC, hematoxylin counterstain). *Slide 10.*

FIGURE 4–2. Pancreatic islet cells show two antigens simultaneously, insulin and glucagon, by use of two chromogens. In the more numerous and centrally located beta cells, the insulin stains red (ABC-PO with AEC). In the less numerous and peripherally located alpha cells, the glucagon stains brown-black (ABC-PO with DAB, hematoxylin counterstain). Reproduced with permission from *Cleve Clin Q* 1981;48:258. *Slide 11.*

FIGURE 4–3. Pancreatic islet. Alpha cells, which contain immunoreactive glucagon (red), are present in lesser numbers than the beta cells (ABC-PO with AEC, hematoxylin counterstain). *Slide 12.*

FIGURE 4–4. Pancreatic islet. Somatostatin (red) is visible in the delta cells (ABC-PO with AEC, hematoxylin counterstain). *Slide 13.*

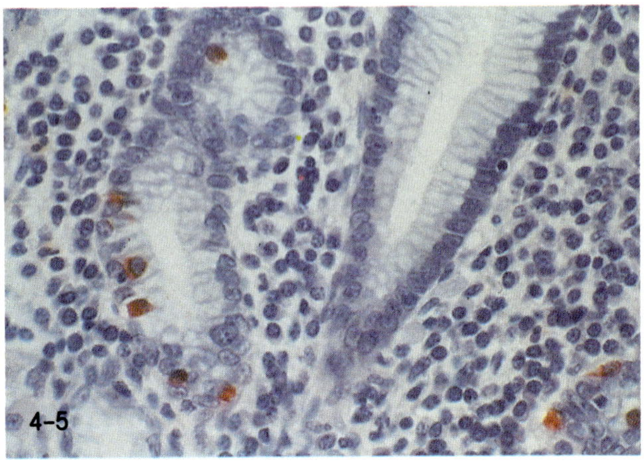

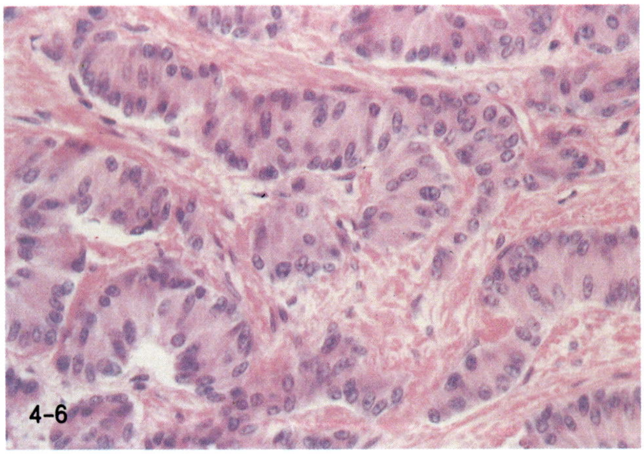

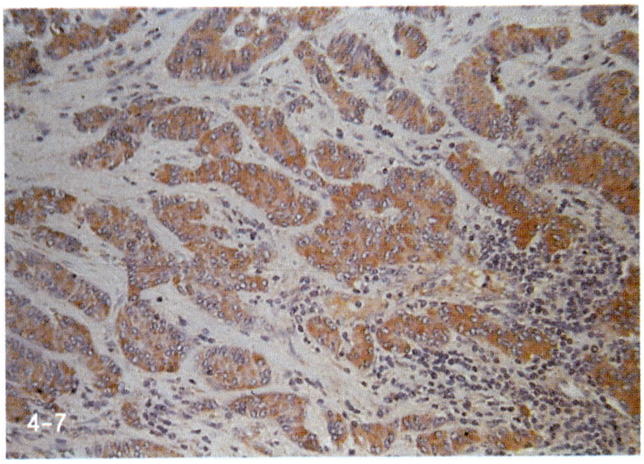

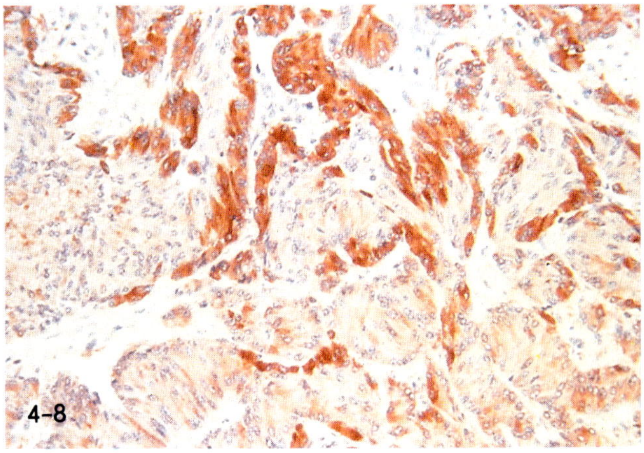

FIGURE 4–5. Gastric antrum control for gastrin. Occasional G-cells stain red (ABC-PO with AEC, hematoxylin counterstain). *Slide 14.*

FIGURE 4–6. Islet cell tumor. Figures 4–6 through 4–8 show sections from the same case. This figure shows the trabecular arrangement of uniform neoplastic cells that is one of the typical patterns seen in islet cell tumors (H & E).

FIGURE 4–7. Same case as 4–6. Immunoreactive vasoactive intestinal polypeptide (red) is visible in almost all the cells (ABC-PO with AEC, hematoxylin counterstain). *Slide 15.*

FIGURE 4–8. Same case as 4–6. Immunoreactive calcitonin (red) is visible in occasional tumor cells (ABC-PO with AEC, hematoxylin counterstain).

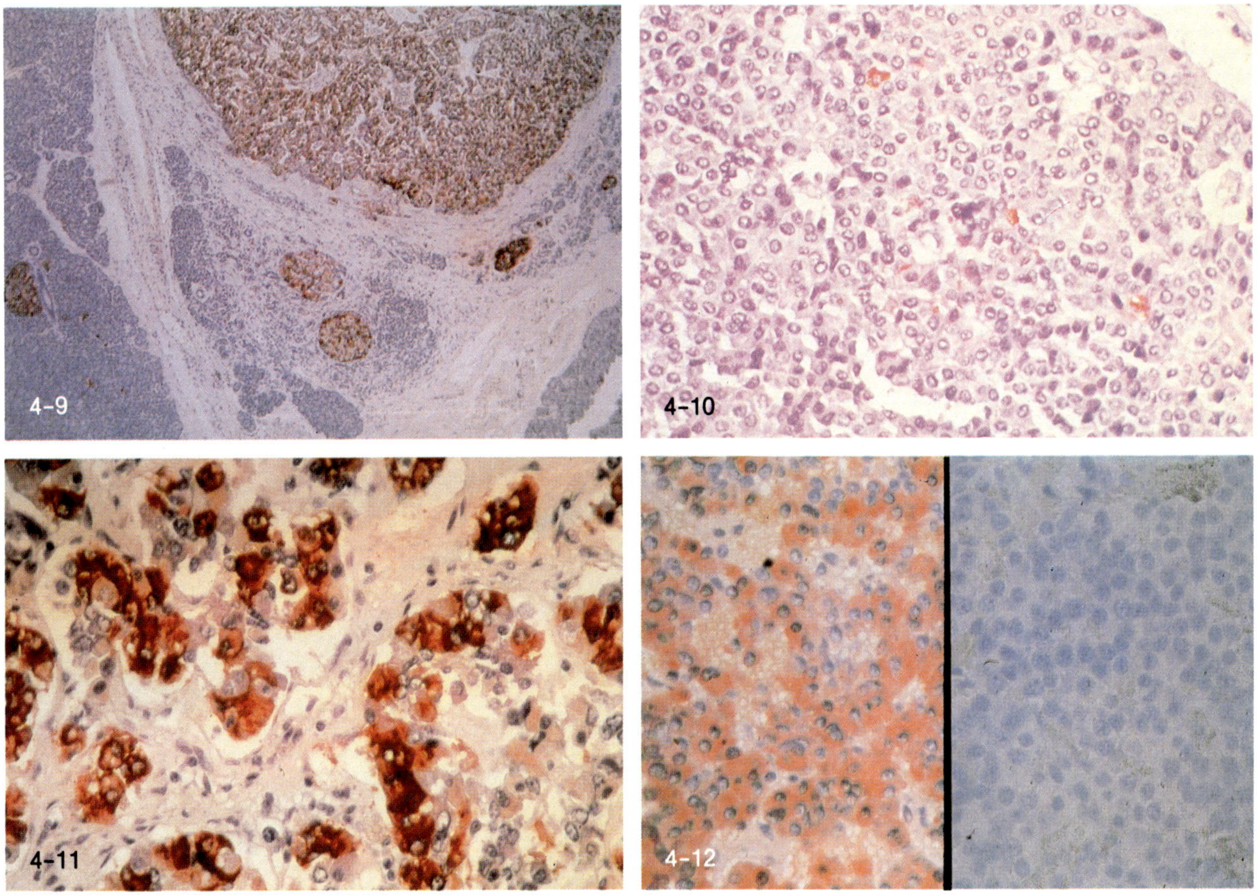

FIGURE 4–9. Small insulinoma. Tumor cells are positive for insulin (red; upper right). If blocks are selected from the interface of the tumor and normal pancreas, the residual islets (lower center and left) can serve as internal positive controls (ABC-PO with AEC, hematoxylin counterstain). Reproduced with permission from *Cleve Clin Q* 1981;48:257.

FIGURE 4–10. Islet cell tumor from a patient with Zollinger-Ellison syndrome stained for gastrin (red). Very few cells are positive (ABC-PO with AEC, hematoxylin counterstain).

FIGURE 4–11. Normal pituitary gland used as a control for ACTH (red-brown; ABC-PO with AEC, hematoxylin counterstain). *Slide 16.*

FIGURE 4–12. Pituitary adenoma stained for immunoreactive growth hormone (red, left). Almost all the cells stain positively and in a diffuse pattern, in contrast with the negative control on the right (ABC-PO with AEC, hematoxylin counterstain).

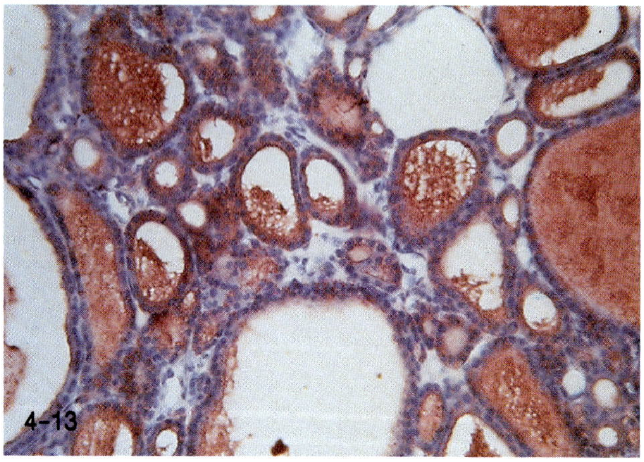

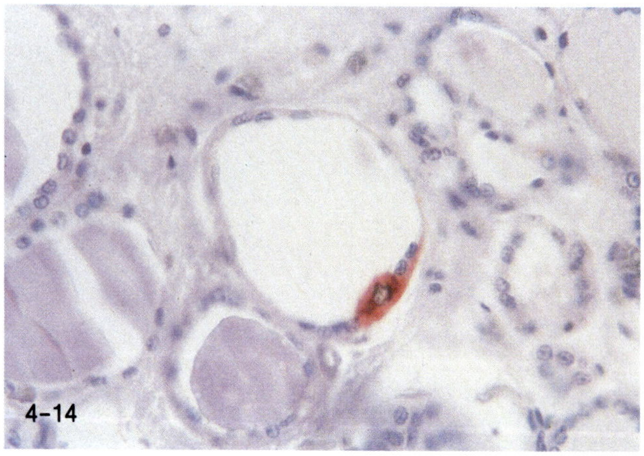

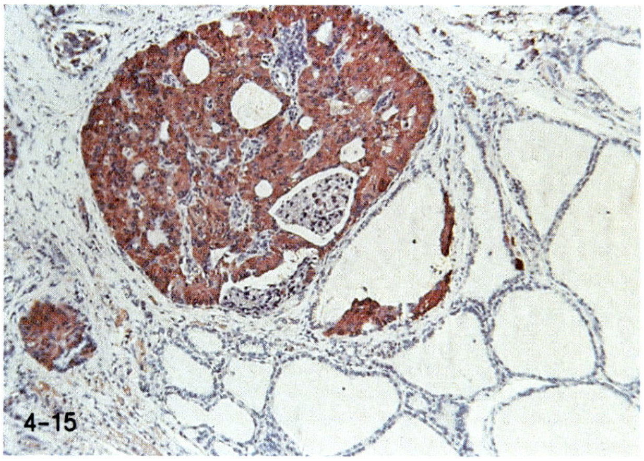

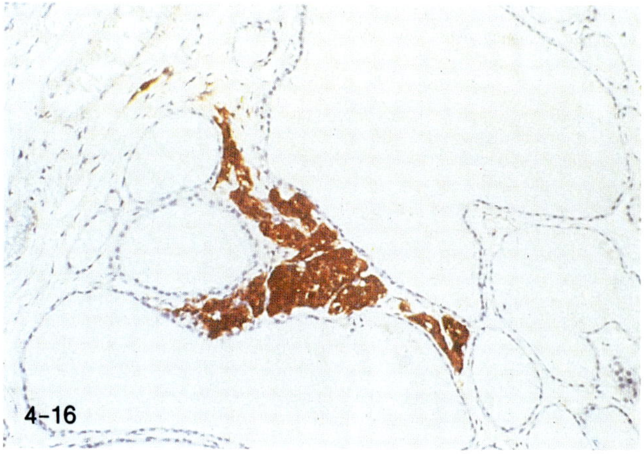

FIGURE 4–13. Nodular colloid goiter stained for thyroglobulin and used as a normal thyroglobulin positive control. Not all the follicular elements or colloid stain positively (red) or with the same intensity (ABC-PO with AEC, hematoxylin counterstain).

FIGURE 4–14. Normal thyroid stained for calcitonin (red). A single C-cell is visible and should not be misinterpreted as cross-reactivity with thyroid follicular epithelial cells (ABC-PO with AEC, hematoxylin counterstain).

FIGURE 4–15. Medullary thyroid carcinoma from a patient with multiple endocrine neoplasia, type II. This section was stained for calcitonin (red) and used as a positive control. Not all tumor cells stain positively or with the same intensity. Invariably, medullary thyroid carcinoma stains much less intensely for calcitonin than will the surrounding normal tissue or hyperplastic C-cells (ABC-PO with AEC, hematoxylin counterstain).

FIGURE 4–16. Thyroid C-cell hyperplasia used as a positive (red) calcitonin control (ABC-PO with AEC, hematoxylin counterstain). *Slide 17.*

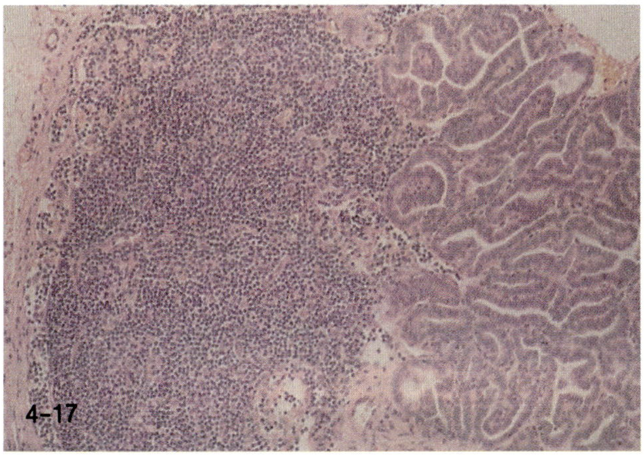

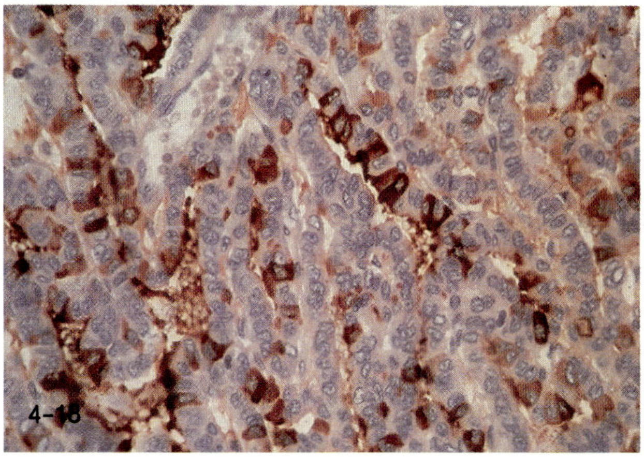

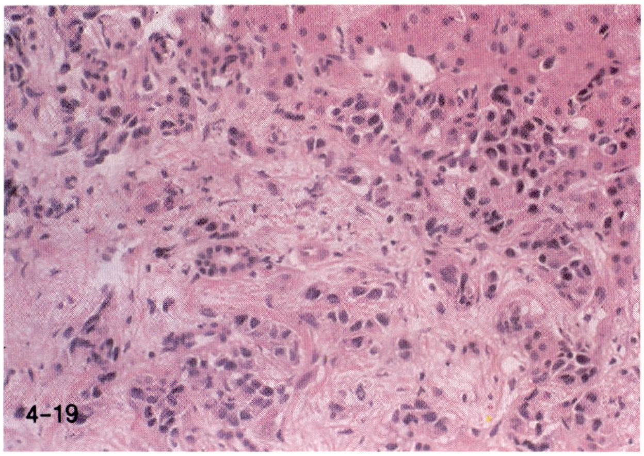

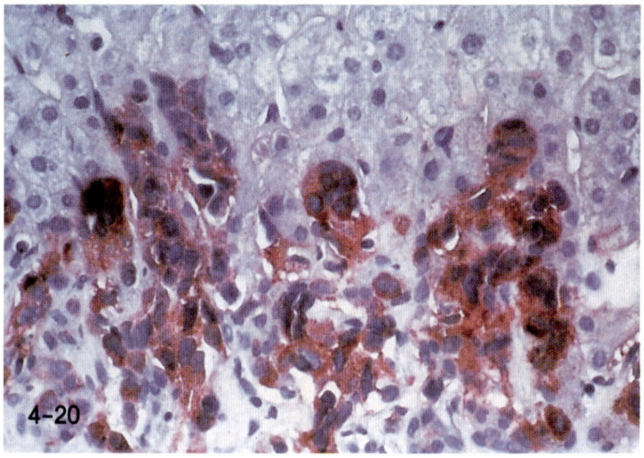

FIGURE 4–17. Metastatic papillary carcinoma in a lymph node. Figures 4–17 and 4–18 are from the same case. This section is stained with H & E.

FIGURE 4–18. Same case as 4–17, lymph node stained for thyroglobulin. The positive reaction (red) establishes that this tumor originated from the thyroid. As with other endocrine neoplasia, not all cells stain positively (ABC-PO with AEC, hematoxylin counterstain). *Slide 18.*

FIGURE 4–19. Medullary thyroid carcinoma metastatic to liver. Figures 4–19 and 4–20 are from the same case. Spindle cell and epithelial components are visible. Stains for amyloid were negative (H & E).

FIGURE 4–20. Same case as 4–19. Staining the tumor tissue for immunoreactive calcitonin (red) establishes this tumor as metastatic medullary thyroid carcinoma (ABC-PO with AEC, hematoxylin counterstain). *Slide 19.*

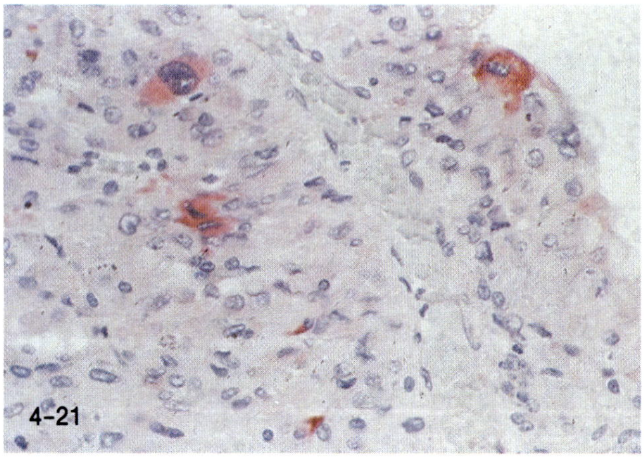

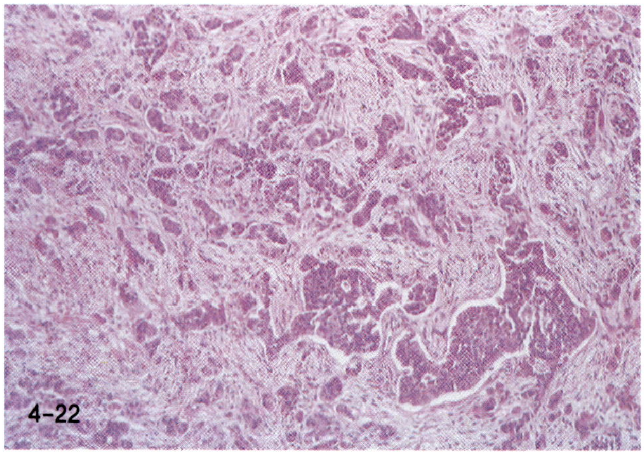

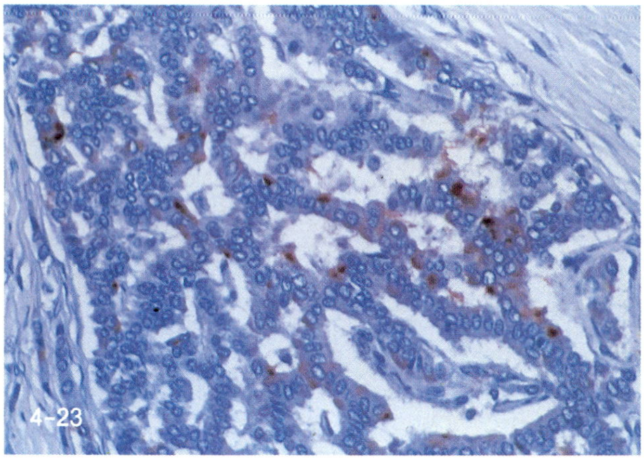

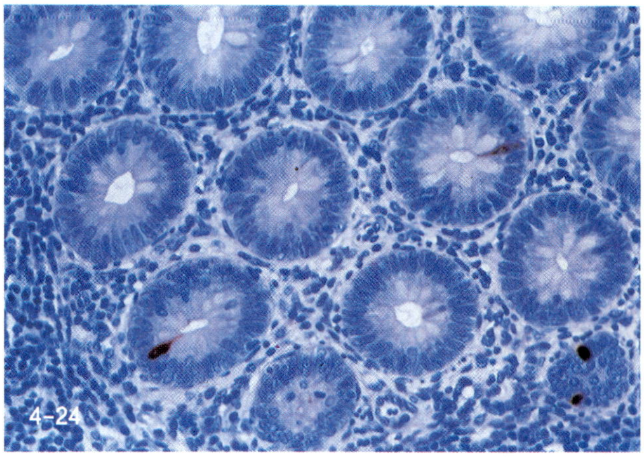

FIGURE 4–21. Pheochromocytoma in a patient presenting with Cushing's syndrome. Focal cells contain ACTH (red; ABC-PO with AEC, hematoxylin counterstain).

FIGURE 4–22. Carcinoid tumor arising in an immature coccygeal teratoma. Figures 4–22 and 4–23 are from the same case. This section is stained with H & E.

FIGURE 4–23. Same case as 4–22. The tumor cells contain serotonin (red; ABC-PO with AEC, hematoxylin counterstain). *Slide 20.*

FIGURE 4–24. A section of appendix serving as serotonin control. Serotonin-containing cells stain red (ABC-PO with AEC, hematoxylin counterstain).

5 Lymphoproliferative Disorders

The past two decades have seen a veritable explosion of information on the functional and antigenic characteristics of lymphoid cell populations. During this time, malignant lymphomas have come to be recognized as neoplasms of the immune system, retaining for the most part functional and antigenic markers for the cell of origin. More recently, hybridoma technology has enhanced the precision of subclassification of these disorders by making available monoclonal antibodies with a variety of specificities. Much has also been learned about nonneoplastic lymphoproliferative disease, including immunodeficiencies and the immunoregulatory abnormalities associated with viral infections and autoimmune diseases, such as rheumatoid arthritis and systemic lupus erythematosus.

Also during the past two decades, morphologic and immunologic approaches to classification of non-Hodgkin's lymphomas have evolved along parallel lines. Only recently has some sort of stability evolved in the classification of non-Hodgkin's lymphoma. Specifically, a study sponsored by the National Cancer Institute has yielded a morphologic working formulation with clinical relevance. For the foreseeable future, this approach will be helpful, at least in ensuring some uniformity of classification so that clinical therapeutic trials can be compared. However, morphologic approaches will probably ultimately be replaced with a classification based on immunotype. Such a classification will relate to the maturation and differentiation stages of T- and B-lymphocytes. Individual maturation stages have been identified by means of a combination of functional markers, such as surface immunoglobulin, and antigenic differentiation markers of both relatively broad and narrow specificity (Table 5–1). Ultimately, these will probably form the subclassification niches in an immunotypic scheme (**FIGURES 5–1** and **5–2**). Some of the subtypes of lymphoma in the International Formulation are composed of one immunotype, but others are heterogeneous (Table 5–2). An immunologic approach would consist of subclasses of lymphomas with specific immunotypes corresponding to differentiation stages.

To classify lymphoproliferative diseases precisely, optimal processing of tissue is required. No longer can the pathologist accept from the operating room lymph nodes immersed in formalin. The pathologist must insist on receiving the fresh specimen as soon as possible from the surgeon, so that properly fixed specimens can be prepared. A protocol for handling lymph node biopsy specimens should be developed along

TABLE 5–1. Primary Specificities of Monoclonal Antibodies for Hematopoietic Cells

Antibody	Detects Cellular Antigens Expressed by:
Pan-T markers	
T11, Leu-5	T-cells forming spontaneous rosettes with sheep erythrocytes, some NK cells
T3, Leu-4	Peripheral T-cells
T1, Leu-1	Thymic and peripheral T-cells, B-CLL cells[a]
T-cell subpopulations	
T4, Leu-3	Helper/inducer T-cells, some macrophages
$T4^+$ Leu 8^-	Helper T-cells
$T4^+$ $2H4^+$	Suppressor inducer T4 subset
$T4^+$ $4B4^+$	Helper inducer T4 subset
T5, T8, Leu-2	Cytotoxic/suppressor T-cells, splenic endothelium
Leu-15	Suppressor T-cells, NK-cells, neutrophils, eosinophils, and monocytes
T6	Immature cortical thymocytes ("common" thymocytes), Langerhan's cells
T9	All cells bearing transferrin receptor (T- and B-cells)
T10	Immature thymocytes, plasma cells
B-cell markers	
Leu-14, B1	Some pre-B, immature, virginal, and secretory blast stage B-cells
Leu-10	B-cells, macrophages
B4	Pre-B, immature, virginal, and some secretory blast stage B-cells
B2	Immature and virginal B-cells, PMNs
I2, HLA-DR, LN3[b]	Most B-cells, macrophages, activated T-cells, and some endothelial cells (those cells that have Ia-like antigens on the surface)
LN1[b]	Immature, virginal, and secretory blast stage B-cells; ductular epithelium; erythrocytic cells and precursors; intrafollicular macrophages
LN2[b]	Pre-B, immature, virginal, and some secretory blast stage B-cells; dendritic reticulum cells
Other markers	
I2, HLA-DR, LN3[b], Leu-M3, Leu-M5, α-1-chymotrypsin and muramidase[b] (polyclonal antibodies)	Macrophages; HLA-DR antigens are present on activated T-cells and most B-cells
NKH-1; Leu-7[b]; Leu-11a, b, c; Leu-15	NK cells; Leu-15 also labels suppressor T-cells

SOURCE: Tubbs RR, Sheibani K: Immunohistology of lymphoproliferative disorders. *Semin Diagn Pathol* 1984;1:275. Used with permission.

Abbreviations: B-CLL = B-cell chronic lymphocytic leukemia, NK = natural killer, PMN = polymorphonuclear leukocyte.

NOTE: The antibodies listed in this table detect only cellular antigens and do not directly profile cell function. Also, other specificities occur for some antibodies, eg, $2H4^+$ B-cells.

[a]Leu-1 and T11 also react with B-cells of B-cell CLL, but not most normal B-cells. Several reports have also identified Leu-1-positive antigen in occasional cases of low-grade follicle center cell lymphomas.

[b]Antibodies that can detect cellular antigens in paraffin-embedded tissue fixed in Bouin's solution or B-5.

TABLE 5–2. Usual Immunotypes of Lymphoproliferative Disorders

Histopathologic Diagnosis	Immunotype
Benign histopathologic findings	Physiologic number and distribution of antigens
Atypical hyperplasia	Variable; some cases have monoclonal[a] immunostaining
Hodgkin's disease	Small lymphocytes principally $T11^+$ $T4^+$.[b] Reed-Sternberg cells and variants Ia^+ $T11^-$ κ^+ λ^+ $LN2^+$ $LN3^+$
Non-Hodgkin's lymphomas[c]	
Low-grade	
Small lymphocytic	Usually monoclonal B-cell (immature stage); some are of T-cell origin
Follicular, small cleaved	Monoclonal B-cell (virginal stage)
Follicular mixed	Monoclonal B-cell (or κ^- λ^- $B1^+$)
Intermediate-grade	
Follicular, large cell	Monoclonal B-cell (secretory blast stage)
Diffuse, small cleaved	Variable
Diffuse, mixed	Variable
Diffuse large cell	
Large-cell, NOS; Large cleaved cell; Large non-cleaved cell	Most cases either monoclonal B-cell (secretory blast stage) or κ^- λ^- $B1^+$ Ia^+
High-grade	
Immunoblastic, NOS	Variable
Plasmacytoid	Usually monoclonal secretory blast B-cell
Clear cell	Usually T-cell (intrathymic or peripheral)
Polymorphous	Usually T-cell (intrathymic or peripheral)
Epithelioid cell component	Variable
Lymphoblastic	Intrathymic T-cell (rarely pre-B)
Small noncleaved cell	Monoclonal B-cell (secretory blast stage)
Miscellaneous	
Mycosis fungoides	Peripheral T-cell (usually $T4^+$ $T8^-$ Leu-9^-)
Extramedullary plasmacytosis	B-cell (monoclonal cytoplasmic immunoglobulin)
Malignant histiocytosis	Tissue macrophage
Not classifiable	Variable

ABBREVIATION: NOS = not otherwise specified.

NOTE: Deletion of an antigen usually expressed in normal lymphocytes at a particular stage is also often seen, especially in T-cell lymphomas.

[a]"Monoclonal" indicates single immunoglobulin light chain (κ or λ). It is recognized that many B-cell lymphomas are better designated as displaying clonal excess and are probably biclonal or oligoclonal.

[b]For most cases (nodular sclerosis, mixed cellularity, and lymphocyte-depleted types); however, the small lymphocytes of lymphocyte-predominant Hodgkin's disease are usually polyclonal B-cells.

[c]International Working Formulation classifications.

the lines specified in **FIGURE 5–3.** Such a protocol ensures that material is available for marker studies using immunocytology, for immunohistochemistry, and for touch preparations using immunocytology or cytochemistry. The protocol also ensures that material well fixed in B-5 is available for accurate histopathologic assessment. Ordinarily, a small amount of tissue should be placed in glutaraldehyde for possible transmission electron microscopy (EM). Usually, EM contributes little to the diagnosis of these diseases. However, on occasion, a poorly differentiated neoplasm may be present in the lymph node, and EM may help differentiate between lymphoma, carcinoma, and melanoma.

Immunotypes can be delineated on frozen tissue sections by immunohistologic methods and on touch and cytocentrifuged preparations from the cell suspension by immunocytologic methods. We have found that a dual approach using frozen tissue sections and air-dried, acetone-fixed, cytocentrifuged preparations is helpful in immunotyping lymphoproliferative diseases. The immunohistologic sections are especially helpful when there is incomplete architectural effacement of the lymph node, especially in follicular lymphomas. The morphologic detail at higher magnification in the frozen tissue sections may be somewhat difficult to interpret. However, immunostained cytocentrifuged preparations correlated with hematoxylin counterstains show superior resolution.

In most cases, the lymphoma is quite uniform with respect to the immunotype displayed by the cells. However, in some, other cell populations may be mixed with the malignant lymphoma cells in the tissue. These subpopulations tend to be overlooked in conventional histopathologic sections, especially in large cell lymphomas where a significant number of smaller lymphoid cells can be identified by careful study. Some mixed lymphomas do bear the same immunotype on both small and large cells. However, a significant number consist of B-cell large cell tumors with extensive infiltration by small T-lymphocytes.

FIGURES 5–4 through **5–61** illustrate the immunohistologic and immunocytologic findings in "reactive" and neoplastic lymphoproliferative lesions. The immunostaining patterns are for fresh-frozen tissue sections or cytocentrifuged preparations made from fresh, single-cell suspensions.

Lymphofollicular hyperplasia is characterized by both κ- and λ-bearing cells (ratio approximately 1:8), in varying numbers in follicular centers and in nearly all the cells of the mantle zone and medullary cords. $T11^+$ cells are located principally in the paracortex and interfollicular zone, but a subpopulation of follicle center cells is also $T11^+$. The intrafollicular component of the T-cell population is primarily $T11^+$ $T4^+$.

Follicular lymphomas are characterized by neoplastic follicles or nodules composed of individual cells staining for only one immunoglobulin light chain, either κ or λ. A variable number of T-cells may be present in the neoplastic follicles, and intervening interfollicular parenchyma usually contains numerous $T11^+$ cells. Lymphomas with diffuse architectural growth patterns of B-cells demonstrate a predominance of one immunoglobulin light chain and variable numbers of $T11^+$ cells and macrophages in the cellular milieu. In most large cell diffuse lymphomas, a combination of immunocytology and immunohistology can be used to discern a differential immunostaining pattern in hematoxylin-counterstained preparations.

Limitations of the procedure include the limited resolution that can be achieved in a frozen tissue section at higher magnification and the invariable adherence to collagen and endothelium of primary antibodies to immunoglobulin heavy and light chains.

Immunocytology is also useful for profiling the immunotypic differentiation of acute leukemia cells. Immunocytologic techniques are applied to cytocentrifuge preparations of cells partially separated over a density sedimentation gradient (**FIGURES 5–46** and **5–47**). Results derived from this method compare favorably with those obtained with flow cytometry. Also, by using enzyme systems other than peroxidase (such as those with alkaline phosphatase (AP), eg, AP–mouse monoclonal AP or ABC–AP systems with levamisole to inhibit endogenous enzyme activity), cellular antigens can be profiled directly in peripheral blood smears.

Immunoglobulin expression by lymphoproliferative disorders is best evaluated using fresh-frozen material or material from cytocentrifuge preparations. However, cytoplasmic immunoglobulin can be accurately assessed in plasma cell myeloma and in some plasmacytoid lymphocytic and some B-immunoblastic lymphomas by the use of paraffin sections (Bouin's fixation preferred), as illustrated in **FIGURE 5–48.**

Currently, tissue macrophages in true histiocytic lymphoma and malignant histiocytosis are best evaluated with material fixed in B-5 or Bouin's solution and immunostained for α-1-chymotrypsin, α-1-antitrypsin, and muramidase (lysozyme), interpreted in conjunction with ultrastructural findings (**FIGURES 5–49** through **5–52**). Other reagents, such as Leu-M5 on frozen sections, may also be helpful.

Immunohistology of Hodgkin's disease usually yields little information of value, with one possible exception. Pleomorphic T-cell lymphomas, especially polymorphous T-cell immunoblastic sarcoma, can mimic Hodgkin's disease. In this case, the absence of expression of T11 or other broadly reactive T-cell antigens on malignant cells may be helpful in confirming the diagnosis of Hodgkin's disease as opposed to T-cell immunoblastic lymphoma (**FIGURES 5–53** through **5–57**). Although there are numerous subpopulations in most cases of Hodgkin's disease, two are of principal concern and bear different immunotypes. In the first, the large, nucleolated, binucleate cell and its mononuclear variants lack T-cell antigens, usually contain polyclonal cytoplasmic immunoglobulins (κ and λ light chains in the same cell), occasionally express S-100 protein (**FIGURE 5–54**), and usually contain polyclonal cytoplasmic light chains and Leu-M1 (**FIGURE 5–57**) and especially LN2 (**FIGURE 5–55**) and surface and cytoplasmic labeling with LN3 (**FIGURE 5–56**). The second major cellular subpopulation in Hodgkin's disease is a small lymphocyte subpopulation, which is admixed with variable numbers of tissue macrophages and eosinophils.

In instances of nodular sclerosis, mixed cellularity, and lymphocyte-depleted variants, the small lymphocyte population consists of $T11^{+}$ $T4^{+}$ cells with only a few $T8^{+}$ cells present. In lymphocyte-predominant Hodgkin's disease, the predominant small lymphocyte component is composed primarily of polyclonal B-cells.

Immunohistology can also be helpful in the evaluation of anterior mediastinal masses. For most such tumors, the light microscopic diagnosis of thymoma, rather than thymic Hodgkin's disease, lymphoblastic lymphoma, or thymic large cell lymphoma, is usually not a problem if the material is well fixed. Immunohistology can play a role in corroborating the light microscopic diagnosis and may be very helpful in cases in which the histopathologic findings are not conclusive.

The immunohistologic findings of a typical thymoma (**FIGURE 5–58**) are illustrated in **FIGURES 5–59** to **5–61**. Thymomas contain varying proportions of lymphoid and epithelial elements. The epithelial elements are identified with cytokeratin antibodies, especially AE1/3, using either pronase-digested paraffin sections of formalin-fixed material or frozen sections. The lymphoid population usually bears the immunotype of the immature cortical thymocyte ($T11^+ T6^+$), as opposed to circulating mature peripheral T-cells ($T11^+ T6^-$).

In some thymomas, spindle cell elements or components composed almost entirely of epithelial cells predominate. In both of these unusual types of thymoma, the spindle or epithelioid elements are $AE1/3^+$ (**FIGURE 5–61**), and usually an immature cortical thymocyte population can be identified in portions of the tumor.

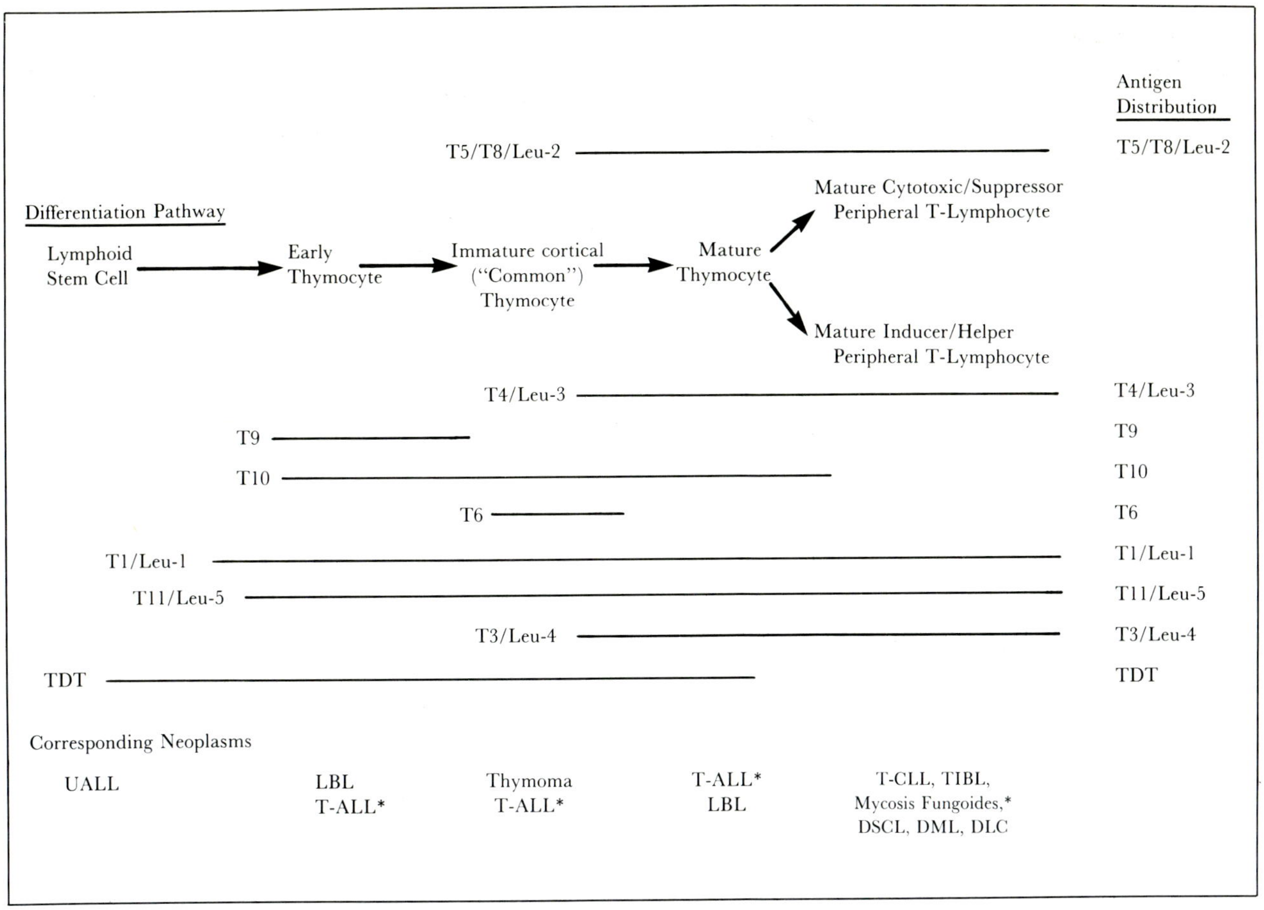

FIGURE 5-1. Stages of T-lymphocyte differentiation with associated antigens and corresponding neoplasms. Source: *Semin Diagn Pathol* 1984;1:276, used with permission.

NOTE: Deletions of individual antigens at a given stage is often seen in T-cell lymphomas.

*Cutaneous T-cell lymphoma (mycosis fungoides) is characterized by lack of expression of 3A1/Leu-9 (not illustrated), monoclonal antibodies which are broadly expressed on most normal T-cells and T-ALL cells.

ABBREVIATIONS: ALL = acute lymphocytic leukemia, DLC = diffuse large cleaved cell lymphoma, DML = diffuse mixed lymphoma, DSCL = diffuse small cleaved cell lymphoma, LBL = lymphoblastic lymphoma, T-ALL = T-cell ALL, T-CLL = T-cell chronic lymphocytic leukemia, TIBL = T-cell immunoblastic lymphoma, UALL = undifferentiated ALL.

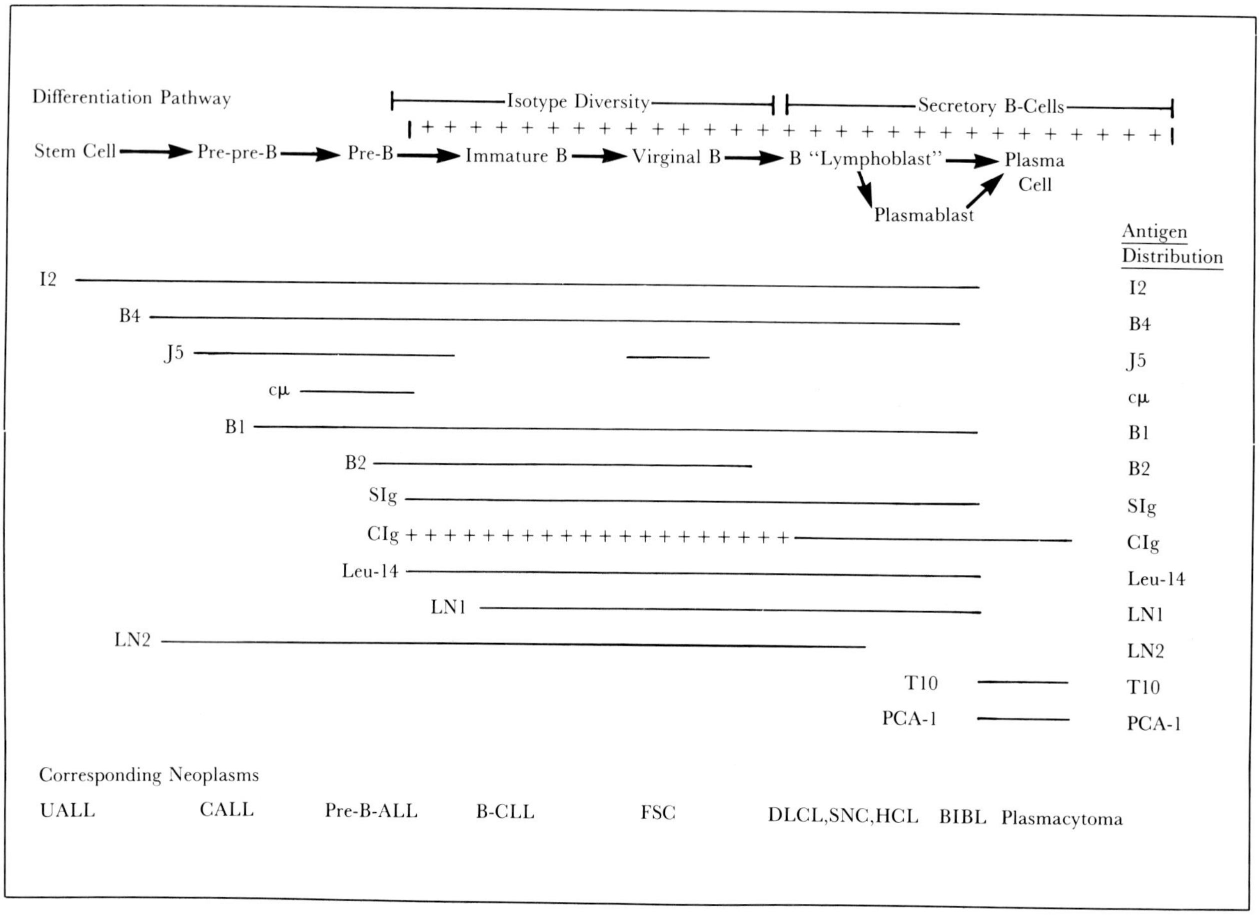

FIGURE 5-2. Stages of B-lymphocyte differentiation with associated antigens and corresponding neoplasms. Source: *Semin Diagn Pathol* 1984;1:277, used with permission.

NOTE: Designations are based on Nadler NL, Anderson KC, Bates MP, et al in Bernard A, Boumsell L, Dausset J, et al (eds): *Leukocyte Typing,* New York, Springer-Verlag, 1984, pp 354-363 and Anderson KC, Bates MP, Slaugherhoupt BL, et al: *Blood* 1984;63:1424-1433.

ABBREVIATIONS: ALL = acute lymphocytic leukemia, B-CLL = B-cell chronic lymphocytic leukemia, BIBL = B-cell immunoblastic lymphoma, CALL = common ALL, CIg = cytoplasmic immunoglobin, cμ = cytoplasmic IgM, DLCL = diffuse large cell lymphoma, FSC = follicular lymphoma, small cleaved cell, HCL = hairy cell leukemia, SIg = surface immunoglobulin, SNC = small noncleaved cell lymphoma, UALL = undifferentiated ALL. |+ + + +| = In our experience using acetone-fixed rather than methanol-fixed cytocentrifuge preparations, monoclonal CIg/secretory B-cells begin earlier in the maturation sequence, ie, in CLL and FSC SIg^+ cells.

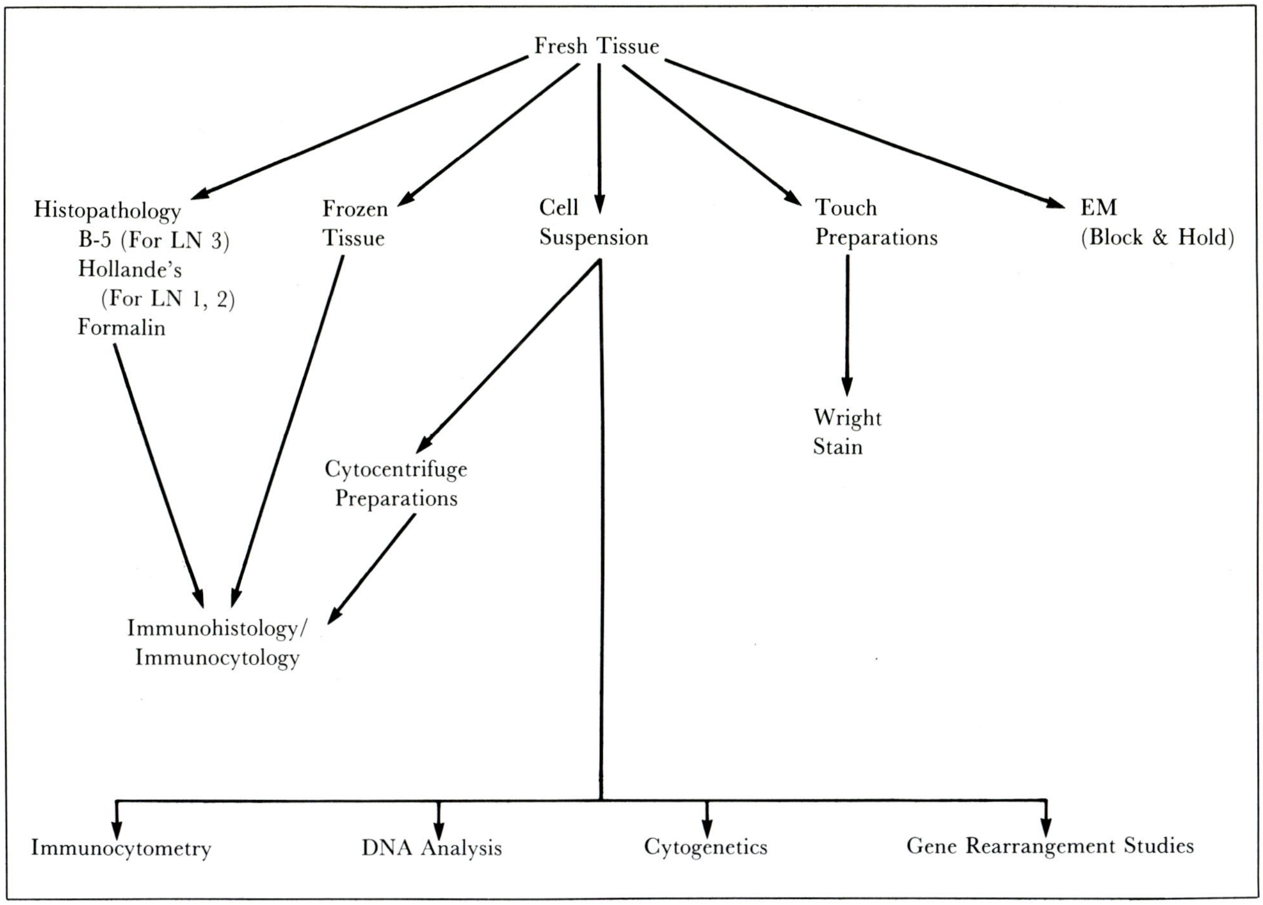

FIGURE 5–3. Processing protocol for lymph node biopsy specimens. Source: *Semin Diagn Pathol* 1984;1:273, used with permission. *Slide 21.*

NOTE: Frozen tissue can also be used for gene rearrangement studies.

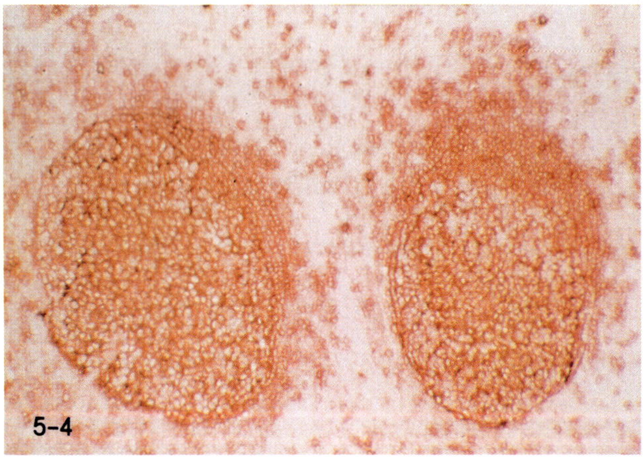

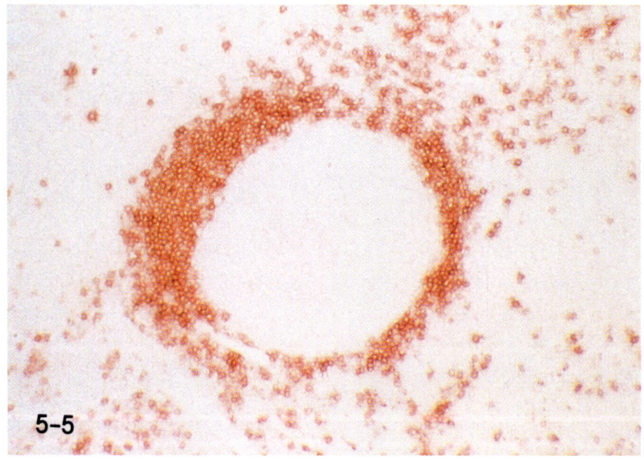

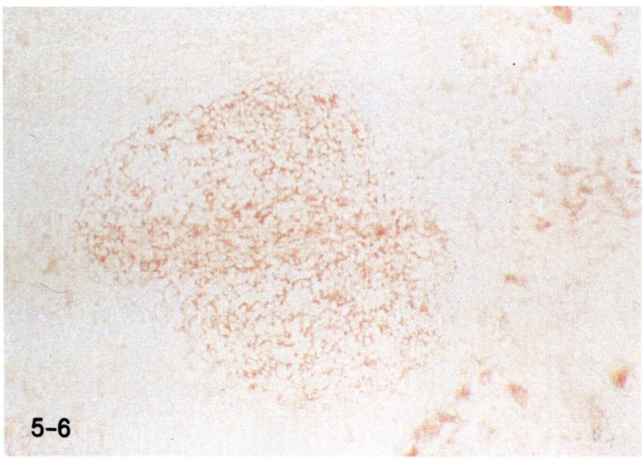

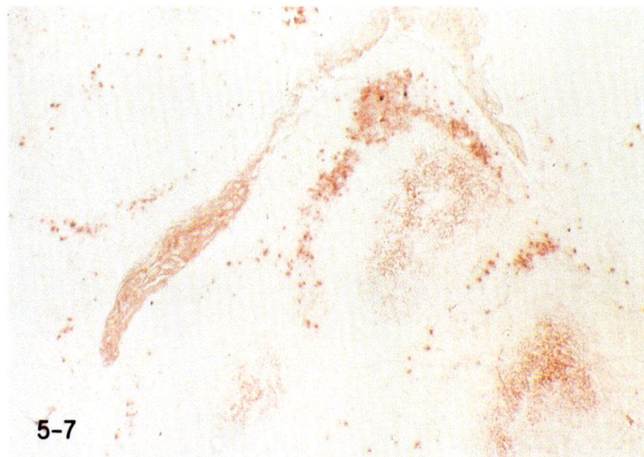

FIGURE 5–4. Tonsil immunostained for IgM (red). Both follicle center cells and the mantle zone lymphocytes are positive (direct IMP with AEC, no counterstain). *Slide 22.*

FIGURE 5–5. Tonsil immunostained for IgD (red). Positive cells are confined to the follicle mantle zones (direct IMP with AEC, no counterstain). *Slide 23.*

FIGURE 5–6. Tonsil immunostained for IgG (red; direct IMP with AEC, no counterstain).

FIGURE 5–7. Tonsil immunostained for IgA (red). The antigen is present in follicle centers and tonsillar epithelium (direct IMP with AEC, no counterstain).

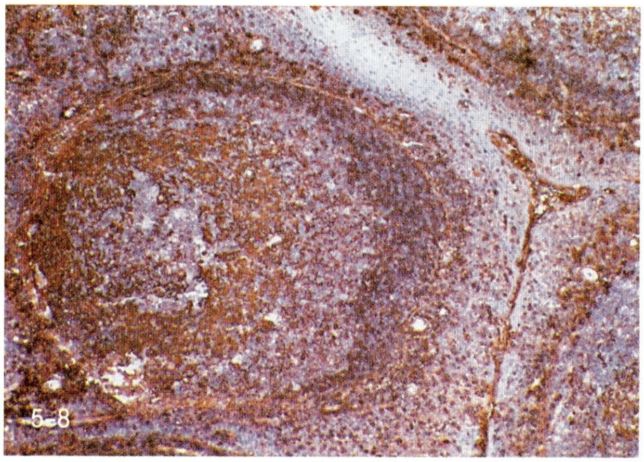

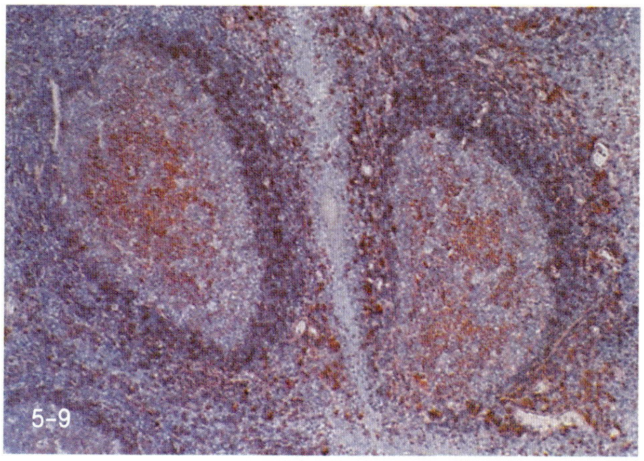

FIGURE 5–8. Tonsil immunostained for κ light chains (direct IMP in a frozen section, hematoxylin counterstain). *Slide 24.*

FIGURE 5–9. Tonsil immunostained for λ light chains (direct IMP in a frozen section, hematoxylin counterstain). *Slide 25.*

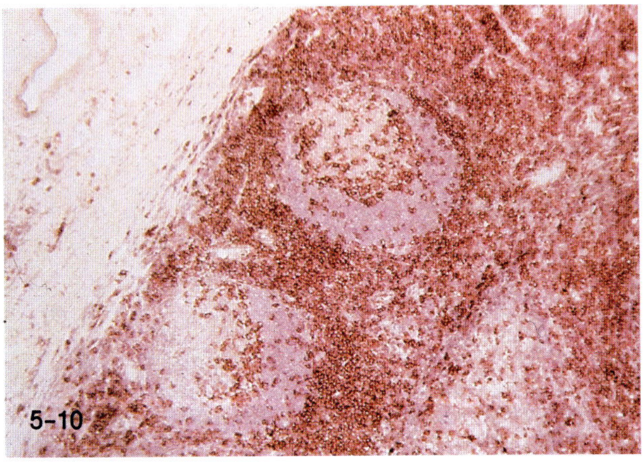

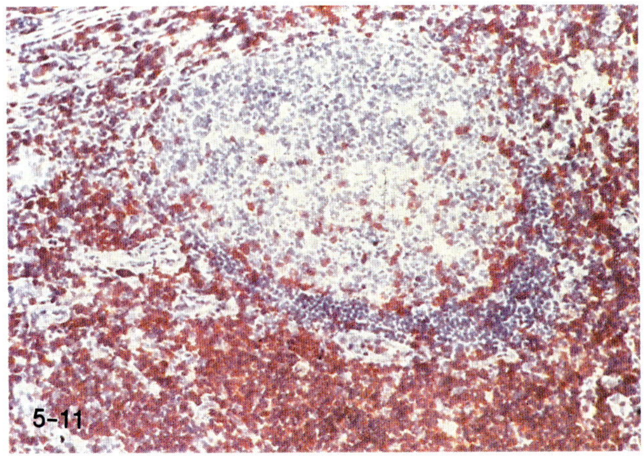

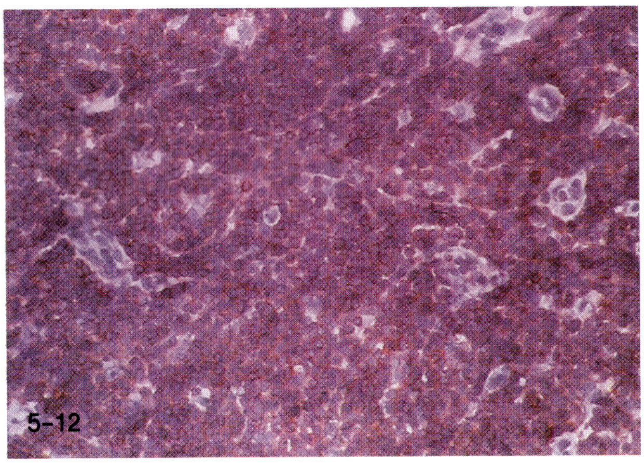

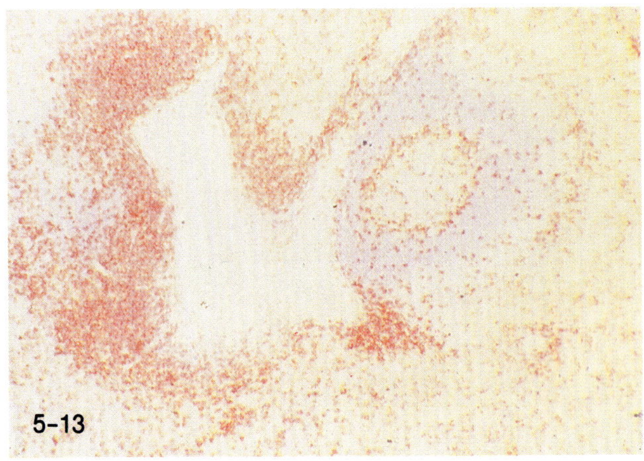

FIGURE 5–10. Tonsil immunostained for a broadly expressed T-cell antigen, T11. Positive cells predominate in the interfollicular areas but are also present in the germinal center (ABC-PO with AEC, hematoxylin counterstain).

FIGURE 5–11. Follicular hyperplasia of lymph node. Distribution of a broadly expressed T-cell antigen, Leu-1 (red) is illustrated (ABC-PO with AEC, hematoxylin counterstain). *Slide 26.*

FIGURE 5–12. Small lymphocytic lymphoma associated with chronic lymphocytic leukemia. Distribution of Leu-1 (red) is illustrated. In such cases, the "pan-T" antigen Leu-1 is coexpressed with monoclonal immunoglobulin (ABC-PO with AEC, hematoxylin counterstain).

FIGURE 5–13. Follicular hyperplasia of spleen. Distribution of a broadly expressed T-cell antigen, T11 (red). The periarteriolar white pulp stains positively, as does an intrafollicular T-cell subpopulation (ABC-PO with AEC, hematoxylin counterstain).

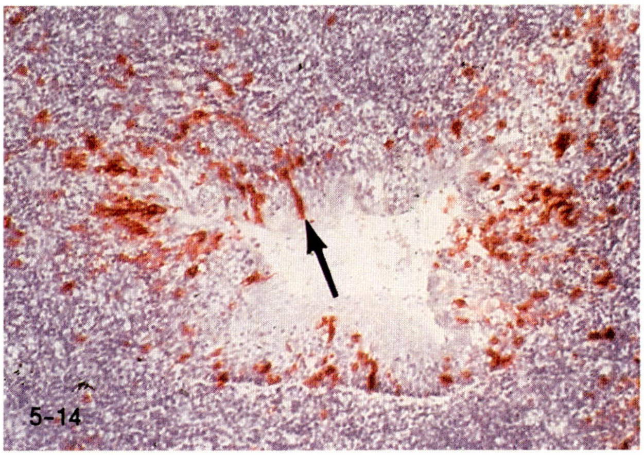

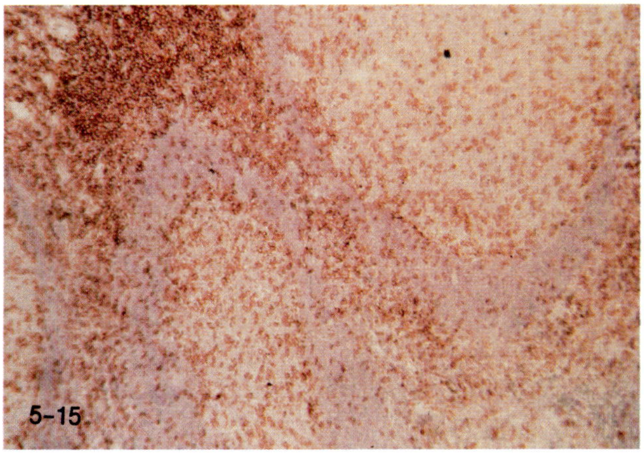

FIGURE 5–14. Tonsil immunostained for the T-cell differentiation antigen, T6. Lymphoid cells are not stained, but Langerhan's cells associated with tonsillar epithelium (arrow) are positive (red; ABC-PO with AEC in a frozen section, hematoxylin counterstain). *Slide 27.*

FIGURE 5–15. Tonsil immunostained for the T-cell differentiation antigen, T4. The T-cell germinal center subpopulation is predominantly $T4^+$ (red). Compare this figure with Figures 5–10, 5–11, and 5–16 (ABC-PO with AEC in a frozen section, hematoxylin counterstain). *Slide 28.*

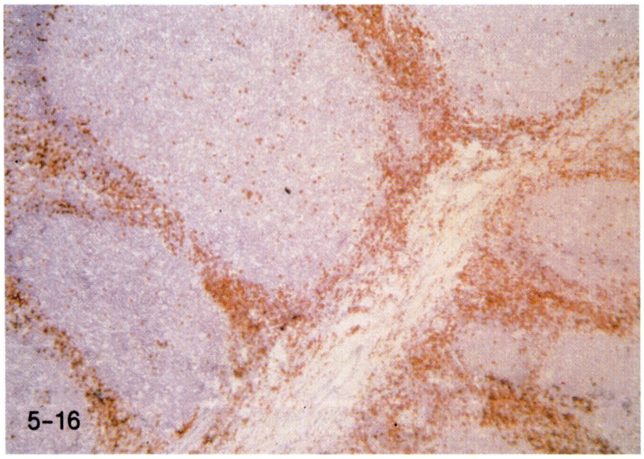

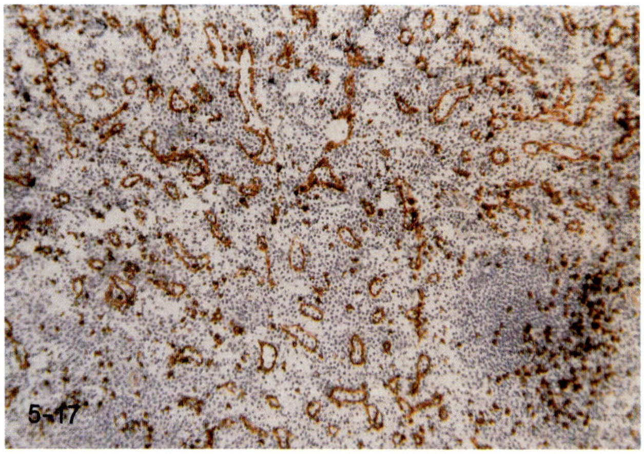

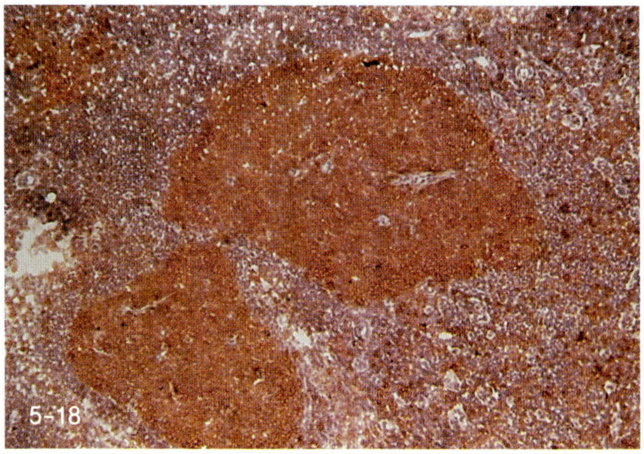

FIGURE 5–16. Tonsil immunostained for the T-cell differentiation antigen, T8. Positive cells (red) are essentially restricted to interfollicular zones (ABC-PO with AEC in a frozen section, hematoxylin counterstain). *Slide 29.*

FIGURE 5–17. Spleen immunostained for the T-cell differentiation antigen, T8. The sinusoidal endothelium is positive (ABC-PO with AEC, hematoxylin counterstain). *Slide 30.*

FIGURE 5–18. Tonsil immunostained for the differentiation antigen, T9 (red). Germinal center cells are positive (ABC-PO with AEC in a frozen section, hematoxylin counterstain).

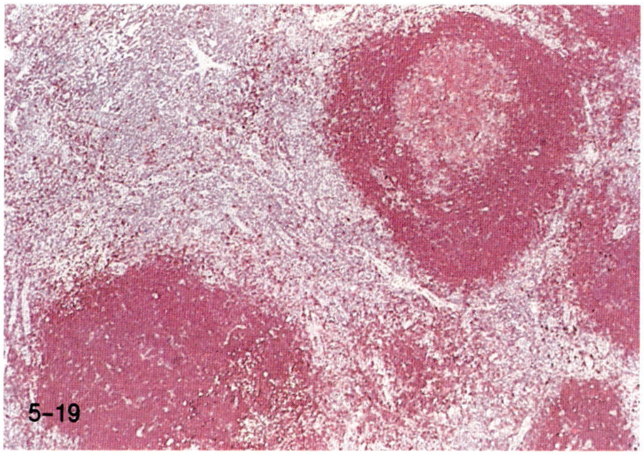

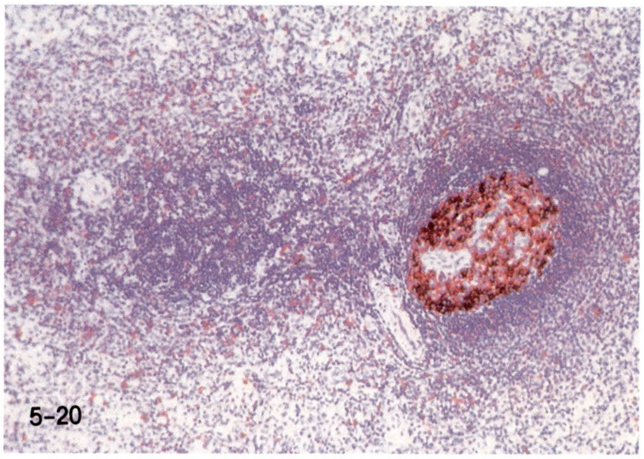

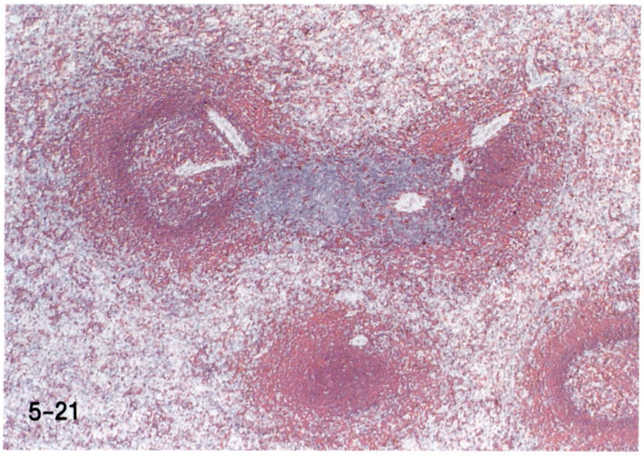

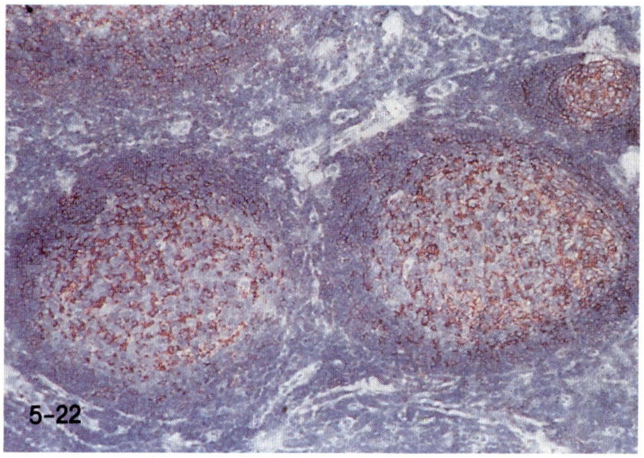

FIGURE 5–19. Follicular hyperplasia of lymph node immunostained for the B-cell differentiation antigen, Leu-14 (red). Both germinal centers and mantle zones are positive (ABC-PO with AEC, hematoxylin counterstain). *Slide 31.*

FIGURE 5–20. Spleen immunostained for the B-cell differentiation antigen, LN1 (red). The germinal center cells are intensely stained (ABC-PO with AEC in a paraffin section of tissue fixed in B-5, hematoxylin counterstain).

FIGURE 5–21. Spleen immunostained for the B-cell differentiation antigen, LN2. The germinal center and mantle zone lymphocytes stain positively, but the periarteriolar sheaths are negative (ABC-PO with AEC in a paraffin section of tissue fixed in B-5, hematoxylin counterstain). *Slide 32.*

FIGURE 5–22. Lymph node immunostained for the B-cell differentiation antigen, B2. Some germinal center and mantle zone cells are positive (ABC-PO with AEC, hematoxylin counterstain).

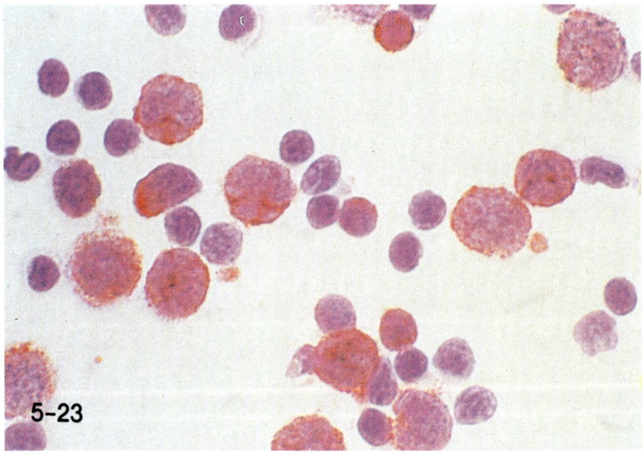

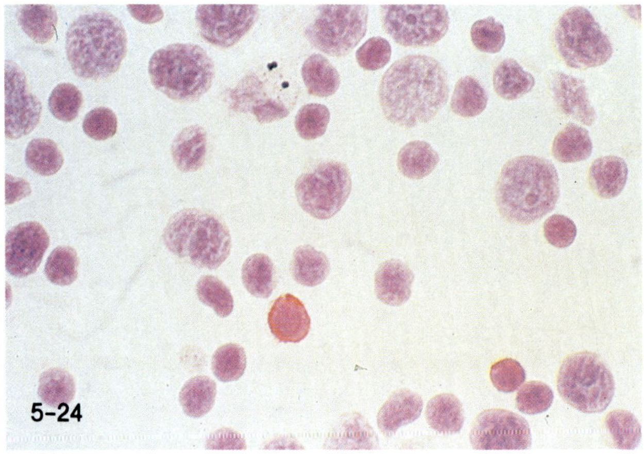

FIGURE 5–23. Follicular large cell lymphoma. Figures 5–23 and 5–24 are from the same case. Here, the κ light chains are immunostained in the large atypical cells (direct IMP with AEC in a cytocentrifuge preparation, hematoxylin counterstain). *Slide 33.*

FIGURE 5–24. Same case as 5–23. This figure shows that the atypical large cell population is negative for λ light chains (direct IMP with AEC in a cytocentrifuge preparation, hematoxylin counterstain). *Slide 34.*

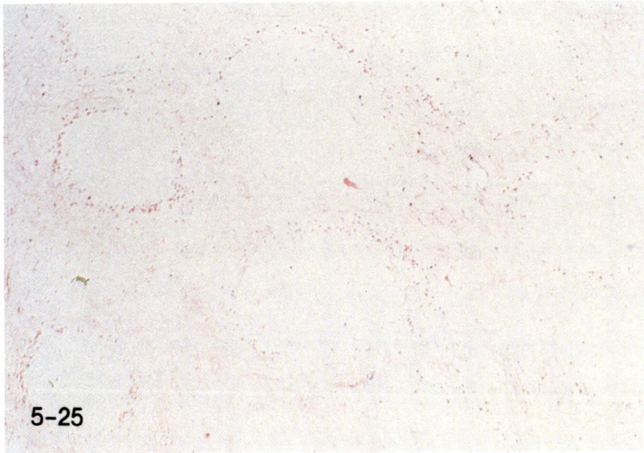

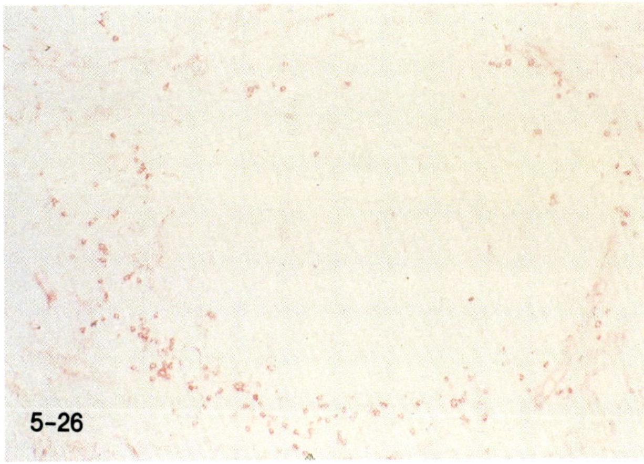

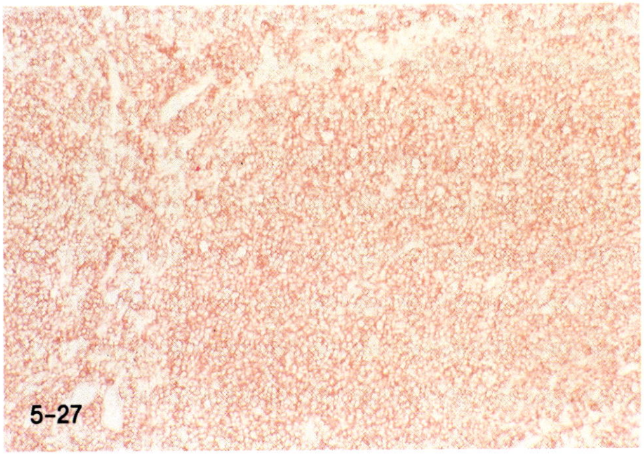

FIGURE 5–25. Follicular small cleaved cell lymphoma, immunotype $\kappa^{-}\lambda^{+}$. Figures 5–25 through 5–27 are from the same case. This figure shows that the tumor nodules are negative for κ light chains (direct IMP with AEC, no counterstain).

FIGURE 5–26. Higher magnification of the same slide as shown in Figure 5–25. The tumor nodules are negative for κ light chains (direct IMP with AEC, no counterstain).

FIGURE 5–27. Same case as 5–25. This section is stained for λ light chains. The tumor nodules are positive for λ light chains (direct IMP with AEC, no counterstain).

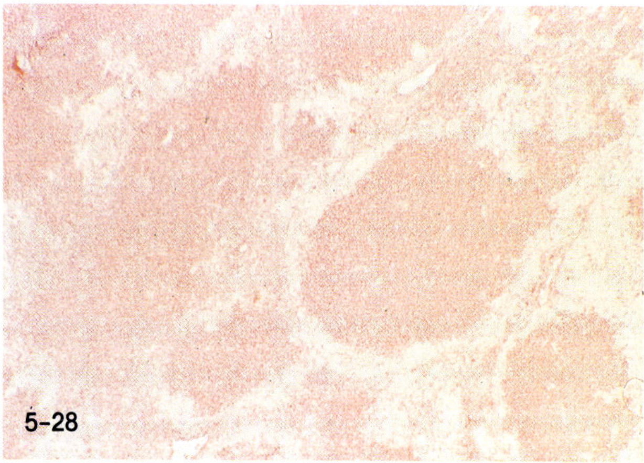

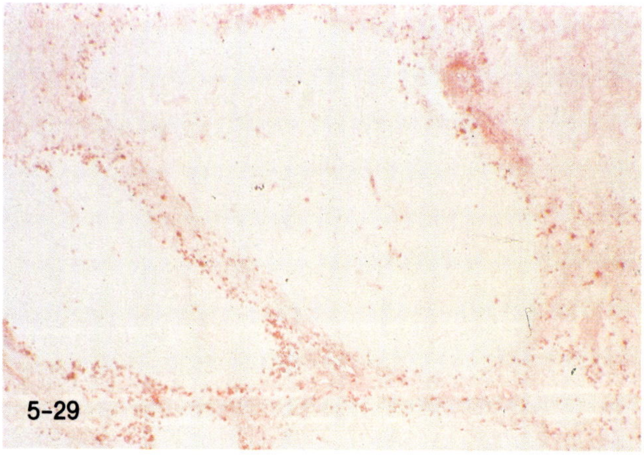

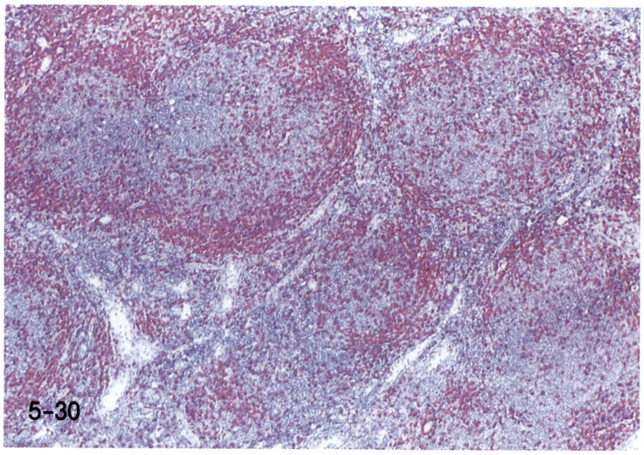

FIGURE 5–28. Another case of follicular predominantly small cleaved cell lymphoma, but with the immunotype $\kappa^+\lambda^-$. Figures 5–28 through 5–33 are from the same case. Here, the neoplastic follicles stain positively for κ light chains (direct IMP with AEC in a frozen section, no counterstain). *Slide 35.*

FIGURE 5–29. Same case as 5–28. Neoplastic follicles do not stain for λ light chains (direct IMP with AEC in a frozen section, no counterstain). *Slide 36.*

FIGURE 5–30. Same case as 5–28. Use of Leu-1 shows T-cells concentrated at the periphery of the neoplastic nodules and in interfollicular areas. Some T-cells infiltrate the neoplastic follicles, but most lie outside, as in this figure (ABC-PO with AEC, hematoxylin counterstain). *Slide 37.*

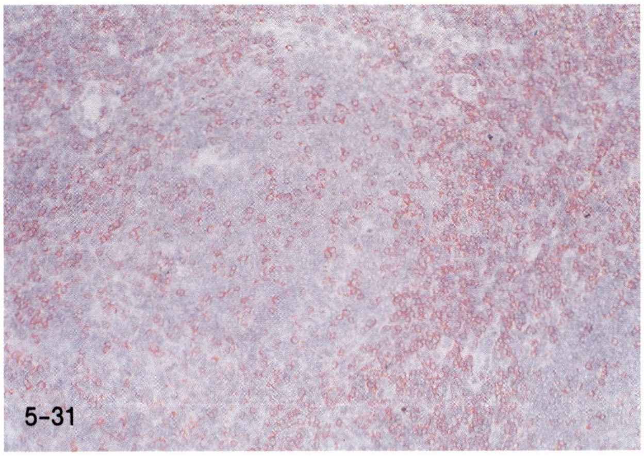

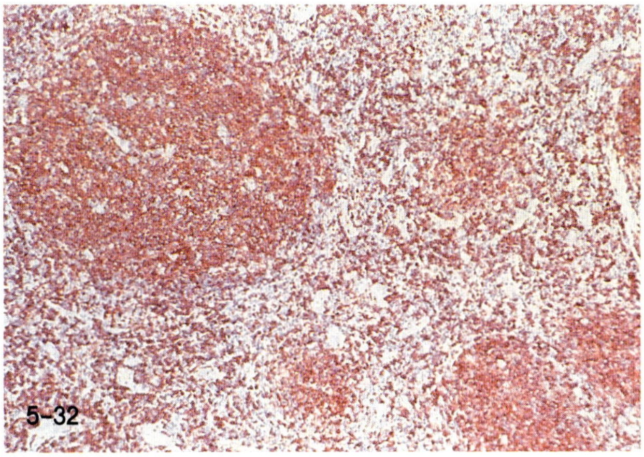

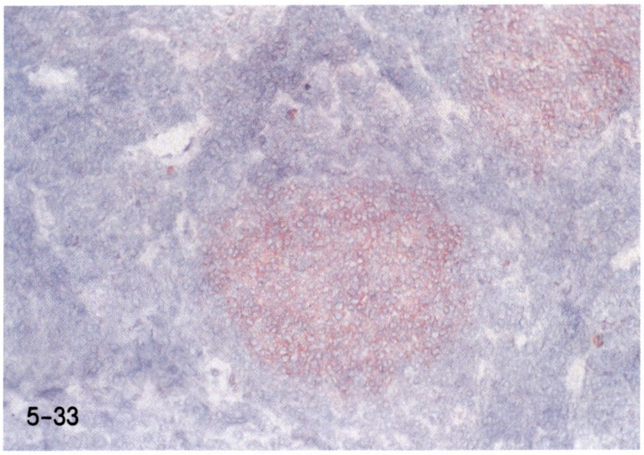

FIGURE 5–31. Same case as 5–28. Use of the T11 differentiation antigen shows that most of the T-cells lie outside the follicles, but an intrafollicular subpopulation of T-cells is also present (ABC-PO with AEC, biotinylated primary modification, in a frozen section, hematoxylin counterstain).

FIGURE 5–32. Same case as 5–28. Neoplastic follicles are positive for the differentiation antigen, B1 (ABC-PO with AEC, biotinylated primary modification, in a frozen section, hematoxylin counterstain). *Slide 38.*

FIGURE 5–33. Same case as 5–28. Use of antibody to J5 (CALLA) differentiation antigen results in weak staining of the neoplastic follicles. The weak staining is characteristic of the virginal stage of the B-cell maturation (ABC-PO with AEC, hematoxylin counterstain).

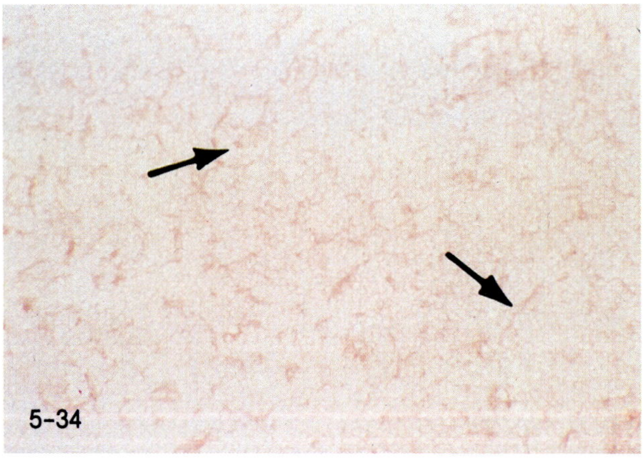

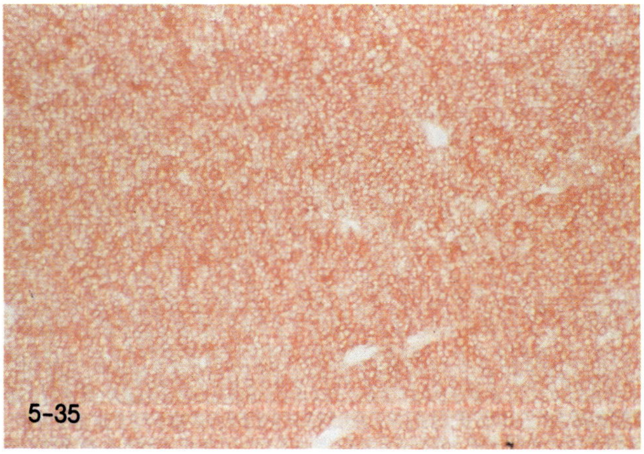

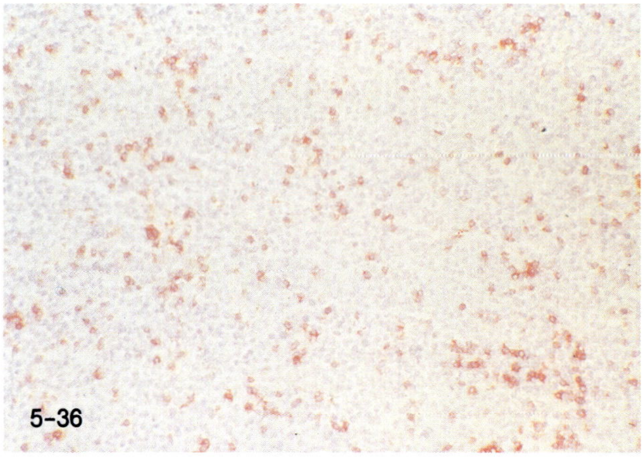

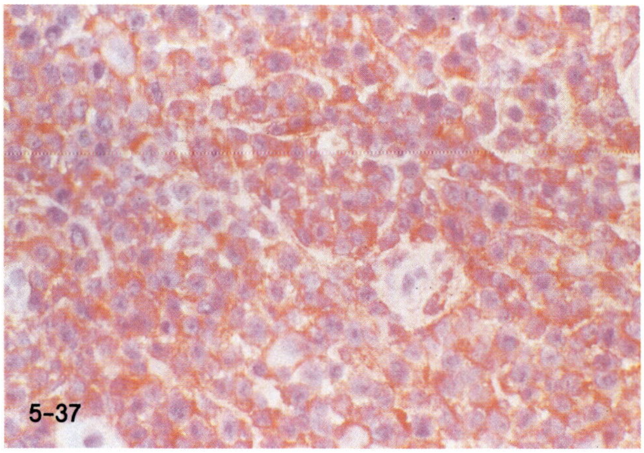

FIGURE 5–34. Small noncleaved cell lymphoma. Figures 5–34 through 5–37 are from the same case. This section is stained for κ light chains. The nonspecific adherence to capillary walls (arrows) is apparent. Similar adherence to collagen occurs in other sites, eg, skin, desmoplastic large cell lymphomas (direct IMP with AEC in a frozen section, no counterstain). *Slide 39.*

FIGURE 5–35. Same case as 5–34. This section is stained for λ light chains. Each individual cell stained positively (direct IMP with AEC in a frozen section, no counterstain). *Slide 40.*

FIGURE 5–36. Same case as 5–34. When the antibody to T11 differentiation antigen is used, an infrequent T-cell subpopulation (red) is identified (ABC-PO with AEC, biotinylated primary modification, in a frozen section, hematoxylin counterstain).

FIGURE 5–37. Same case as 5–34. When stained with B1 differentiation antigen, the cells are diffusely positive (ABC-PO with AEC, biotinylated primary modification, in a frozen section, hematoxylin counterstain). *Slide 41.*

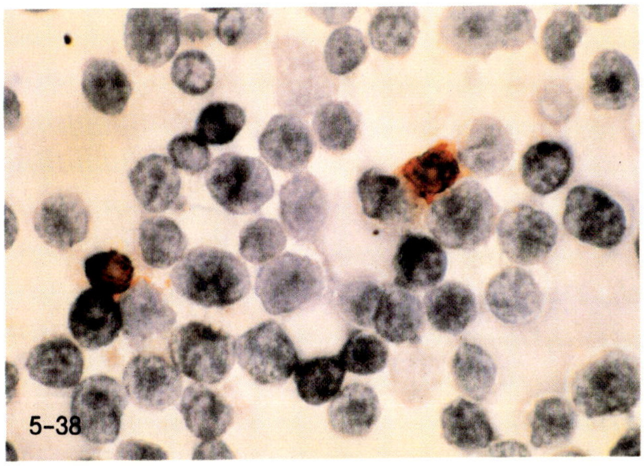

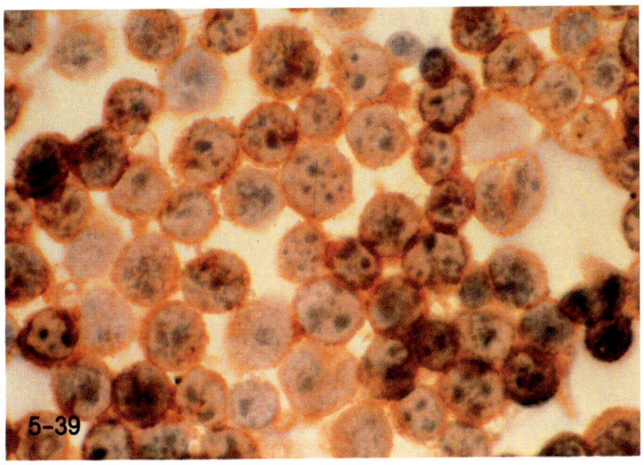

FIGURE 5–38. Another small noncleaved cell lymphoma. Figures 5–38 and 5–39 are from the same case. Here the rare, nonnucleolated small lymphocytes are positive (red) for κ light chains. The nucleolated tumor cells are negative (direct IMP with AEC in a cytocentrifuge preparation, hematoxylin counterstain). *Slide 42.*

FIGURE 5–39. Same case as 5–38. This section is stained for λ light chains (red). The nucleolated tumor cells are positive (direct IMP with AEC, hematoxylin counterstain). *Slide 43.*

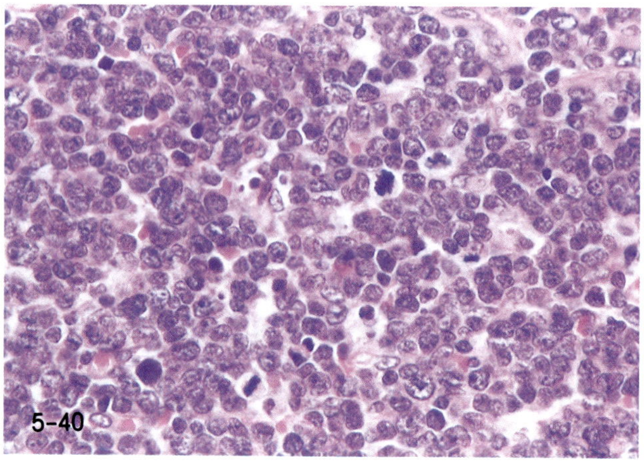

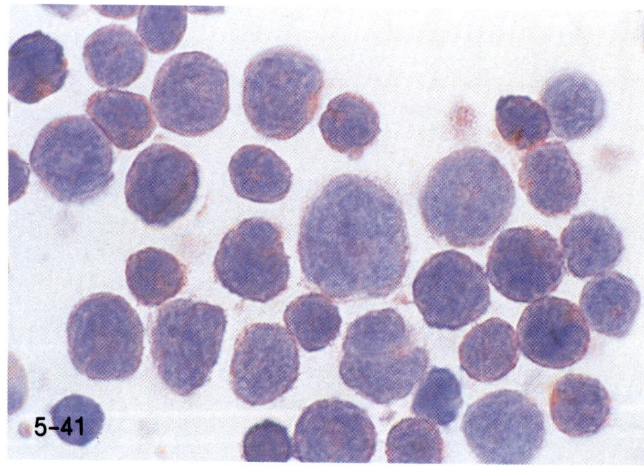

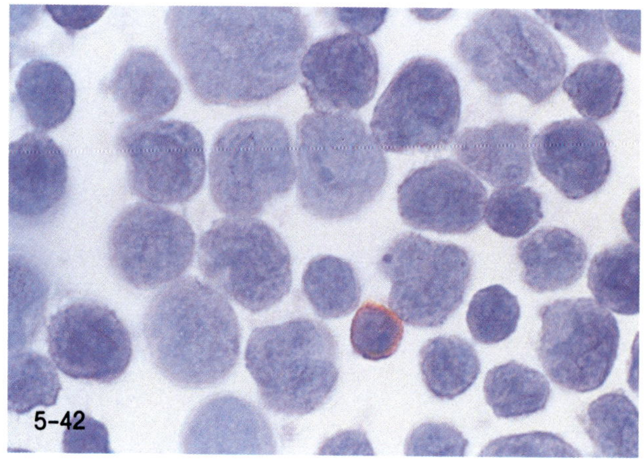

FIGURE 5–40. Lymphoblastic (convoluted cell) lymphoma. Figures 5–40 through 5–45 are from the same case. This tissue section is stained with H & E.

FIGURE 5–41. Same case as 5–40. When immunostained for the T-cell antigen, Leu-1, the atypical convoluted cells are positive (ABC-PO with AEC in a cytocentrifuge preparation, hematoxylin counterstain). *Slide 44.*

FIGURE 5–42. Same case as 5–40. When immunostained for κ light chains, the residual B-cells contaminating the suspension show positive cytoplasmic staining, but the atypical larger convoluted cells are negative (direct IMP with AEC, hematoxylin counterstain).

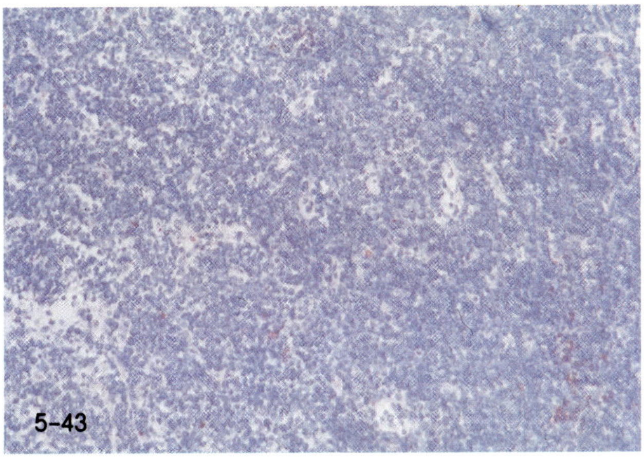

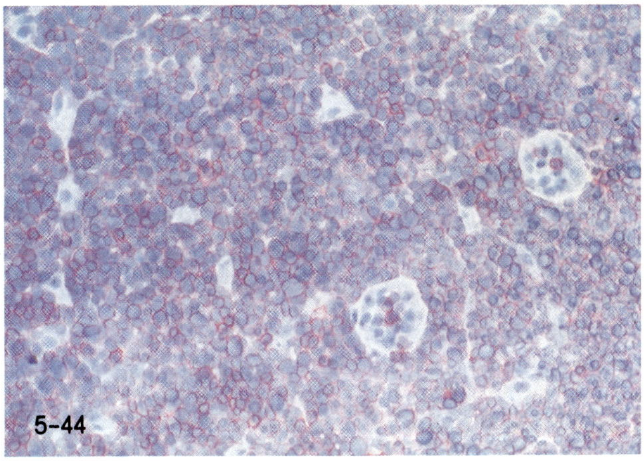

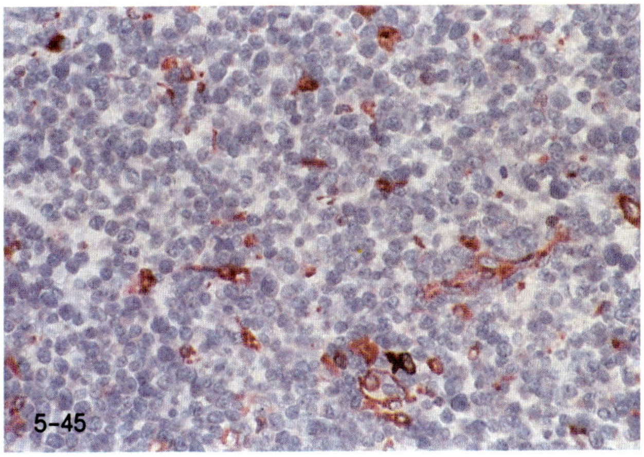

FIGURE 5–43. Same case as 5–40. When immunostained for the B-cell differentiation antigen, Leu-14, a few residual B-cells are positive (lower right), but most of the cells are negative (ABC-PO with AEC in a frozen section, hematoxylin counterstain). *Slide 45.*

FIGURE 5–44. Same case as 5–40. When immunostained for the T-cell differentiation antigen, T11, most of the cells are positive, but the intensity varies (ABC-PO with AEC in a frozen section, hematoxylin counterstain). *Slide 46.*

FIGURE 5–45. Same case as 5–40. When stained for the differentiation antigen, LN2, the macrophages are positive, but the tumor cells are negative (ABC-PO with AEC in a paraffin section of tissue fixed in B-5, hematoxylin counterstain). *Slide 47.*

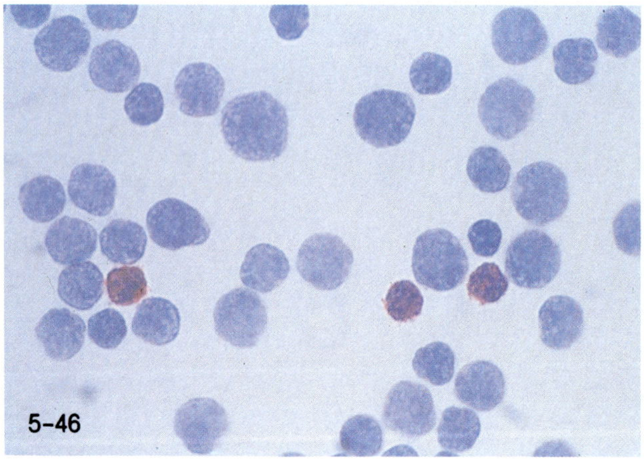

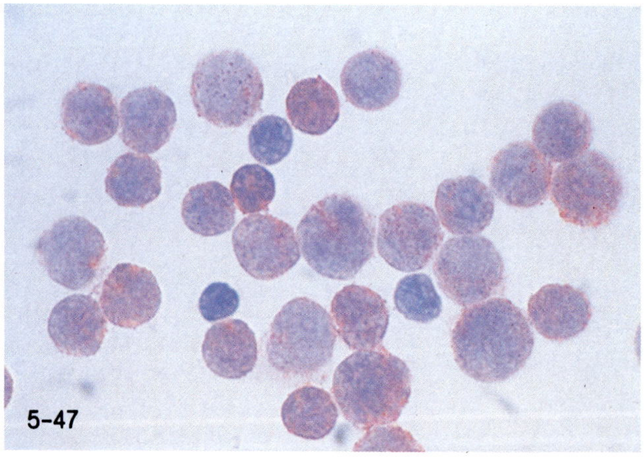

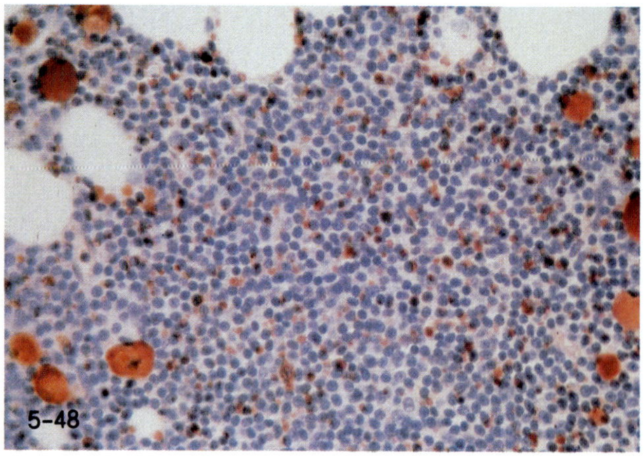

FIGURE 5–46. Acute leukemia. Figures 5–46 and 5–47 are from the same case. When immunostained for the T-cell differentiation antigen, T11, the small lymphocytes are $T11^+$ and the large blasts are $T11^-$ (ABC-PO with AEC in a cytocentrifuge preparation, hematoxylin counterstain). Figure courtesy of Andrew Fishleder, MD, and Richard A. Savage, MD. *Slide 48.*

FIGURE 5–47. Same case as 5–46. When stained for the differentiation antigen, J5 (CALLA), the blasts are $J5^+$ and the small lymphocytes are $J5^-$ (ABC-PO with AEC in a cytocentrifuge preparation, hematoxylin counterstain). Figure courtesy of Andrew Fishleder, MD, and Richard A. Savage, MD. *Slide 49.*

FIGURE 5–48. Plasmacytoid lymphocytic lymphoma, bone marrow biopsy specimen showing many Russell bodies. Cytoplasmic immunoglobulin (red), indicated by κ light chain staining, is visible in the Russell bodies and lymphoid cells (ABC-PO with AEC in a paraffin section of tissue fixed in Zenker's solution, hematoxylin counterstain).

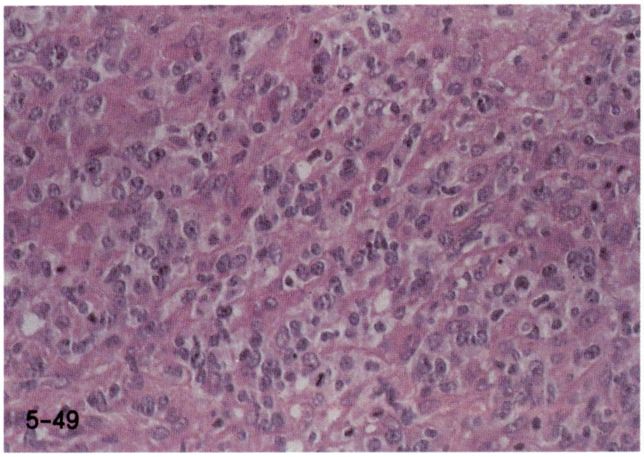

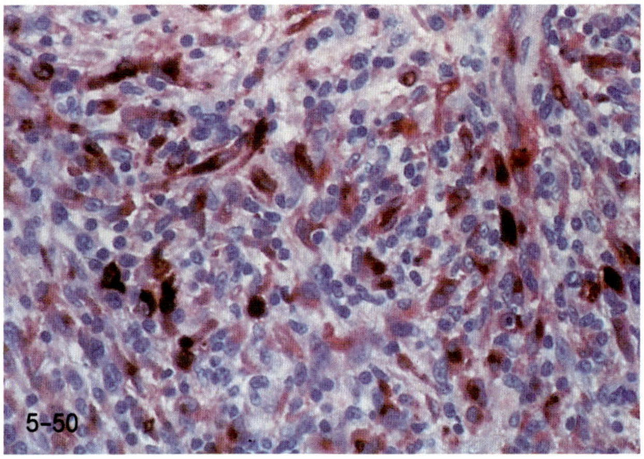

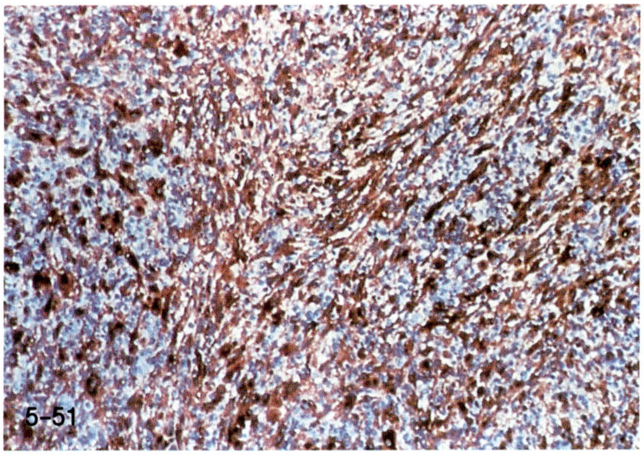

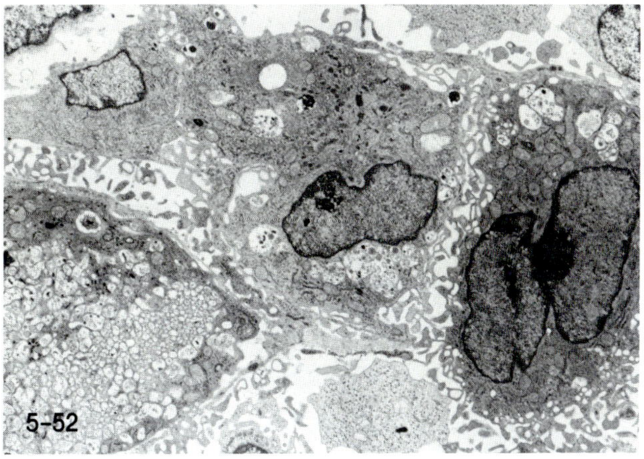

FIGURE 5–49. True histiocytic lymphoma in an axillary lymph node. Figures 5–49 through 5–52 are from the same case. In this section, a spindle cell component is visible (H & E).

FIGURE 5–50. Same case as 5–49. When stained for muramidase, mainly the spindle cells are positive (ABC-PO with AEC in a paraffin section of tissue fixed in B-5, hematoxylin counterstain).

FIGURE 5–51. Same case as 5–49. When stained for α-1-chymotrypsin, both the spindle cell and round cell components are positive (ABC-PO with AEC in a paraffin section of tissue fixed in Bouin's solution, hematoxylin counterstain).

FIGURE 5–52. Same case as 5–49. Electron micrograph. Complex surface projections, abundant phagolysosomes, and vacuoles are visible (lead citrate and uranyl acetate).

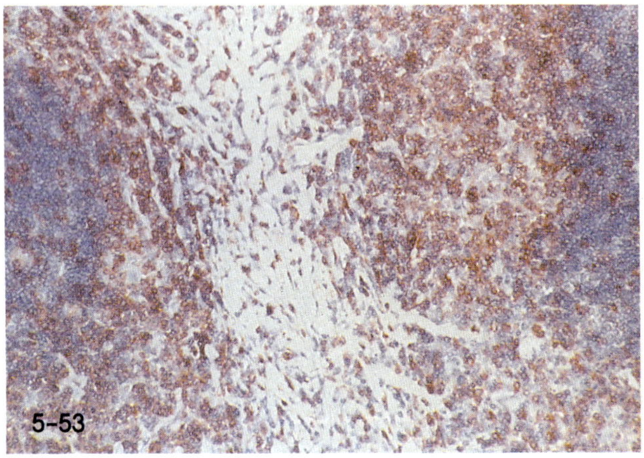

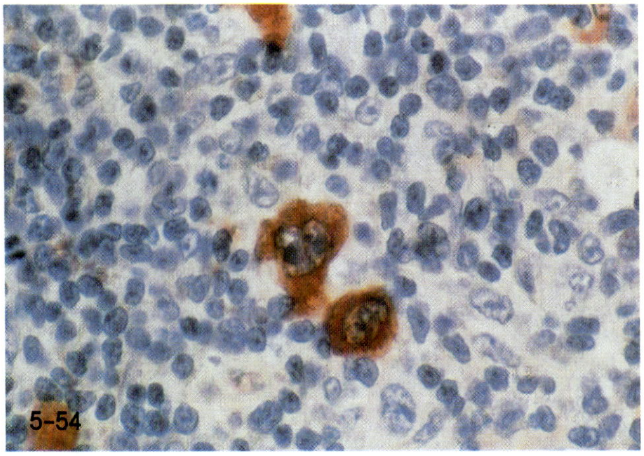

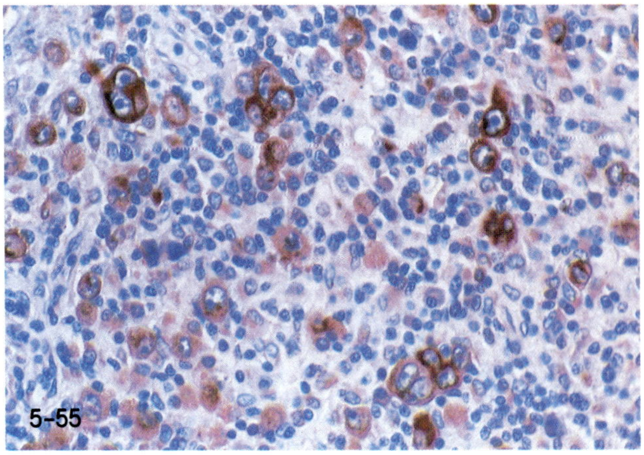

FIGURE 5–53. Hodgkin's disease. When stained for the T-cell antigen, Leu-1, the predominant small lymphocyte population is positive (ABC-PO with AEC in a frozen section, hematoxylin counterstain).

FIGURE 5–54. Hodgkin's disease. As illustrated here, when immunostained for S-100 protein, some cases show positive staining in the Reed-Sternberg cells and mononuclear variants (ABC-PO with AEC in a paraffin section of tissue fixed in Bouin's solution, hematoxylin counterstain).

FIGURE 5–55. Hodgkin's disease. When immunostained for the differentiation antigen, LN2, the neoplastic cells are positive. A positive Reed-Sternberg cell (red) is visible in the upper left corner (ABC-PO with AEC in a paraffin section of tissue fixed in B-5, hematoxylin counterstain). *Slide 50.*

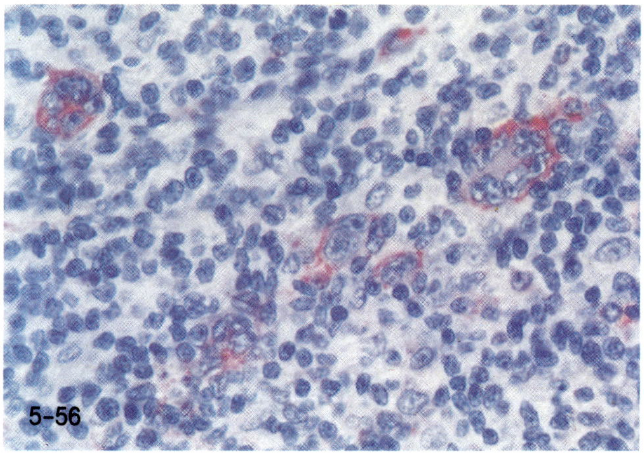

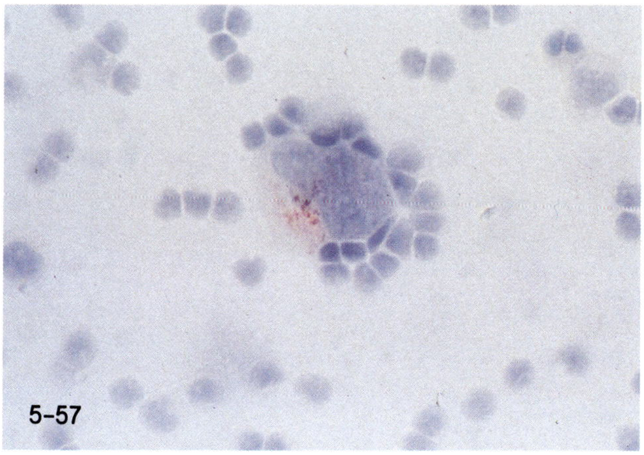

FIGURE 5–56. Hodgkin's disease. When immunostained for the differentiation antigen, LN3, the neoplastic cells show mostly surface staining but some cytoplasmic staining (ABC-PO with AEC in a paraffin section of tissue fixed in B-5, hematoxylin counterstain).

FIGURE 5–57. Hodgkin's disease. When immunostained for Leu-M1, a Reed-Sternberg cell in a cytocentrifuge preparation is positive (red granules in left center; ABC-PO with AEC in a cytocentrifuge preparation, hematoxylin counterstain). Note the lymphoctye auto rosette surrounding the atypical large cell.

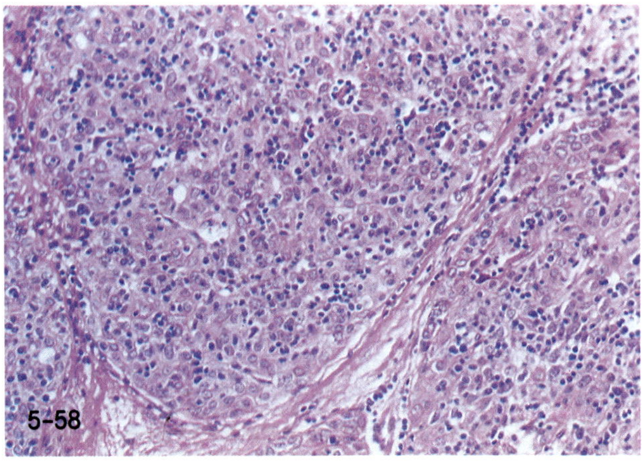

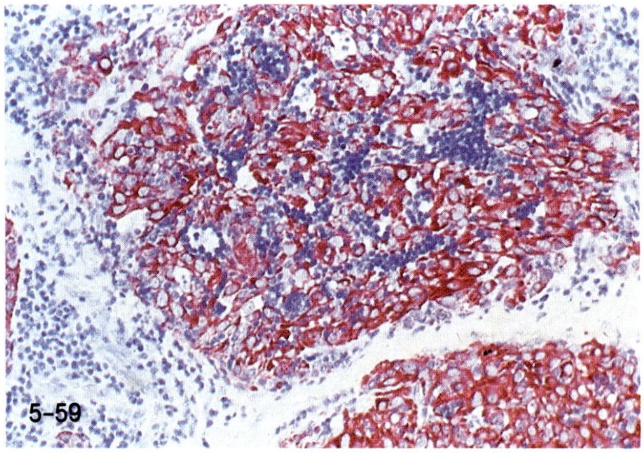

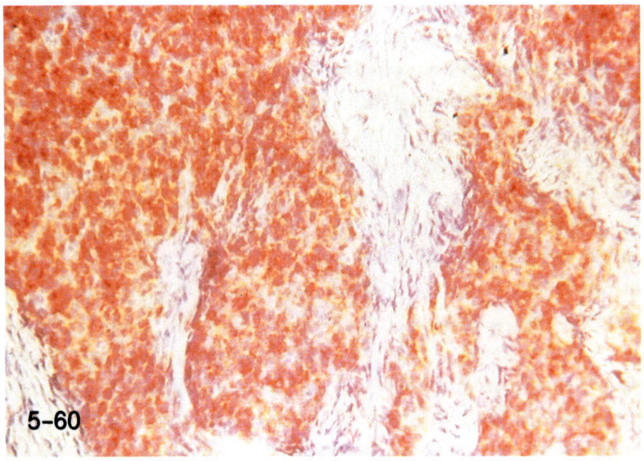

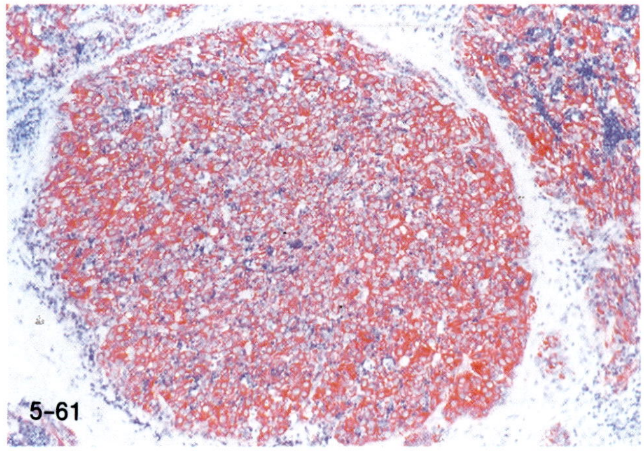

FIGURE 5–58. Mixed cell thymoma. Figures 5–58 through 5–60 are from the same case. This section is stained with H & E.

FIGURE 5–59. Same case as 5–58. When immunostained with AE1/3 for cytokeratins (red), the epithelial elements are positive (ABC-PO with AEC in a frozen tissue, hematoxylin counterstain). *Slide 51.*

FIGURE 5–60. Same case as 5–58. When stained for the T-cell antigen, T6, the lymphoid cells are positive. The lymphoid elements of thymomas usually bear the immunotype of immature cortical thymocytes: $T11^+T6^+$ (ABC-PO with AEC in a frozen section, hematoxylin counterstain).

FIGURE 5–61. Predominantly epithelial cell thymoma. When stained with AE1/3, the large tumor cells express abundant cytokeratins (ABC-PO with AEC in a frozen tissue section, hematoxylin counterstain).

6 Nephropathology

In our laboratory all renal biopsy specimens are processed by the direct immunoperoxidase technique using Hanker-Yates reagent (*p*-phenylenediamine and pyrocatechol) as the chromogen, with and without the PAS counterstain (IMP/IMPAS), and evaluated for the presence or absence of IgG, IgA, IgM, and C3. Other antigens, such as viral, bacterial, epithelial, hormonal, and oncodevelopmental antigens, may also be identified and localized by the IMP/IMPAS technique. The IMP/IMPAS methods provide permanent preparations. The PAS counterstain demonstrates histologic detail of renal structures and allows localization of antigens in various renal structures. **FIGURES 6–1** through **6–3** illustrate the histologic detail in the IMPAS sections.

The IMPAS sections allow for localization of antigens in various renal structures, including glomeruli, tubules, and vessels. Table 6–1 summarizes patterns of deposits in various types of renal disease. With the IMPAS technique, deposits of IgM and C3 are readily localized in collapsed or uncollapsed segments of glomeruli in cases of focal and segmental glomerulosclerosis (**FIGURES 6–4** and **6–5**). The PAS counterstain helps demonstrate segmental sclerosis, which may not be evident in the routine histologic or electron microscopic sections (**FIGURES 6–1** and **6–4**). Mesangial deposits are clearly defined by the IMPAS technique in cases of mesangiopathic glomerulonephritis (**FIGURES 6–6** through **6–8**). In the majority of these cases, the peripheral glomerular basement membrane exhibits no deposit. In some cases, the PAS counterstain may obscure faint mesangial deposits, illustrating the importance of performing IMP without the PAS counterstain.

Epimembranous and intramembranous deposits are readily demonstrated by the IMPAS technique. These deposits are usually diffuse and may vary in size (**FIGURES 6–9** through **6–13**). Confluent and finely granular "pseudolinear" deposits are observed in some cases of membranous glomerulonephritis in which the epimembranous deposits are so extensive that IMP demonstrates diffuse deposits that appear continuous over most of the glomerular basement membrane (**FIGURES 6–14** and **6–15**). The IMPAS technique also demonstrates subendothelial deposits; however, in some cases of membranoproliferative glomerulonephritis (Type 1) and "diffuse" lupus glomerulonephritis, subendothelial deposits may be so prominent and extensive that demonstration of subendothelial localization may be difficult (**FIGURES 6–16** through **6–23**).

TABLE 6–1. Typical Patterns of Deposits in Renal Diseases Evaluated by Immunoperoxidase Techniques

	Location of Deposits					
Type of Renal Disease	EPM	IMB	SE	MES	AR/AD	TBM
Minimal change/no lesion	−	−	−	−	−	−
Focal-segmental glomerulosclerosis	−	−	−	−	(+)	−
Membranous GN stage I	+	−	−	−	−	−
Membranous GN stage II	+	−	−	−	−	−
Membranous GN stages III to IV	+	+	−	−	−	−
Membranous lupus GN	+	+	−	(+)	−	(+)
IgA nephropathy	−	−	−	+	−	−
Henoch-Schönlein-associated GN	−	−	(+)	+	−	−
Mesangiopathic lupus GN	−	−	−	+	−	(+)
Membranoproliferative GN type I	−	−	+	(+)	−	−
Diffuse lupus GN	(+)	(+)	+	+	−	(+)
Membranoproliferative GN type II (dense deposit disease)	−	+	−	(+)	−	+
Diffuse GN (poststreptococcal type)	+	(+)	+	+	−	−
Anti-GBM disease/Goodpasture's syndrome	−	+	−	−	−	(+)
Amyloidosis	−	+	−	+	+	+
κ light chain deposition disease	−	+	(+)	(+)[c]	(+)	+
λ light chain deposition disease	−	+	(+)	(+)[c]	(+)	+
Arteriolosclerosis and arterio-sclerosis	−	−	−	−	+	−
Tubulointerstitial nephritis (immune complex type)	−	−	−	−	−	+

SOURCE: Tubbs RR, Gephardt GN: Use and interpretation of immunoperoxidase procedures in renal disease, in Rosen S (ed): *Pathology of Glomerular Disease.* New York, Churchill Livingstone, 1983, p 21. Used with permission.

ABBREVIATIONS: AR/AD = arteriolar-arterial deposits, EPM = epimembranous, GBM = glomerular basement membrane, GN = glomerulonephritis, IMB = intramembranous, MES = mesangial, SE = subendothelial, TBM = tubular basement membrane, κ = κ light chain, λ = λ light chain, + indicates present, − indicates absent, (+) indicates variably present.

[a]C1q and C4 may be detected in membranoproliferative GN type I but usually not in membranoproliferative GN type II (dense deposit disease). C1q, C3, and C4 are frequently detected in diffuse lupus nephritis.

[b]The composition of deposits in amyloidosis depends on the composition of amyloid protein.

[c]Nodular mesangial deposits of light chains may be detected in cases of κ and λ light chain deposition disease.

Composition of Deposits						
IgG	IgA	IgM	C3	κ	λ	Characteristics of Deposits
−	−	−	−	−	−	No deposits (no segmental sclerosis in IMPAS)
−	−	+	+	+	+	Focal-segmental, granular in sclerotic segments
+	−	−	+	+	+	Diffuse, generalized, confluent, finely granular
+	−	−	+	+	+	Diffuse, generalized, granular
+	−	−	+	+	+	Diffuse, generalized, granular
+	+	+	+	+	+	Diffuse, generalized, granular
+	+	−	+	+	+	Diffuse, generalized, granular
+	+	−	+	+	+	Diffuse, generalized, granular
+	+	+	+	+	+	Diffuse, generalized, granular
+	(+)	(+)	+	+	+	Diffuse, generalized, granular with segmental accentuation[a]
+	+	+	+	+	+	Diffuse, generalized, granular with segmental accentuation[a]
−	−	−	(+)	−	−	Diffuse, generalized, granular[a]
+	−	−	+	+	+	Diffuse, generalized, granular
+	−	−	+	+	+	Diffuse, generalized, linear
(+)	(+)	(+)	(+)	(+)	(+)	Diffuse, homogeneous (if deposits present)[b]
−	−	−	−	+	−	Diffuse, generalized, linear[c]
−	−	−	−	−	+	Diffuse, generalized, linear[c]
−	−	−	+	−	−	Granular
+	−	−	+	+	+	Granular

In cases of crescentic glomerulonephritis, the IMP/IMPAS technique demonstrates the presence or absence of granular or linear deposits of immunoglobulin and complement (**FIGURES 6–24** through **6–26**). The PAS counterstain demonstrates crescent formation. In cases of acute renal failure, the IMP/IMPAS sections may be prepared within one to two hours after the biopsy specimen is taken. Not only is the presence or absence and pattern of immunoglobulin and complement deposits demonstrated, but the presence or absence of glomerular crescents may be demonstrated as well.

Abnormal proteins, such as κ or λ immunoglobulin light chains in light chain deposition disease, may be demonstrated by the immunoperoxidase technique (**FIGURES 6–27** through **6–30**). Light chain deposition disease is characterized by diffuse granular deposits of κ or λ immunoglobulin light chains in the glomerular basement membrane, mesangium, tubular basement membranes, and vessels. In some cases of renal amyloidosis, deposits of immunoglobulins and light chains may be detected. These may exhibit a diffuse pattern without distinct localization (**FIGURES 6–31** through **6–33**).

Fibrin/fibrinogen may be demonstrated in the kidney by the IMP/IMPAS technique in such diseases as crescentic glomerulonephritis and microangiopathy/hemolytic uremic syndrome (**FIGURES 6–34** and **6–35**).

Tubular basement membranes exhibit deposits of immunoglobulin and complement in many cases of systemic lupus erythematosus, usually in association with glomerular deposits of immunoglobulin and complement. These deposits contain immunoglobulin and complement and are easily localized in the tubular basement membrane with the PAS counterstain (**FIGURES 6–36** and **6–37**). Other patterns of deposits, such as those in light chain deposition disease, may also be detected (**FIGURES 6–27** and **6–29**).

Vascular deposits of immunoglobulins and complement are frequently detected in hypertensive states regardless of the etiology of the hypertension, in lupus nephritis (**FIGURE 6–38**), and in vasculitis (**FIGURE 6–39**). The PAS counterstain is helpful in defining deposits as vascular or tubular.

Lymphocyte differentiation antigens in interstitial cellular infiltrates may be demonstrated by the immunoperoxidase technique. These studies are appropriate in interstitial nephritis and in acute transplant rejection characterized by interstitial lymphocytic infiltrates (**FIGURE 6–40**).

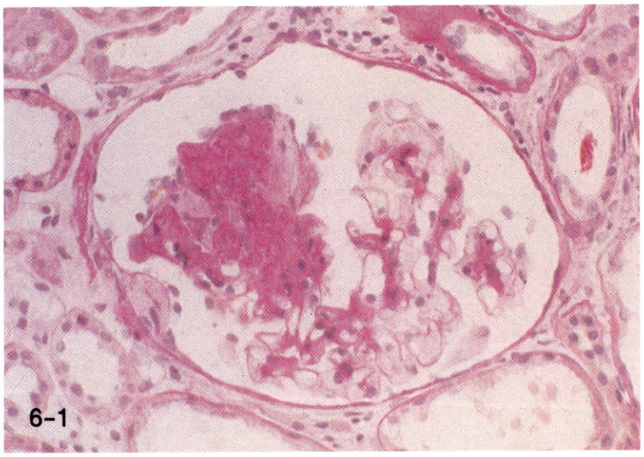

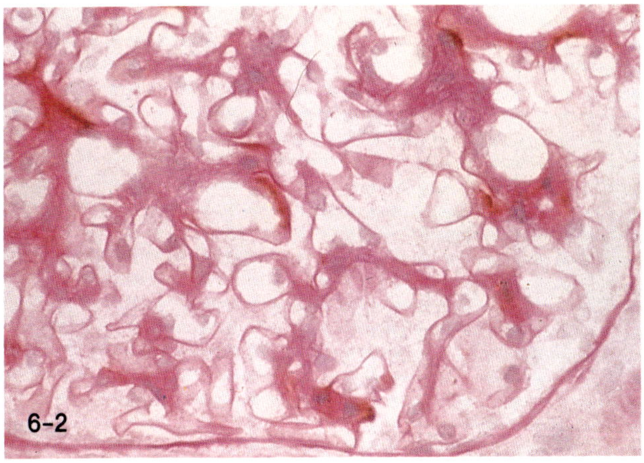

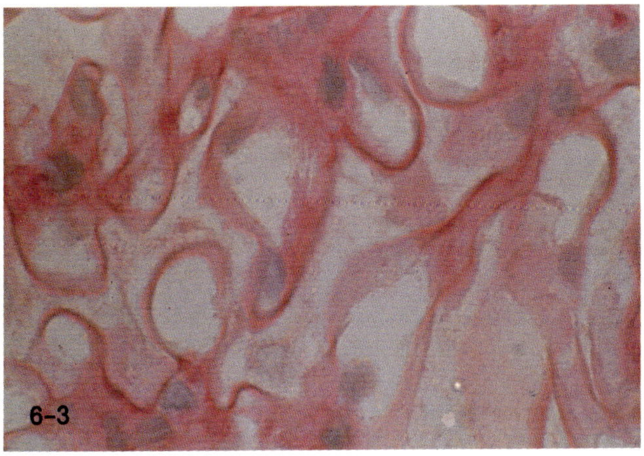

FIGURE 6–1. Focal and segmental sclerosis. The segmental sclerosis is clearly demonstrated by the PAS counterstain. No deposits of IgA are present, but the sclerotic area contained IgM and C3 deposits (IMPAS for IgA, hematoxylin counterstain).

FIGURE 6–2. Renal amyloidosis. Figures 6–2 and 6–3 are from the same case. This figure shows glomerular detail. Faint deposits of IgA are identified in the mesangial regions (IMPAS for IgA, hematoxylin counterstain).

FIGURE 6–3. Same case as 6–2. Fine detail of glomerular structures shows well-defined capillary loops and mesangial regions. No deposits of IgM are present (IMPAS for IgM, hematoxylin counterstain).

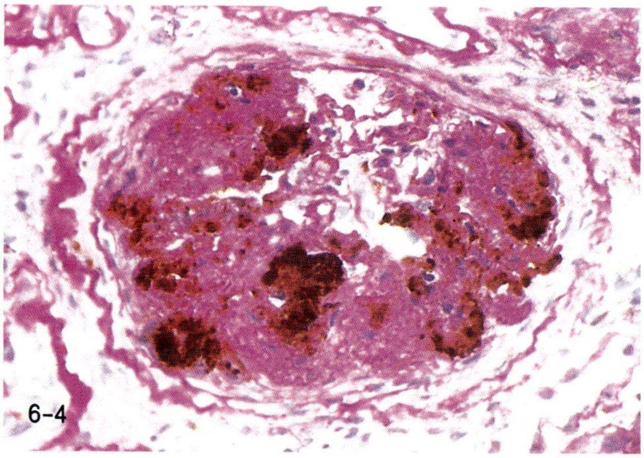

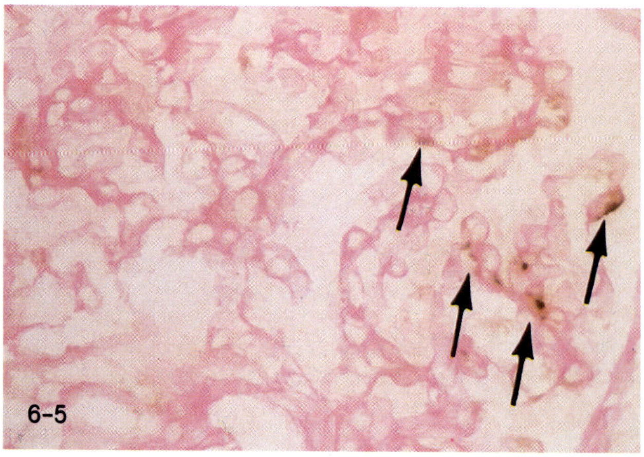

FIGURE 6–4. Focal and segmental sclerosis. This figure shows deposits of C3 in sclerotic segments of a glomerulus. The nonsclerotic portion is clearly visible (IMPAS for C3, hematoxylin counterstain). *Slide 52.*

FIGURE 6–5. Focal and segmental sclerosis. Deposits of C3 (arrows) are visible in nonsclerotic segments of the glomerulus. Segmental collapse and hyaline deposits were demonstrated in other glomeruli (IMPAS for C3).

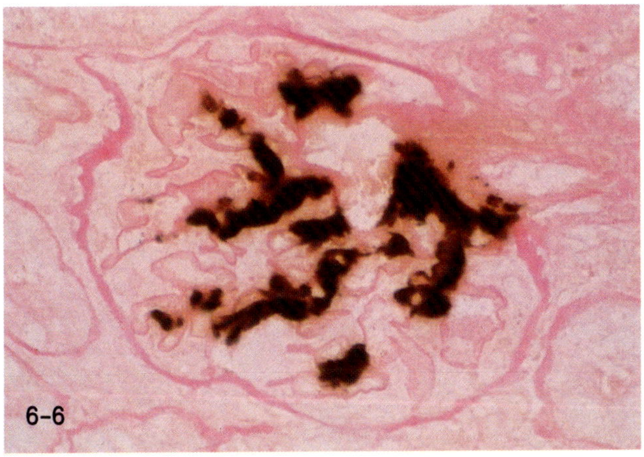

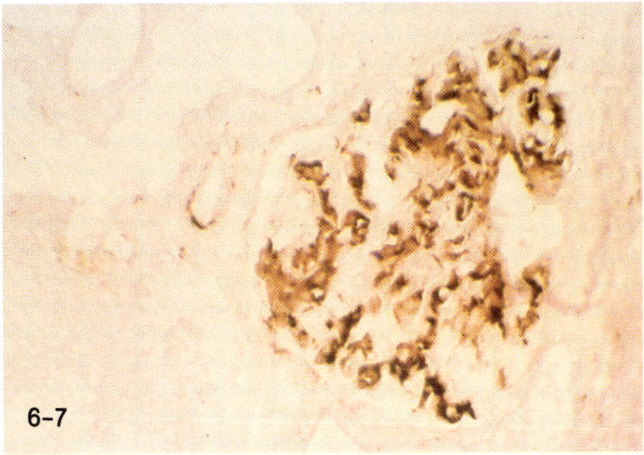

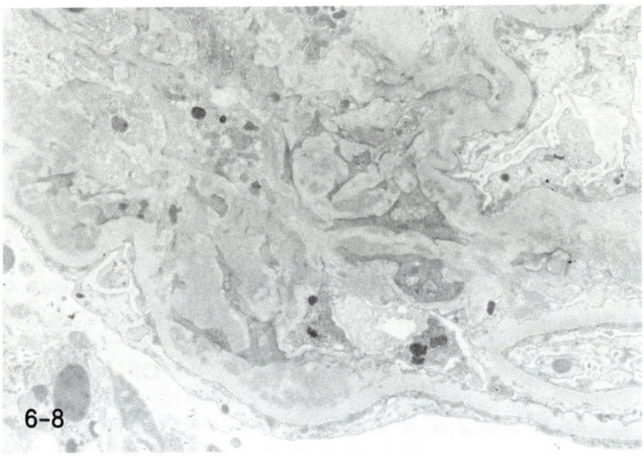

FIGURE 6–6. Mesangiopathic glomerulonephritis. Deposits of IgA are confined to the mesangial region (IMPAS for IgA).

FIGURE 6–7. Mesangial glomerulonephritis. Figures 6–7 and 6–8 are from the same case. The mesangial pattern of C3 deposits is visible. A vessel adjacent to the glomerulus also shows deposits of C3 (IMP for C3).

FIGURE 6–8. Same case as 6–7. Electron micrograph. Mesangial dense deposits are visible (lead citrate and uranyl acetate).

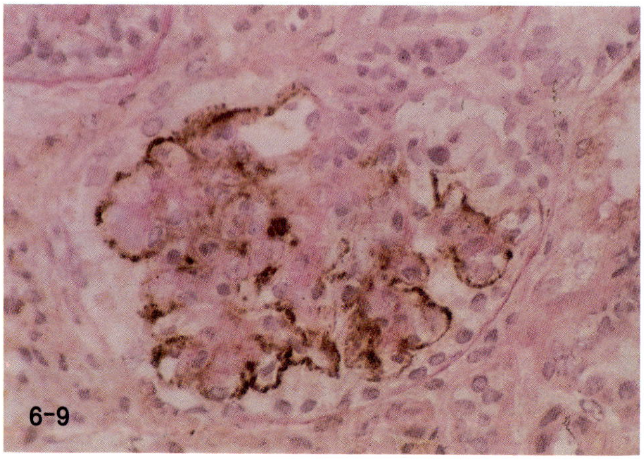

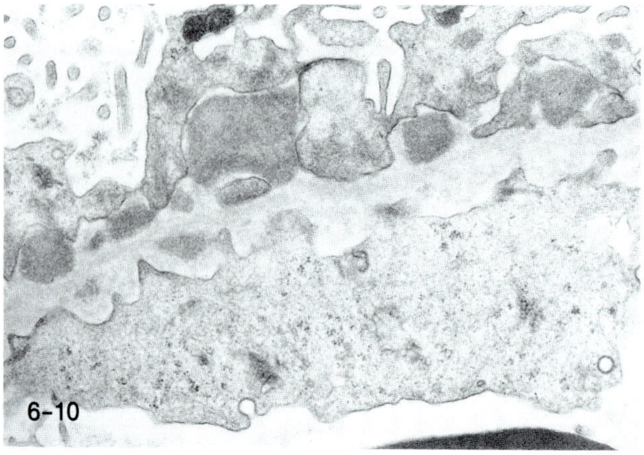

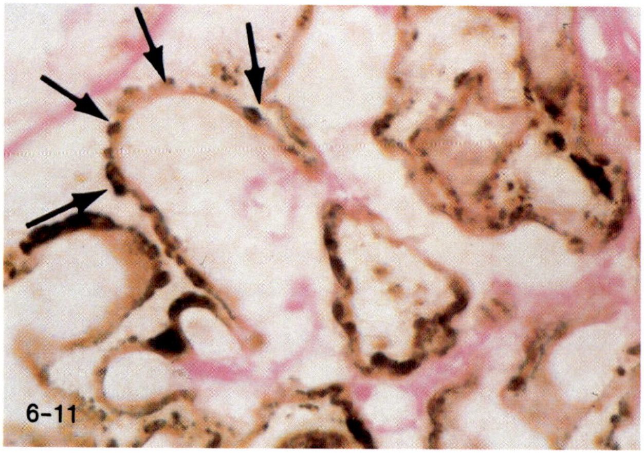

FIGURE 6–9. Poststreptococcal glomerulonephritis. Figures 6–9 and 6–10 are from the same case. Epimembranous and mesangial deposits of C3 are visible (IMPAS for C3, hematoxylin counterstain). *Slide 53.*

FIGURE 6–10. Same case as 6–9. Electron micrograph shows epimembranous and small intramembranous deposits (lead citrate and uranyl acetate).

FIGURE 6–11. Membranous glomerulonephritis. The generalized deposits of C3 (arrows) are clearly localized in the epimembranous area (IMPAS for C3). *Slide 54.*

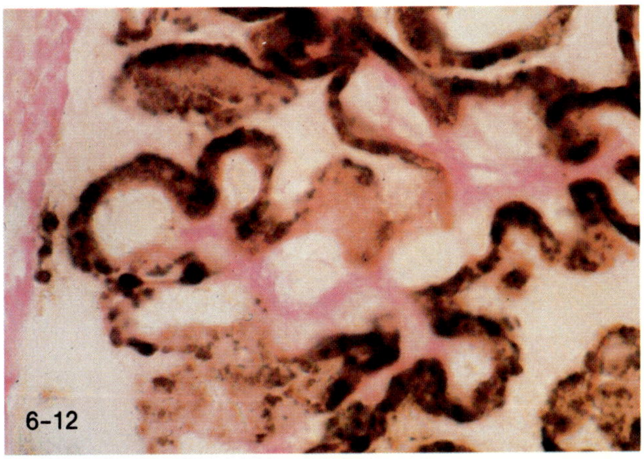

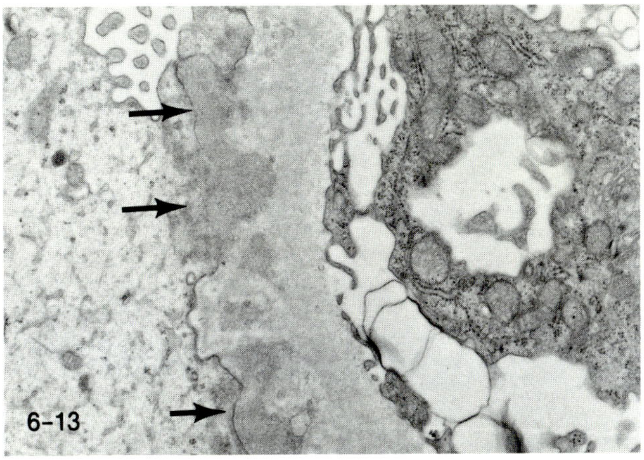

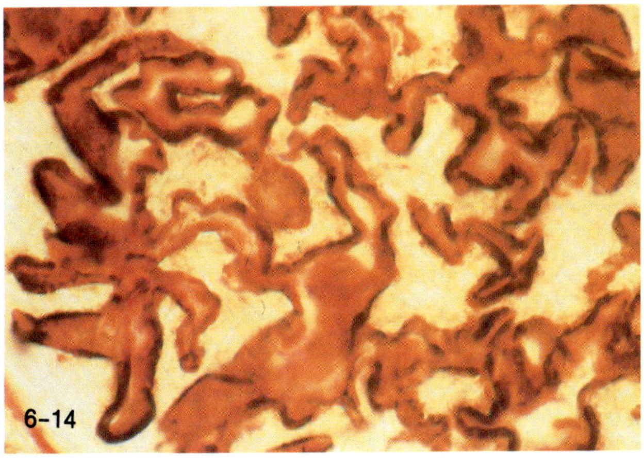

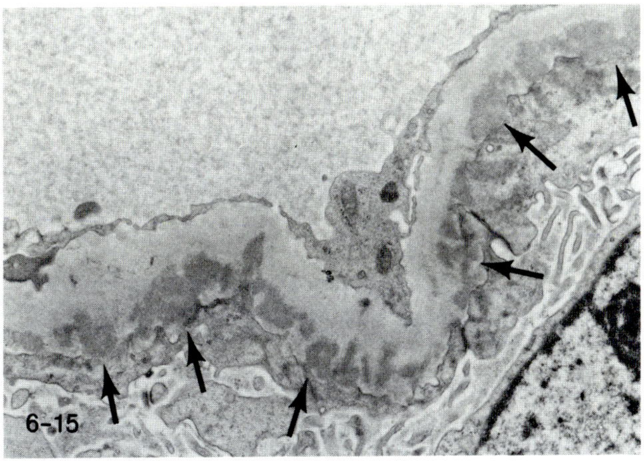

FIGURE 6–12. Membranous glomerulonephritis. Figures 6–12 and 6–13 are from the same case. The generalized prominent granular deposits of C3 in the glomerular basement membrane are both intramembranous and epimembranous (IMPAS for C3).

FIGURE 6–13. Same case as 6–12. Electron micrograph shows epimembranous dense deposits (arrows; lead citrate and uranyl acetate).

FIGURE 6–14. Membranous glomerulonephritis. Figures 6–14 and 6–15 are from the same case. Continuous deposits of C3 in a "pseudolinear" (confluent finely granular) pattern. In this case, the granular or discreet nature of the deposits is difficult to discern (IMPAS for C3).

FIGURE 6–15. Same case as 6–14. Electron micrograph shows epimembranous dense deposits (arrows). Some deposits are confluent, which correlates with the "pseudolinear" pattern observed by the immunoperoxidase stain (lead citrate and uranyl acetate).

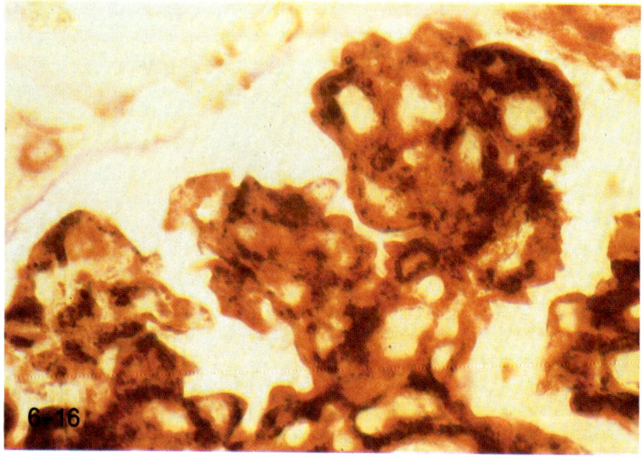

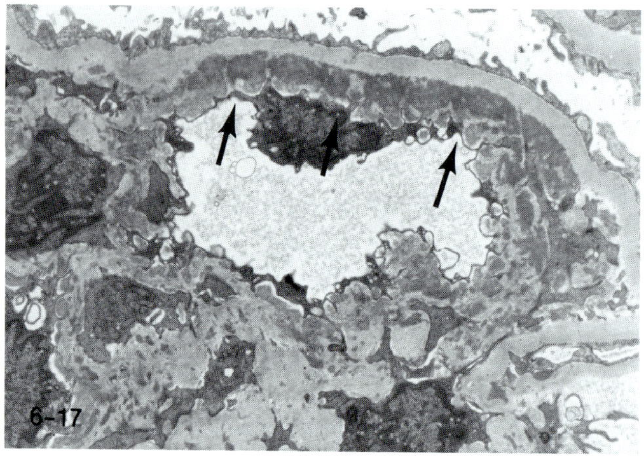

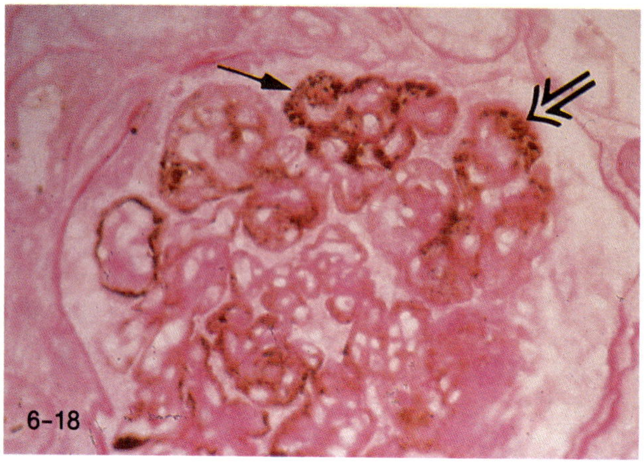

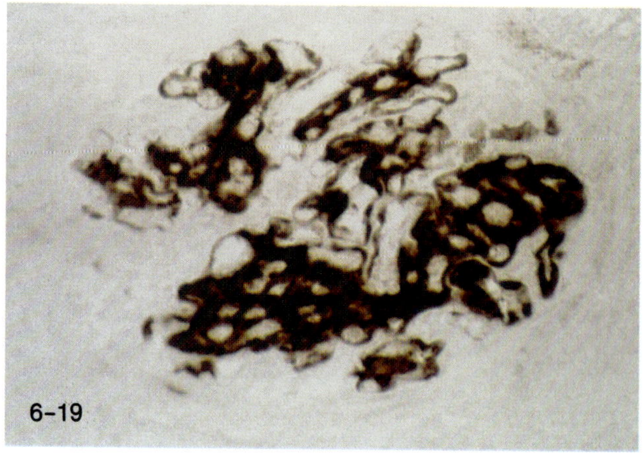

FIGURE 6–16. Diffuse lupus glomerulonephritis. Figures 6–16 and 6–17 are from the same case. Massive mesangial and glomerular basement membrane deposits of C3 are visible. Here, precise localization of the peripheral glomerular basement membrane deposits is difficult (IMPAS for C3).

FIGURE 6–17. Same case as 6–16. Electron micrograph shows subendothelial (arrows) and mesangial dense deposits (lead citrate and uranyl acetate).

FIGURE 6–18. Membranoproliferative glomerulonephritis. Subendothelial (double arrows) and epimembranous deposits (single arrow) of C3 are visible (IMPAS for C3). *Slide 55.*

FIGURE 6–19. Diffuse lupus glomerulonephritis. Figures 6–19 through 6–21 are from the same case. Granular deposits of C3 in mesangial regions and peripheral glomerular basement membrane are visible (IMP for C3).

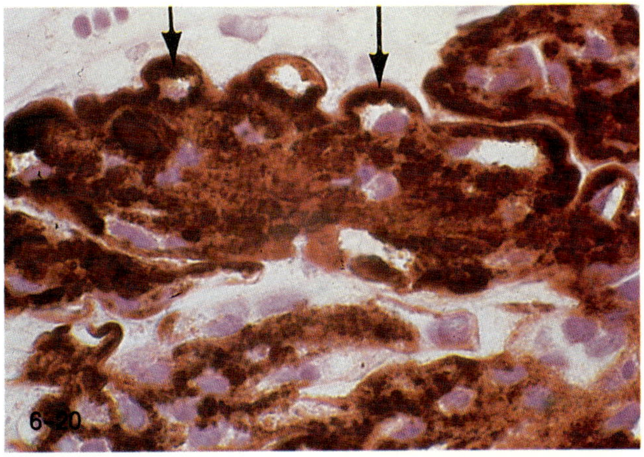

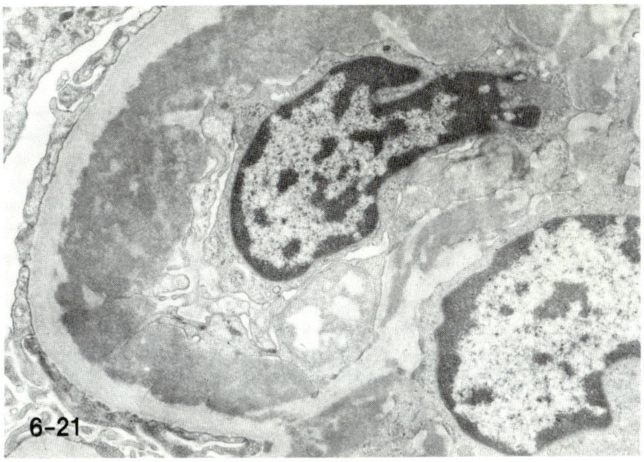

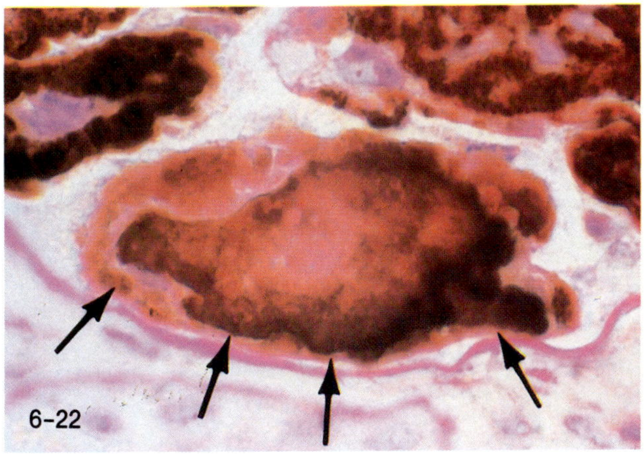

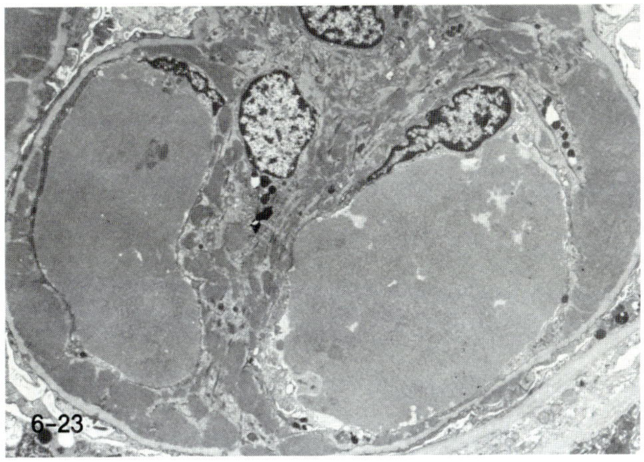

FIGURE 6–20. Same case as 6–19. Subendothelial dense deposits of C3 (arrows) and prominent mesangial deposits are visible (IMPAS for C3, hematoxylin counterstain). *Slide 56.*

FIGURE 6–21. Same case as 6–19. Electron micrograph shows prominent subendothelial dense deposits (lead citrate and uranyl acetate). *Slide 57.*

FIGURE 6–22. Diffuse lupus glomerulonephritis. Figures 6–22 and 6–23 are from the same case. Prominent intraluminal/ subendothelial deposits of C3 (arrows) are visible. Adjacent capillary loops also exhibit subendothelial deposits of C3 (IMPAS for C3, hematoxylin counterstain). *Slide 58.*

FIGURE 6–23. Same case as 6–22. Electron micrograph shows prominent intraluminal, subendothelial, and mesangial deposits (lead citrate and uranyl acetate). *Slide 59.*

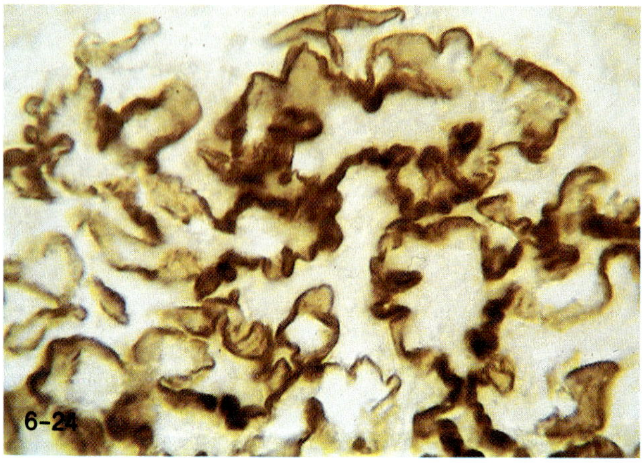

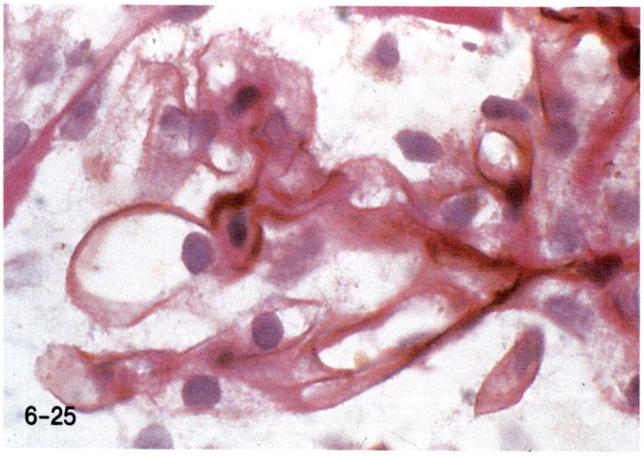

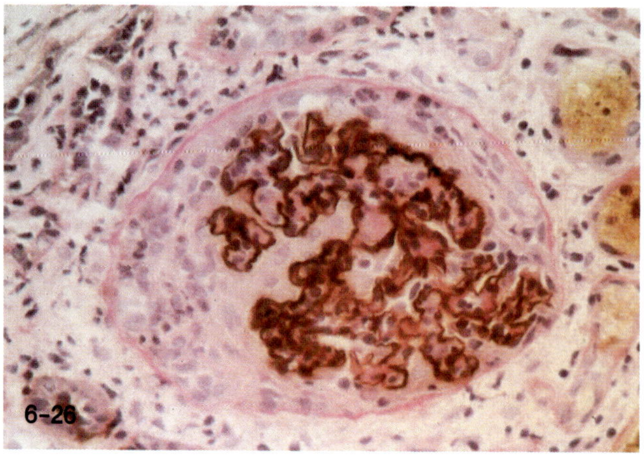

FIGURE 6–24. Anti–glomerular basement membrane disease. Linear deposits of IgG are visible in the peripheral glomerular basement membrane (IMP for IgG). *Slide 60.*

FIGURE 6–25. Anti–glomerular basement membrane disease. Linear deposits of IgG (brown) are visible in the glomerular basement membrane (IMPAS for IgG, hematoxylin counterstain). *Slide 61.*

FIGURE 6–26. Anti–glomerular basement membrane disease. Linear deposits of IgG and associated crescent formation (IMPAS for IgG, hematoxylin counterstain).

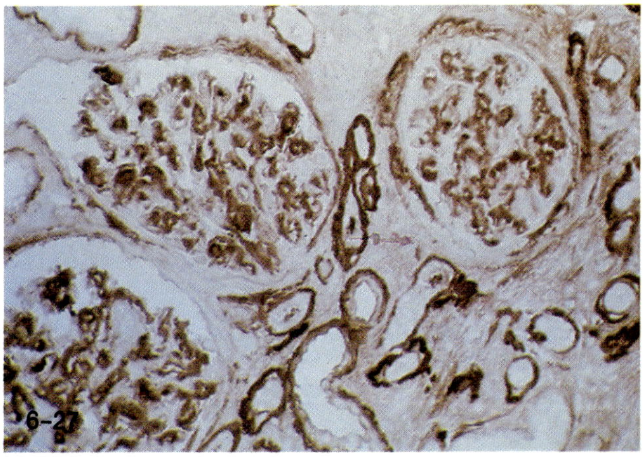

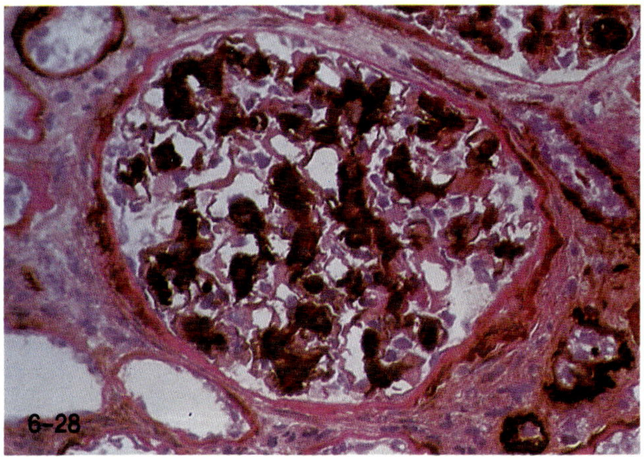

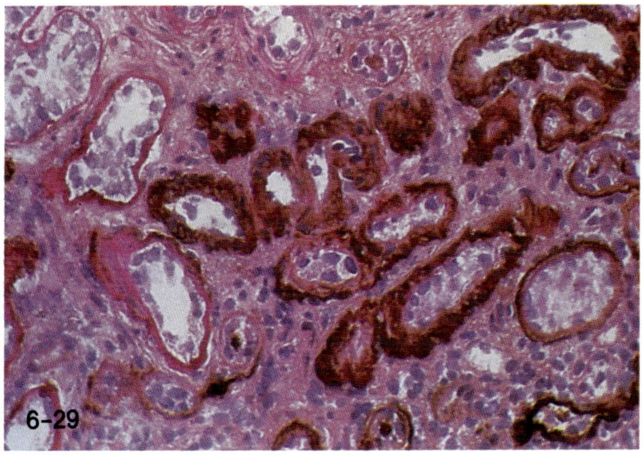

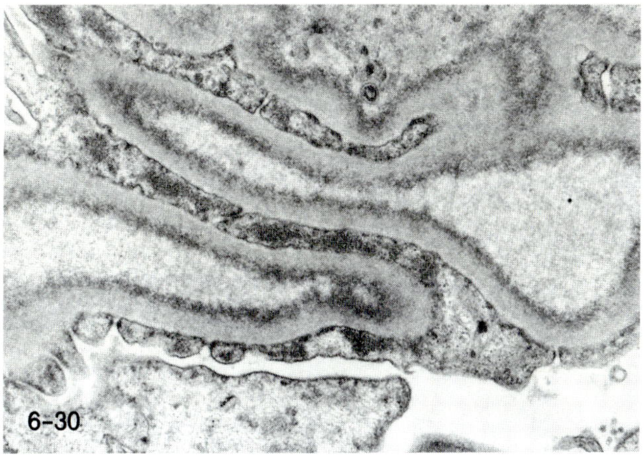

FIGURE 6–27. κ light chain deposition disease. Figures 6–27 through 6–30 are from the same case. Diffuse deposits of κ immunoglobulin light chains in glomeruli, vessels, and tubular basement membranes are visible (IMP for κ immunoglobulin light chains). *Slide 62.*

FIGURE 6–28. Same case as 6–27. Diffuse deposits of κ immunoglobulin light chains are visible in a glomerulus and adjacent tubular basement membranes (IMPAS for κ immunoglobulin light chains, hematoxylin counterstain). *Slide 63.*

FIGURE 6–29. Same case as 6–27. Diffuse deposits of κ immunoglobulin light chains are visible in tubular basement membranes (IMPAS for κ immunoglobulin light chains, hematoxylin counterstain).

FIGURE 6–30. Same case as 6–27. Electron micrograph shows continuous, finely granular, dense deposits concentrated in the internal aspect of the glomerular basement membrane (lead citrate and uranyl acetate). *Slide 64.*

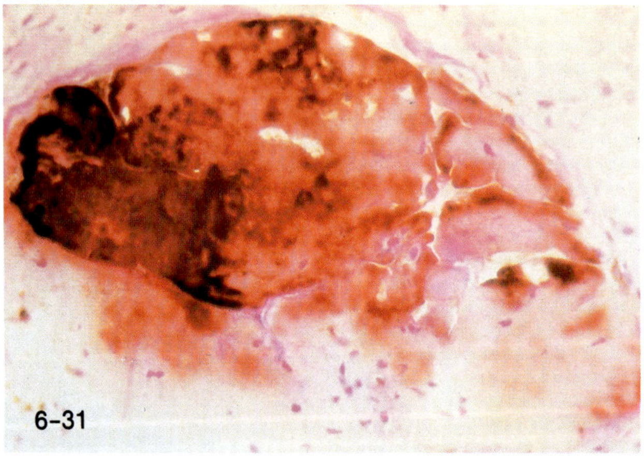

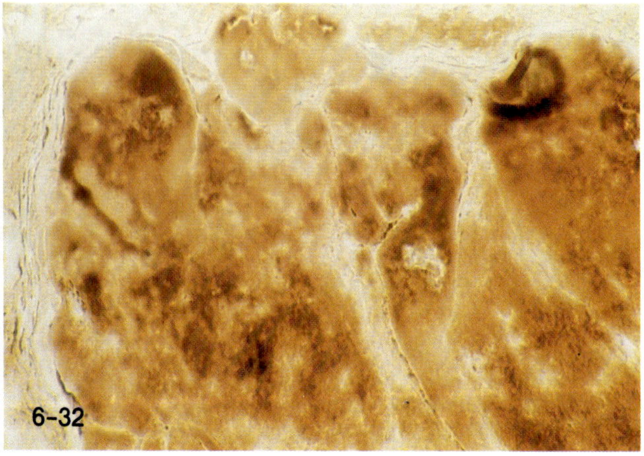

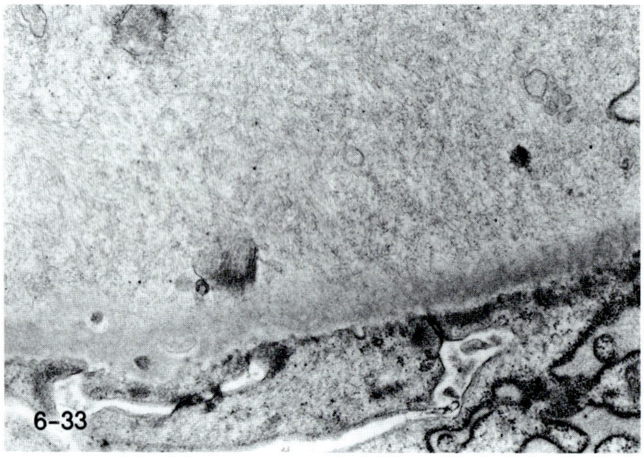

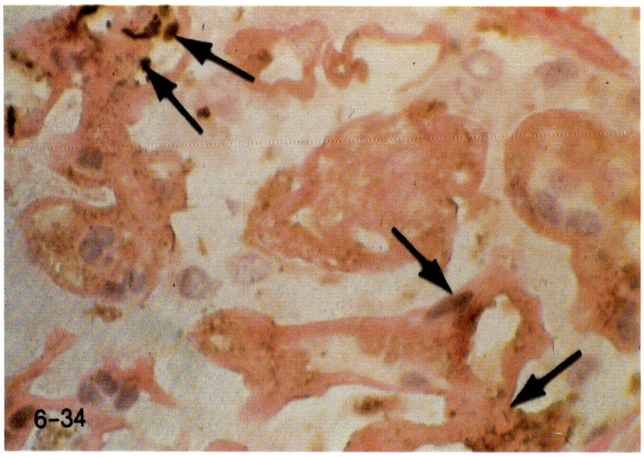

FIGURE 6–31. Renal amyloidosis. Figures 6–31 through 6–33 are from the same case. Generalized granular to homogeneous glomerular deposits of IgM are visible (IMPAS for IgM, hematoxylin counterstain). *Slide 65.*

FIGURE 6–32. Same case as 6–31. Generalized glomerular staining for κ immunoglobulin light chains (IMP for κ immunoglobulin light chains, no counterstain). *Slide 66.*

FIGURE 6–33. Same case as 6–31. Electron micrograph shows detail of amyloid deposits (lead citrate and uranyl acetate).

FIGURE 6–34. Microangiopathy. Figures 6–34 and 6–35 are from the same case. Glomerulus shows deposits of fibrinogen (arrows; IMPAS for fibrinogen, hematoxylin counterstain).

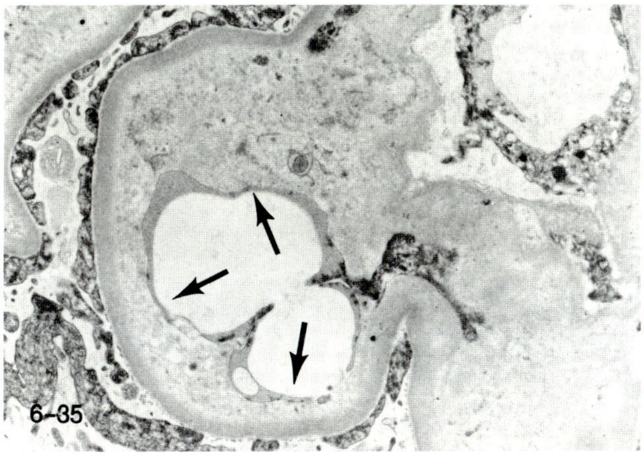

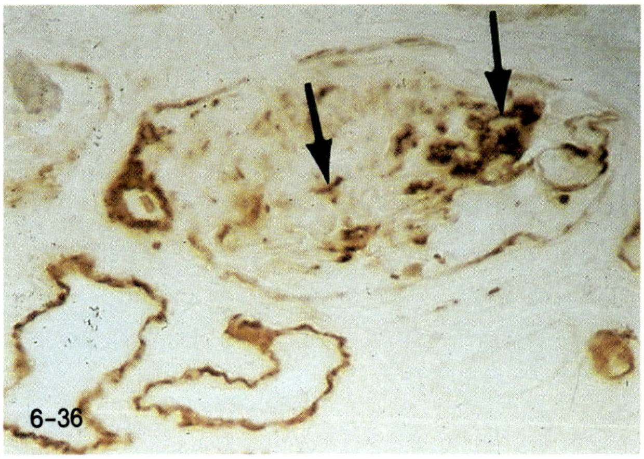

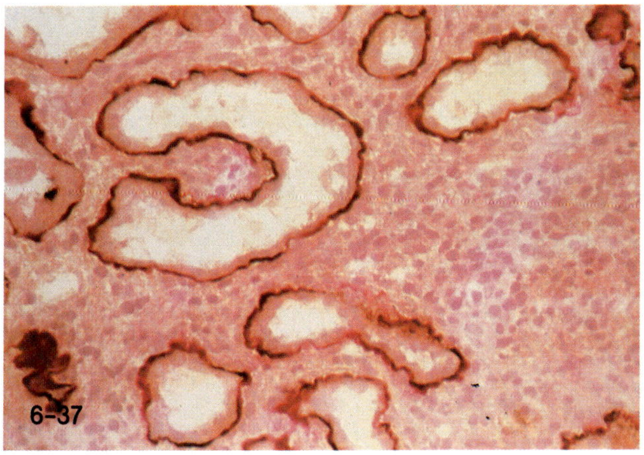

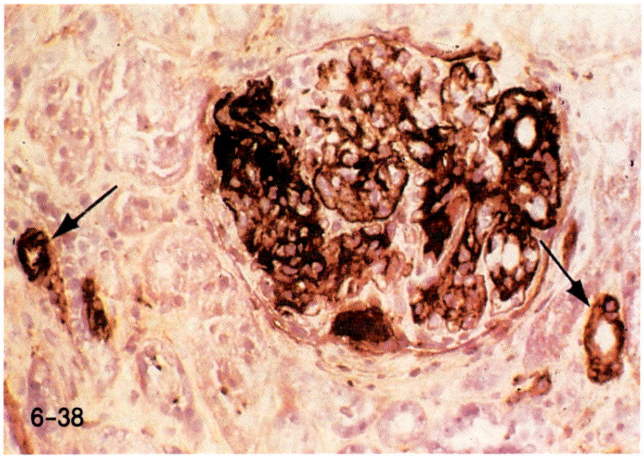

FIGURE 6–35. Same case as 6–34. Electron micrograph shows flocculent material in lucent subendothelial areas (arrows). Occasional fibrillar deposits typical of fibrin were demonstrated in other foci (lead citrate and uranyl acetate).

FIGURE 6–36. Lupus nephritis. Prominent tubular deposits of C3 are visible. Glomerular deposits of C3 (arrows) are also present in this photograph (IMP for C3, no counterstain). *Slide 67.*

FIGURE 6–37. Lupus nephritis. Deposits of C3 in tubular basement membranes. Interstitial cellular infiltrates are also present (IMPAS for C3, hematoxylin counterstain). *Slide 68.*

FIGURE 6–38. Lupus nephritis. Vascular deposits (arrows) and mesangial and peripheral glomerular basement membrane deposits of IgG in severe diffuse lupus nephritis (IMPAS for IgG, hematoxylin counterstain). *Slide 69.*

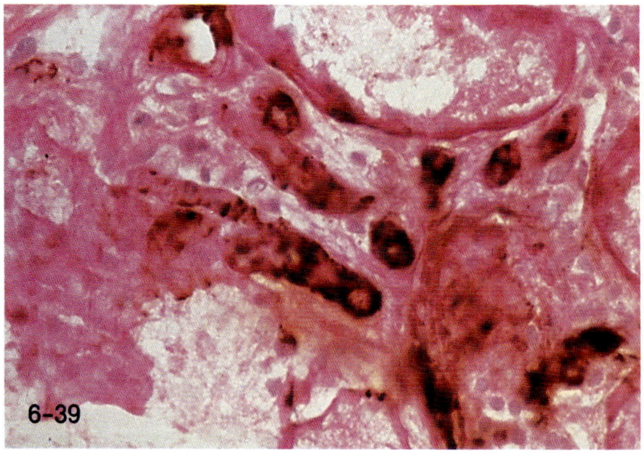

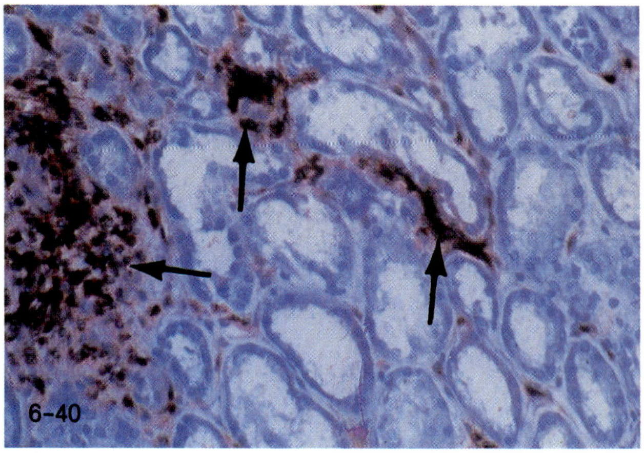

FIGURE 6–39. Vasculitis in kidney. Granular deposits of C3 in vessels (IMPAS for C3).

FIGURE 6–40. Acute cellular rejection. The majority of mononuclear (lymphocytic) interstitial infiltrates are positive for T11 (arrows), a pan-T-cell marker (IMP, hematoxylin counterstain). *Slide 70.*

7 Diseases of the Lung and Pleura

Immune Deposits

Deposits of immunoglobulin and complement may be identified in the lung with the immunoperoxidase (IMP) technique and localized in alveolar septa and larger vessels with PAS (IMPAS) or hematoxylin or both as counterstains. The method of analysis for the presence and localization of the deposits is similar to that employed in renal biopsy material (Chapter 6). Our experience with immune complex deposits in the lung has been limited to lupus pneumonitis, in which granular deposits of immunoglobulin and complement may be detected (**FIGURES 7–1** and **7–2**).

Linear deposits of IgG and complement in alveolar septa may be detected in cases of Goodpasture's syndrome with anti-glomerular basement membrane disease (Chapter 6). We have not had the opportunity to use the IMP technique in studying lung tissue in Goodpasture's syndrome. Deposits of immunoglobulin and complement have been reported in cases of fibrosing interstitial pneumonitis; however, we have not observed them in 14 cases.

Pulmonary Vasculitis

In cases of pulmonary vasculitis (Wegener's granulomatosis) the immunoperoxidase technique with PAS or hematoxylin or both as counterstains may be used to demonstrate the presence or absence of immunoglobulin or complement in vessels, as well as to investigate the type of cells composing the vascular infiltrates. In two cases of Wegener's granulomatosis, we have observed no deposits of IgG, IgA, IgM, or C3 in the lung. The cellular infiltrates in the vessels were a mixture of polyclonal B-cells, T-cells, and monocytes/macrophages (**FIGURES 7–3** and **7–4**).

Lymphoid Neoplasms and Lymphoid Infiltrates

Immunoperoxidase techniques are especially valuable in diagnosing lymphoid neoplasms and infiltrates involving a variety of tissues, including the lung (Chapter 5). The majority of lymphocyte differentiation antigens can be detected only in frozen tissue. The determination of surface immunoglobulin light chains (κ and λ) in paraffin-embedded material is not reliable.

Pseudolymphoma is characterized by polyclonal B-cell infiltrates exhibiting κ and λ immunoglobulin light chains, as well as T-cells (**FIGURES 7–5** through **7–9**). B-cell lymphomas are characterized by monoclonal B-cell infiltrates, exhibiting either κ or λ immunoglobulin light chain staining, but not both (**FIGURES 7–10** through **7–12**). We have found that immunoperoxidase is especially helpful in differentiating pseudolymphoma from B-cell lymphoma in infiltrates composed predominantly of "small" lymphocytes.

We have studied one T-cell lymphoma that was not angiocentric (**FIGURES 7–13** and **7–14**). In our experience with two cases of lymphomatoid granulomatosis, the atypical angiocentric infiltrates contained predominantly T-cells (**FIGURES 7–15** through **7–17**). These two cases of lymphomatoid granulomatosis, characterized by abundant vascular and perivascular T-cells, raise the possibility that this lesion is simply a T-cell lymphoma.

Detection of lymphocytic/leukocytic markers (LN-1, LN-2, and common leukocyte antigen) in paraffin-embedded tissue is diagnostic of lymphoma when the infiltrate exhibits cytologic malignancy (**FIGURES 7–18** and **7–19**). Detection of these markers is especially helpful if frozen tissue is not available for evaluation of lymphocyte differentiation markers. Immunoperoxidase techniques may also be used to identify and subtype mononuclear/lymphocytic infiltrates in a variety of lung diseases, including interstitial pneumonitis.

Nonlymphoid Neoplasms

If the history or histologic appearance of the pulmonary neoplasm suggests a metastatic carcinoma, certain antigens may be sought, such as prostatic antigen, prostatic acid phosphatase, or S-100 protein for melanoma. We anticipate a wider application of immunoperoxidase techniques for selected tumor-specific antigens to determine whether a neoplasm is primary or metastatic. Carcinoembryonic antigen (CEA) may be sought in small cell undifferentiated carcinoma to predict those cases in which plasma levels of this antigen may be useful in follow-up studies. Lymphocyte differentiation antigens, CEA, cytokeratins, and the common leukocyte antigen may be used in the diagnosis of undifferentiated small or large cell neoplasms of the lung (**FIGURES 7–20** through **7–23**).

Immunohistochemistry may demonstrate peptide hormones in neoplasms associated with ectopic hormone production (**FIGURES 7–24** and **7–25**).

Currently, one of the most promising applications of immunoperoxidase techniques is the separation of malignant mesothelioma from primary lung carcinomas or from metastatic carcinomas involving the pleura, especially in the differential diagnosis of malignant epithelioid mesothelioma versus metastatic adenocarcinoma. Although the pattern of antigen expression may suggest the diagnosis of either adenocarcinoma or mesothelioma, it is premature to assume that these patterns are definitive. The patient's history (especially history of occupational, medical, or other exposure to carcinogenic substances), as well as evaluation of routinely stained paraffin-embedded tissue, histochemistry, and electron microscopy (including elemental analysis and electron diffraction) remain essential in the evaluation of pleural tumors, especially if associated with occupational exposure to asbestos.

In general, mesotheliomas exhibit absent or minimal cellular staining for CEA but prominent cytoplasmic staining for cytokeratins (**FIGURES 7–26** through **7–29**). Pronase digestion enhances the expression of keratin antigens (**FIGURES 7–28** and **7–29**). Typically, but not always, metastatic adenocarcinomas and primary lung adenocarcinomas involving the pleura exhibit prominent cytoplasmic staining for CEA and variable staining for cytokeratins (**FIGURES 7–30** and **7–31**).

Cytokeratins are a related family of intermediate filaments with a variable distribution in normal and neoplastic tissue. Because keratins of different molecular weights are present in different pulmonary and pleural neoplasms, the molecular weight of the cytokeratin antigens being studied should be determined. The molecular weights of the cytokeratins to which commercially available antibodies react is usually not stated by the manufacturer. Said et al have demonstrated that a cytokeratin with a molecular weight of 63,000 daltons is present in mesotheliomas, but not in adenocarcinomas.

Caution should be exercised because some adenocarcinomas involving the pleura are negative for CEA. Battifora has demonstrated the presence of human milk fat globulin in all metastatic carcinomas involving the pleura, but this protein was absent in all mesotheliomas studied; however, Marshall et al reported contradictory findings.

Other Applications

Immunoperoxidase techniques may also be used to identify a variety of infectious agents; however, we have not done so on a routine basis. Study of various collagen types in lung biopsy specimens from patients with cryptogenic fibrosing alveolitis may also be of value. Antigens of epithelial and macrophagic/leukocytic origin demonstrate typical staining patterns in fibrosing alveolitis and desquamative interstitial pneumonia. The epithelial membrane antigen is typically localized to the cells lining the alveoli; whereas muramidase and α-antichymotrypsin are localized in the alveolar macrophages (**FIGURES 7–32** through **7–35**).

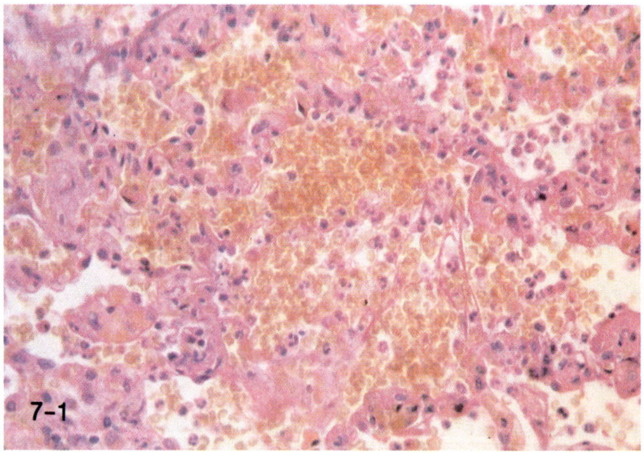

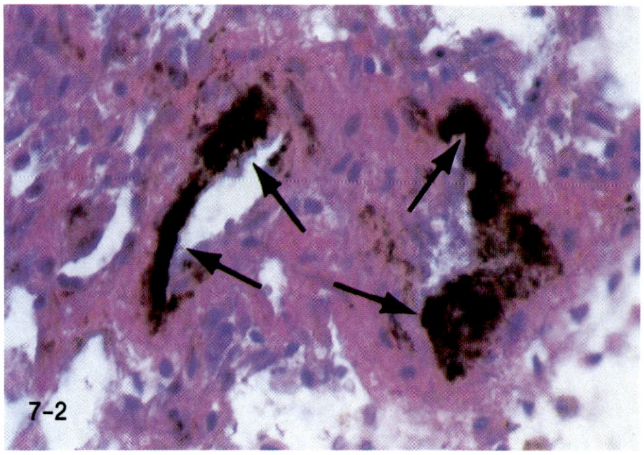

FIGURE 7–1. Lupus pneumonitis. Figures 7–1 and 7–2 are from the same case. In this figure, extensive alveolar hemorrhage is present (H & E).

FIGURE 7–2. Same case as 7–1. Prominent vascular deposits of C3 (arrows) are visible. (IMPAS for C3 with hematoxylin counterstain). *Slide 71.*

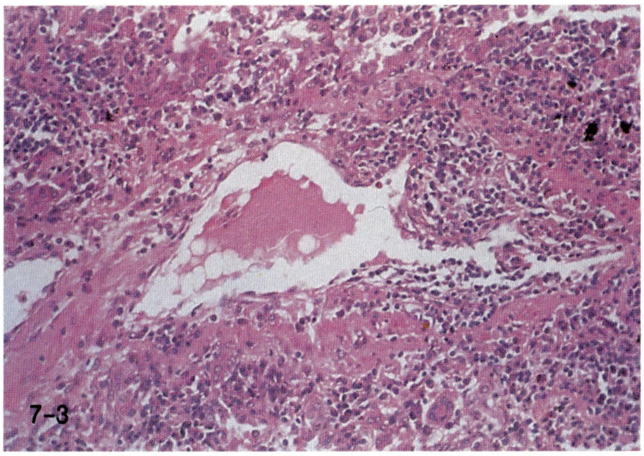

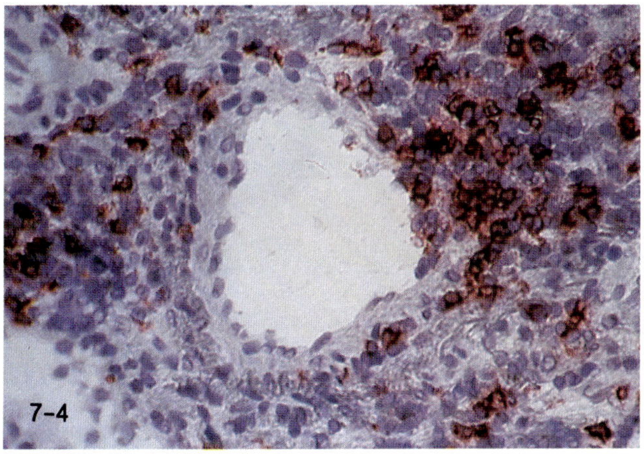

FIGURE 7–3. Pulmonary vasculitis/Wegener's granulomatosis. Figures 7–3 and 7–4 are from the same case. In this figure, cellular infiltrates are present in a pulmonary vessel (H & E).

FIGURE 7–4. Same case as 7–3. $T8^{+}$ cells (cytotoxic/suppressor subset of T-cells) are visible in the vascular infiltrate (ABC-PO with AEC, hematoxylin counterstain). *Slide 72.*

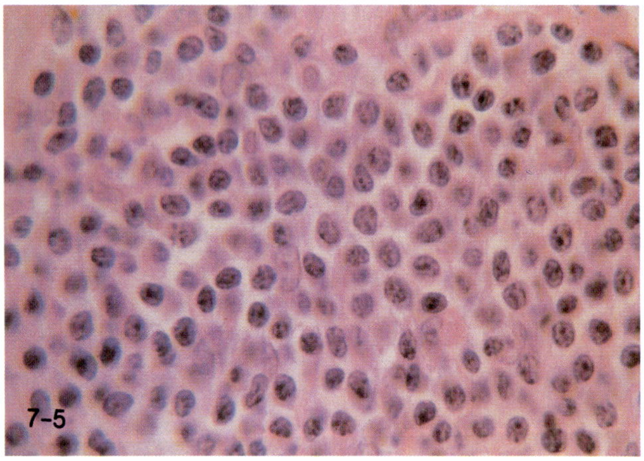

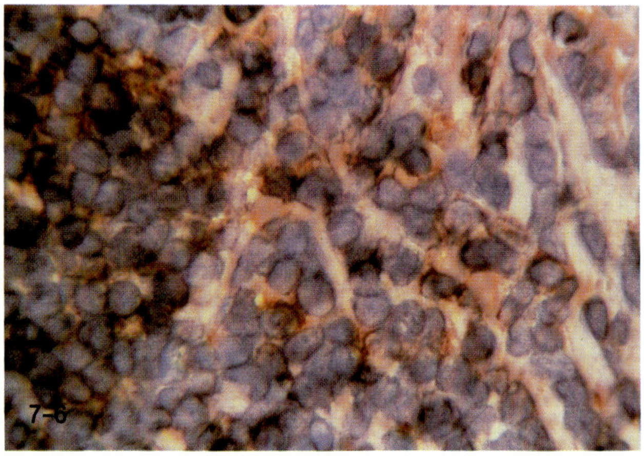

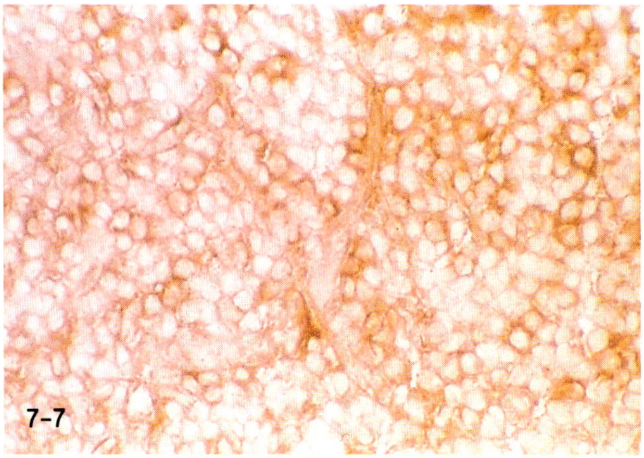

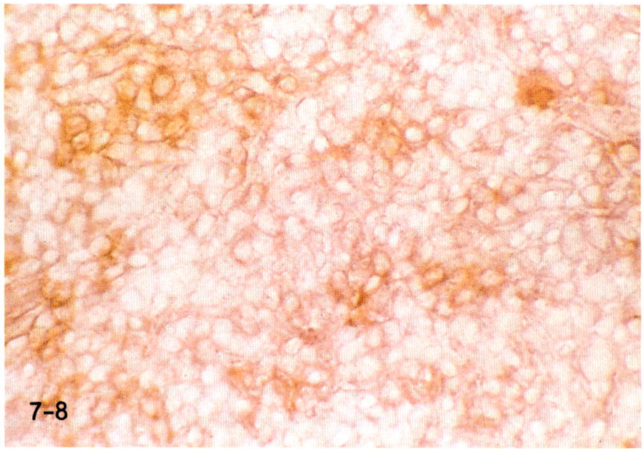

FIGURE 7–5. Pulmonary pseudolymphoma. Figures 7–5 through 7–9 are from the same case. In this figure, small lymphocytes predominate (H & E).

FIGURE 7–6. Same case as 7–5. This section is positive for the B1 differentiation antigen (ABC-PO with AEC, hematoxylin counterstain).

FIGURE 7–7. Same case as 7–5. Some cells are positive and some are negative for κ immunoglobulin light chains (IMP with AEC, no counterstain).

FIGURE 7–8. Same case as 7–5. Some cells are positive and some are negative for λ immunoglobulin light chains (IMP with AEC, no counterstain).

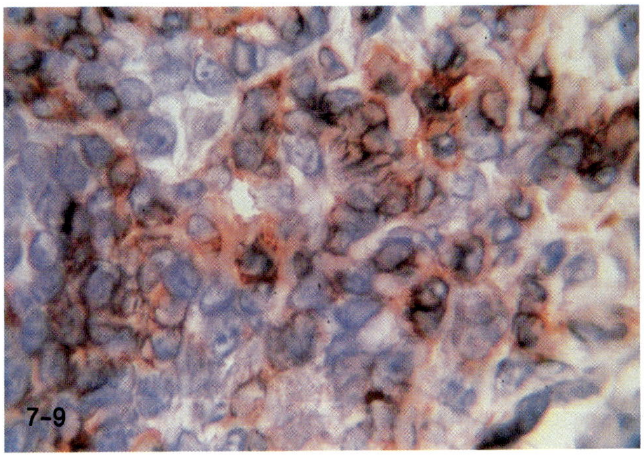

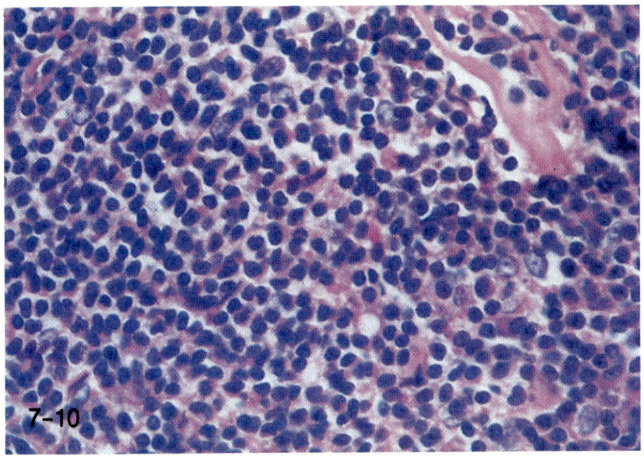

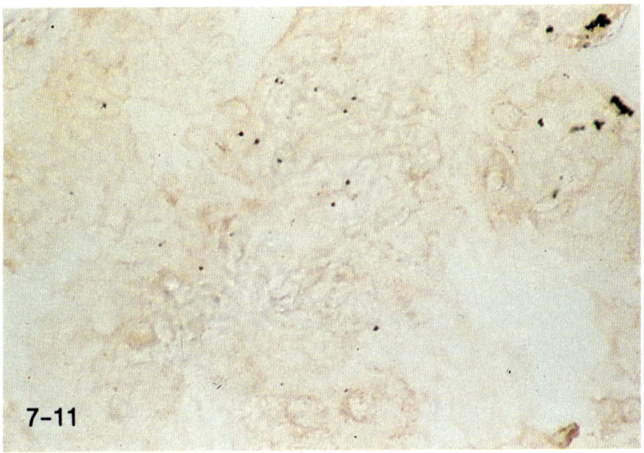

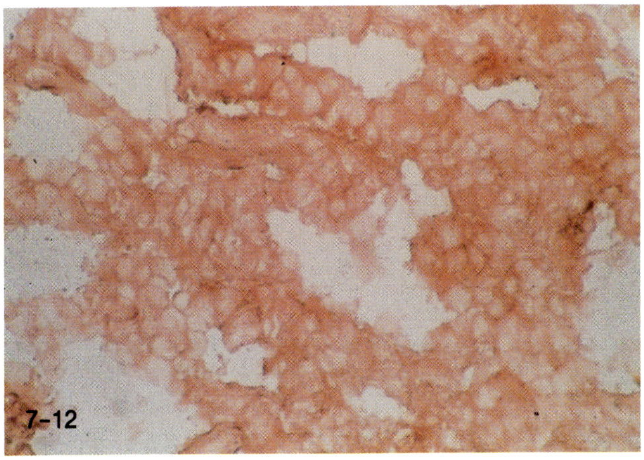

FIGURE 7–9. Same case as 7–5. $T11^+$ cells (pan T-cell marker) are visible (ABC-PO with AEC, hematoxylin counterstain).

FIGURE 7–10. Pulmonary B-cell lymphoma. Figures 7–10 through 7–12 are from the same case. The tumor is predominantly composed of small lymphocytes. In this figure, plasma cells are also present (H & E).

FIGURE 7–11. Same case as 7–10. κ immunoglobulin light chains were not detected. The lymphoma was positive when stained for λ immunoglobulin light chains (see 7–12). Anthracotic pigment is present (direct IMP with AEC, no counterstain).

FIGURE 7–12. Same case as 7–10. Positive staining for λ immunoglobulin light chains is visible (IMP with AEC, no counterstain).

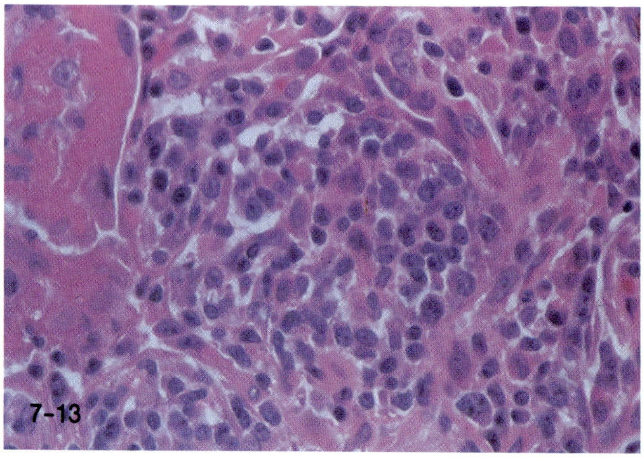

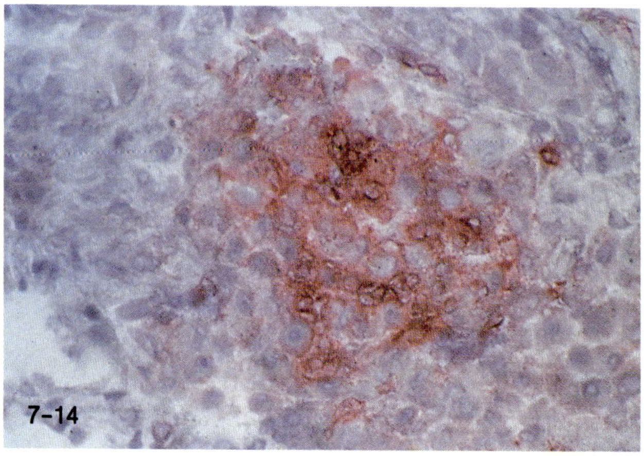

FIGURE 7–13. Pulmonary T-cell lymphoma. Figures 7–13 and 7–14 are from the same case. The patient presented with lymphoma involving peripheral lymph nodes, and one year later developed pulmonary infiltrates, which are demonstrated in this biopsy specimen (H & E).

FIGURE 7–14. Same case as 7–13. Cells positive for T11 (pan T-cell marker) are visible (ABC-PO with AEC, hematoxylin counterstain). Surrounding lung parenchyma is negative.

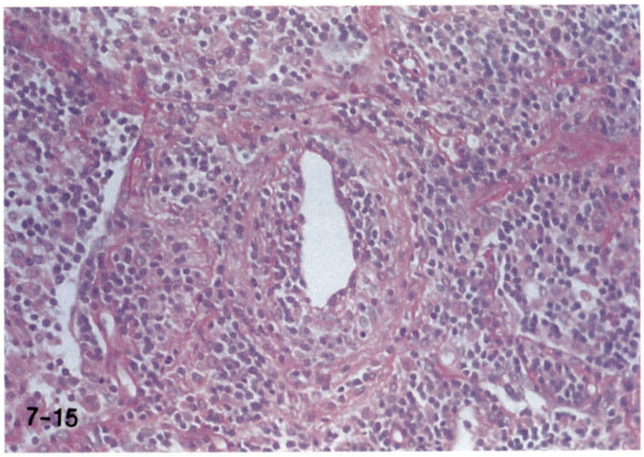

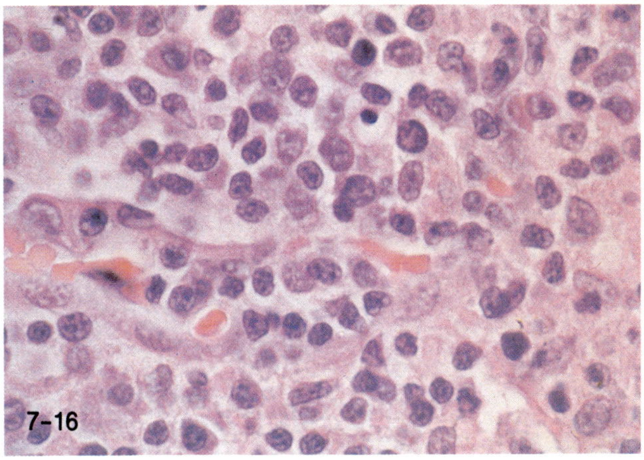

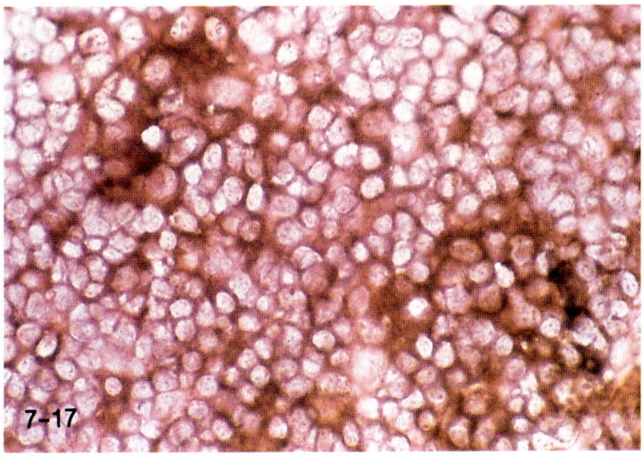

FIGURE 7–15. Lymphomatoid granulomatosis. Figures 7–15 through 7–17 are from the same case. In this figure, vascular and perivascular mononuclear infiltrates are present (PAS with hematoxylin counterstain).

FIGURE 7–16. Same case as 7–15. Atypical lymphoid cells are visible (H & E).

FIGURE 7–17. Same case as 7–15. T3 antigen is present on most of the cells (ABC-PO with AEC, hematoxylin counterstain).

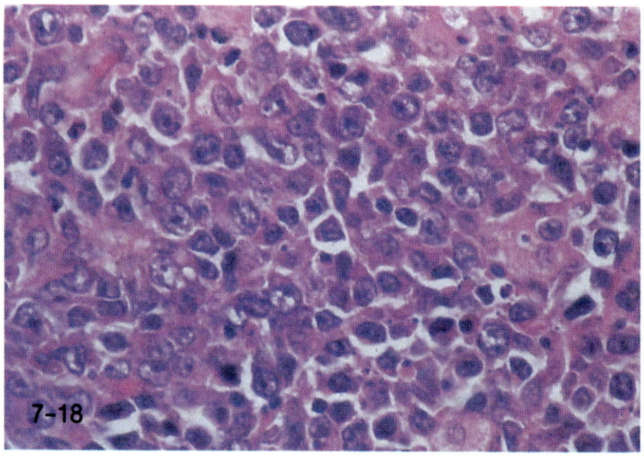

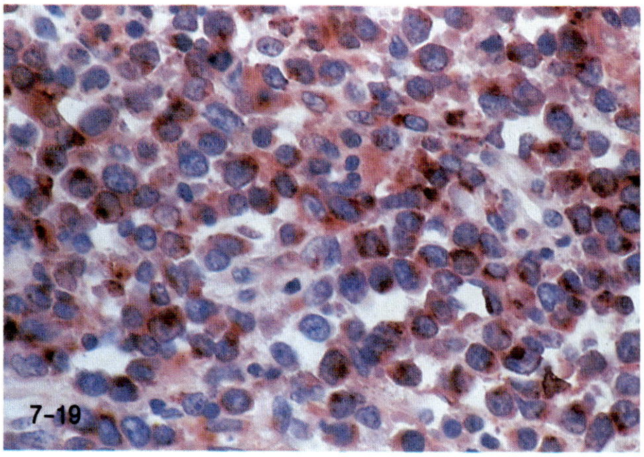

FIGURE 7–18. Immunoblastic sarcoma, primary in the lung. Figures 7–18 and 7–19 are from the same case. This tissue section is stained with H & E.

FIGURE 7–19. Same case as 7–18. The majority of cells exhibit the LN2 antigen, indicating B-lymphocytic origin of the cytologically malignant cells (ABC-PO with AEC in a paraffin section of Hollande's-fixed tissue, hematoxylin counterstain). *Slide 73.*

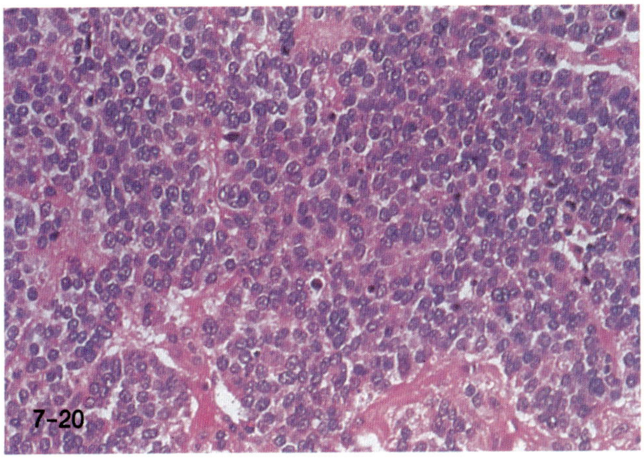

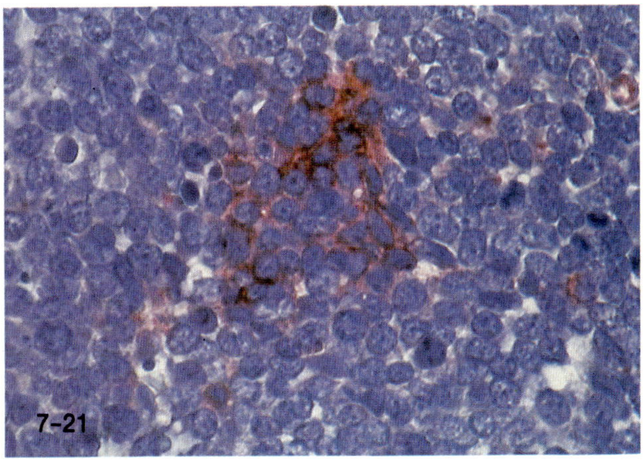

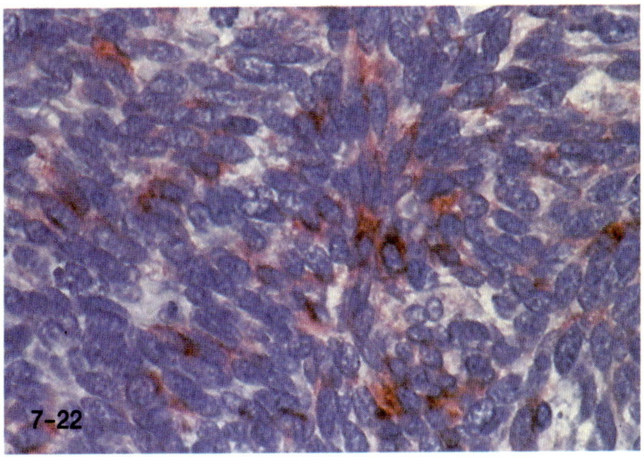

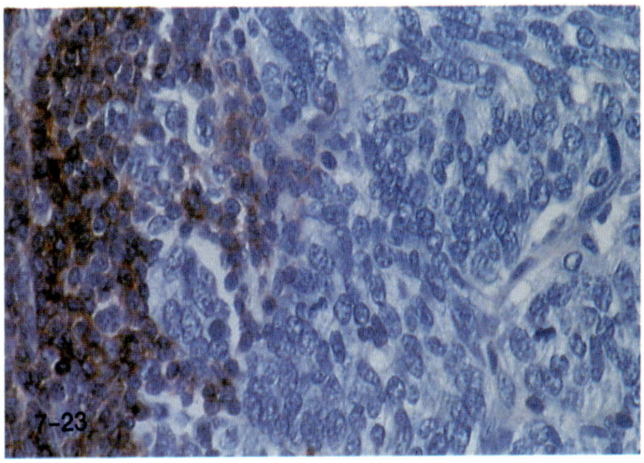

FIGURE 7–20. Small cell undifferentiated carcinoma of the lung. Figures 7–20 through 7–23 are from the same case. This tissue section is stained with H & E.

FIGURE 7–21. Same case as 7–20. Carcinoembryonic antigen (CEA) is present in a cluster of cells (center; ABC-PO with AEC, hematoxylin counterstain).

FIGURE 7–22. Same case as 7–20. CEA is expressed in scattered cells (ABC-PO with AEC, hematoxylin counterstain). *Slide 74.*

FIGURE 7–23. Same case as 7–20. Lymphocytes adjacent to the undifferentiated small cell carcinoma (left) are positive for common leukocyte antigen, whereas the carcinoma (center and right) is negative for this antigen (ABC-PO with AEC, hematoxylin counterstain). *Slide 75.*

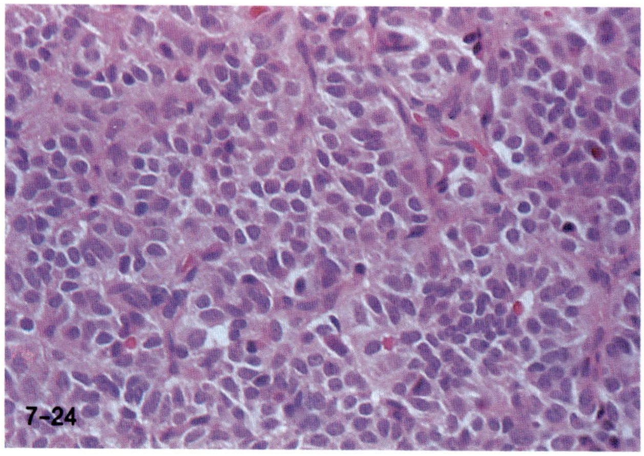

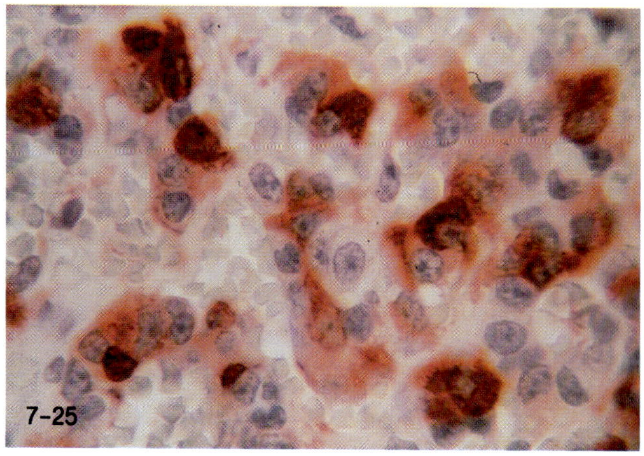

FIGURE 7–24. Carcinoid tumor of the lung. Figures 7–24 and 7–25 are from the same case. This tissue section is stained with H & E.

FIGURE 7–25. Same case as 7–24. Cells are positive for ACTH. This patient had Cushing's syndrome, which was cured following resection of the tumor (ABC-PO with AEC, hematoxylin counterstain). *Slide 76.*

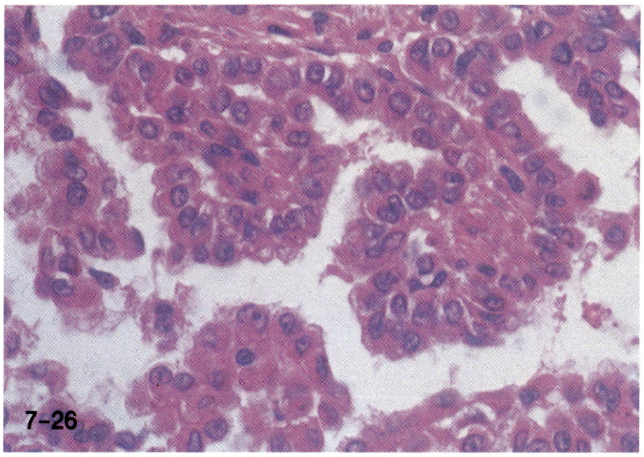

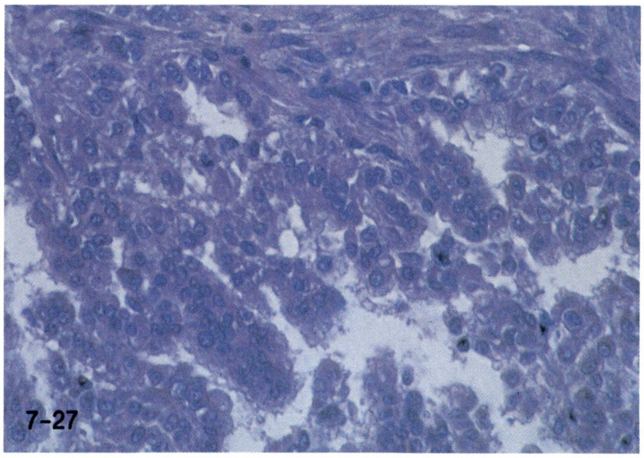

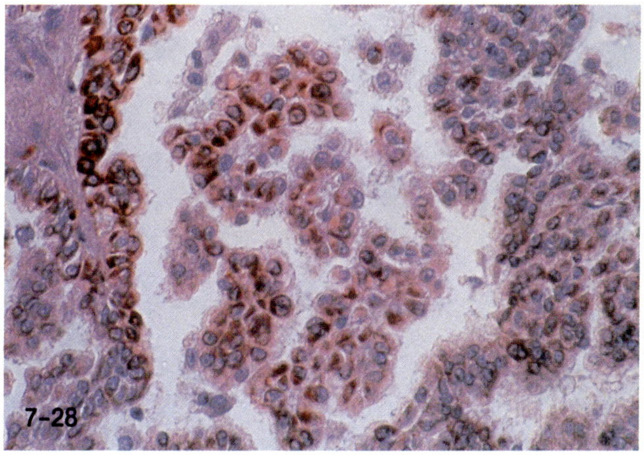

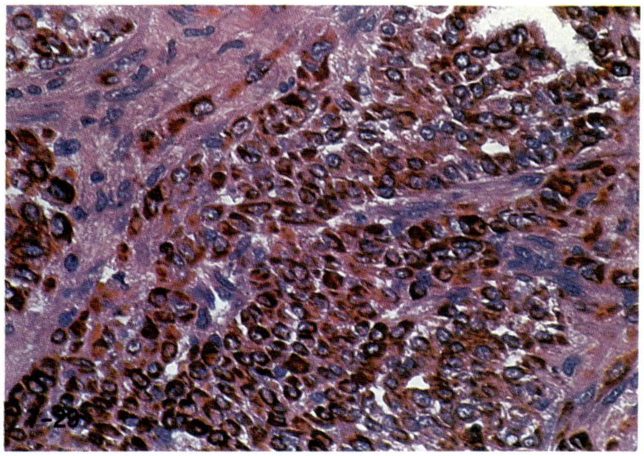

FIGURE 7–26. Malignant mesothelioma diffusely involving the pleura. Figures 7–26 through 7–29 are from the same case. The patient had a history of asbestos exposure. The mesothelioma, visible in this figure, is of the epithelioid type (H & E).

FIGURE 7–27. Same case as 7–26. This section shows negative staining for CEA (ABC-PO with AEC, hematoxylin counterstain). *Slide 77.*

FIGURE 7–28. Same case as 7–26. Cytokeratins (detected with AE1/3, an antibody to low molecular weight cytokeratins) are present in some but not all cells (ABC-PO with AEC in a paraffin section without pronase, hematoxylin counterstain).

FIGURE 7–29. Same case as 7–26. Cytokeratins (detected with AE1/3) are present in a majority of neoplastic cells (ABC-PO with AEC in a pronase-digested paraffin section, hematoxylin counterstain). *Slide 78.*

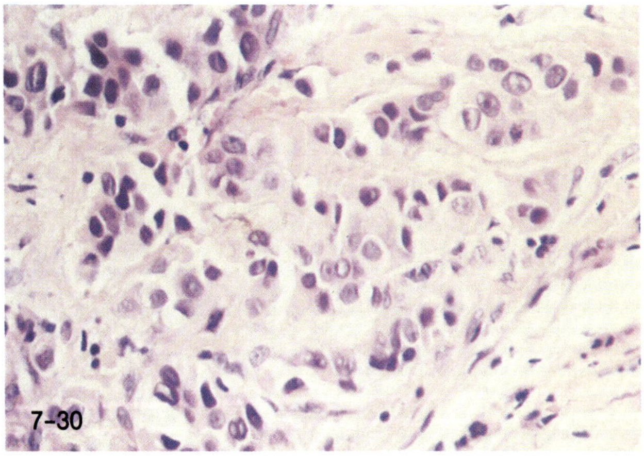

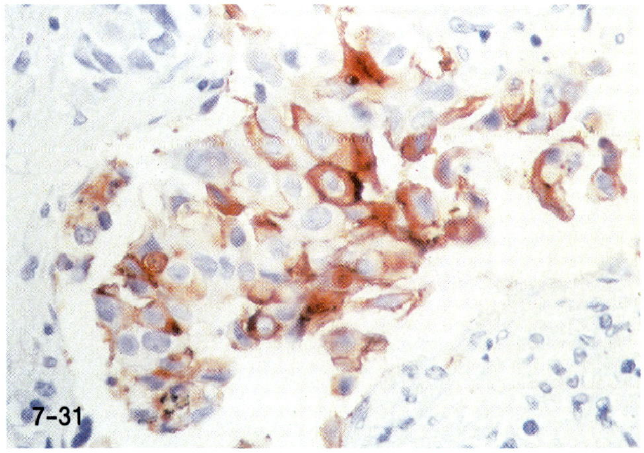

FIGURE 7–30. Metastatic adenocarcinoma involving the pleura. Figures 7–30 and 7–31 are from the same case. This tissue section is stained with H & E.

FIGURE 7–31. Same case as 7–30. CEA is present in most of the cells. The majority of neoplastic cells were also positive when stained for cytokeratins with AE1/3, an antibody to low molecular weight cytokeratins (ABC-PO with AEC for CEA, hematoxylin counterstain). *Slide 79.*

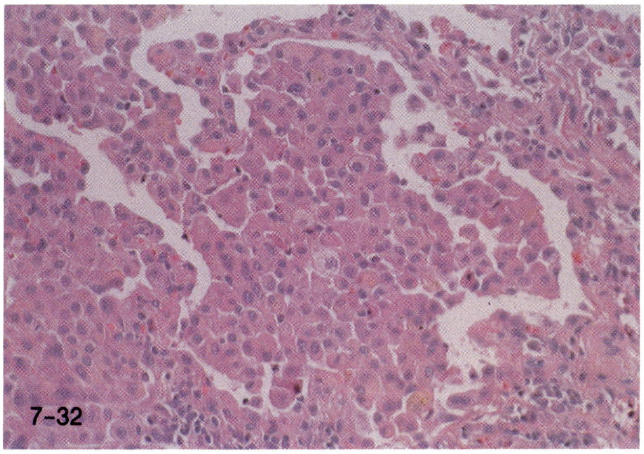

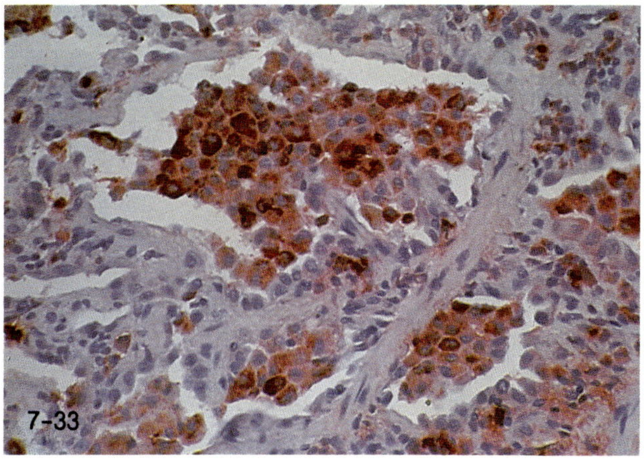

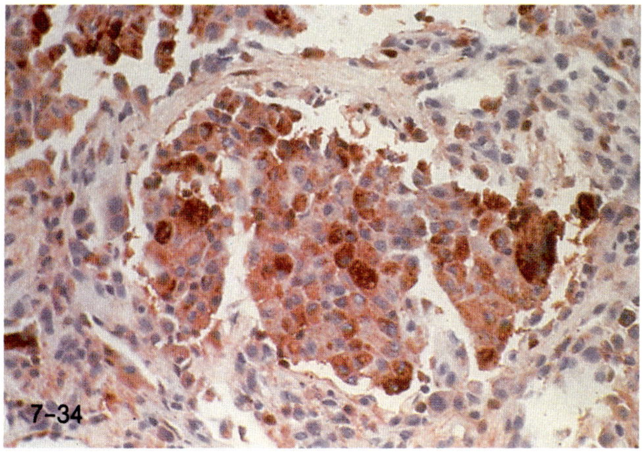

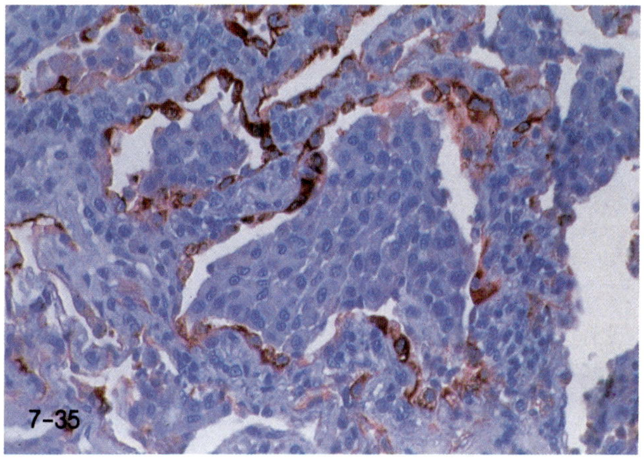

FIGURE 7–32. Desquamative interstitial pneumonia with prominent alveolar macrophages. Figures 7–32 through 7–35 are from the same case. This tissue section is stained with H & E.

FIGURE 7–33. Same case as 7–32. Muramidase activity in alveolar macrophages is visible (ABC-PO with AEC in a paraffin section, hematoxylin counterstain). *Slide 80.*

FIGURE 7–34. Same case as 7–32. α-1-Chymotrypsin is demonstrated in alveolar macrophages (ABC-PO with AEC in a paraffin section, hematoxylin counterstain).

FIGURE 7–35. Same case as 7–32. Epithelial membrane antigen is limited to alveolar lining cells. Alveolar macrophages are negative (ABC-PO with AEC, hematoxylin counterstain). *Slide 81.*

8 Genitourinary Pathology

In this chapter, antigen systems applicable to genitourinary pathology will be briefly overviewed. The applications of immunohistochemistry to genitourinary pathology are principally (1) classification of germinal tumors of ovary and testis, (2) delineation of prostatic origin of metastases, (3) documentation of renal origin of metastatic carcinoma, and (4) recognition of blood group antigen deletion as a marker for biologic potential of bladder tumors.

Germinal and Epithelial Tumors

The role of immunohistochemistry in evaluating germ cell tumors is to confirm the findings of light microscopy (**FIGURES 8–1** and **8–2**) and to recognize cell types that may not be obvious by light microscopy. These tumors often consist of multiple cell types. Thus, a given neoplasm may contain components of embryonal carcinoma, choriocarcinoma, endodermal sinus tumor, and teratoma. Using a combination of antibodies to oncodevelopmental antigens, immunohistochemistry can be used to help recognize different elements in a mixed germ cell tumor, as outlined in Table 8–1. Also, the use of monoclonal antibodies to cytoskeletal keratin can facilitate distinguishing between so-called anaplastic seminoma and embryonal carcinoma. Furthermore, immunohistochemistry with antibody to the β subunit of human chorionic gonadotropin may facilitate the recognition of syncytial trophoblastic giant cells in seminoma. Some investigators have suggested that seminomas with syncytial trophoblastic giant cells may have a more aggressive clinical course than those without such cells.

In addition to a role in the subclassification of germ cell tumors, immunohistochemistry may also predict serum markers useful in monitoring patients for the recurrence of germ cell neoplasia. However, syncytial trophoblastic giant cells may sometimes be found in germ cell tumors without a corresponding elevation of serum human chorionic gonadotropin. Also, very high levels of serum α-fetoprotein may occur in the absence of immunostainable α-fetoprotein in paraffin tissue sections even when the morphology is typical of endodermal sinus tumor. The role of fixation and processing in such situations remains undefined.

Immunohistochemistry may also be used to profile the relative expression of β-HCG and placental lactogen in syncytiotrophoblasts and "intermediate" trophoblasts (**FIGURES 8–3** through **8–5**). This information may be helpful in recognizing placental site trophoblastic tumor and classifying trophoblastic neoplasms.

TABLE 8–1. Differential Immunostaining in Germ Cell Tumors

Tissue Antigen	Type of Section	Seminoma[a]	Responses to Immunostaining for Antigen: Seminoma with STGC	Embryonal Carcinoma	Entodermal Sinus	Chorio-carcinoma	Teratoma
Keratin[b]	F[c]	−	+[d]	+	+	+	+[e]
β-HCG	F, P	−	+[d]	(+)[d]	−	+	−
α-FP	F, P	−	−	(+)	+	−	−

ABBREVIATIONS: α-FP = α-fetoprotein, β-HCG = β subunit of human chorionic gonadotropin, F = frozen, P = paraffin, STGC = syncytial trophoblastic giant cells, + indicates present, − indicates absent, (+) indicates variably present.

[a]Seminomas usually contain immunoreactive ferritin.

[b]Cytokeratins are defined in frozen sections by monoclonal antibody AE1/3.

[c]Best results with frozen tissue sections, tissues well-fixed in absolute ethanol, or pronase-digested sections of formalin-fixed tissue.

[d]In these tumors, syncytial trophoblastic giant cells, which occur rarely, are positive.

[e]In the epithelial components.

Immunohistochemical study of the steroid hormones expressed by Sertoli-Leydig cell tumors and granulosa cell tumors has limited practical usefulness, since in most instances the histopathologic features are typical and predictive of given clinical syndromes. Also, in our experience, available antibodies to steroid hormones require relatively high concentrations of primary antibody, so that nonspecific adherence and background staining is a problem with such preparations. In the rare instances in which such tumors present as poorly differentiated metastases, immunohistochemistry may provide some additional corroboration for the origin of the tumor. However, great care must be exercised to exclude nonspecific binding of the immunoglobulin moieties in this setting. Orchiectomy specimens removed for the purpose of managing prostate carcinoma serve well as positive controls (**FIGURE 8–6**).

The combined use of S-100 protein, keratins, and carcinoembryonic antigen may help in classifying intraepithelial neoplasms of the vulva (**FIGURES 8–7** through **8–11**).

Prostatic Neoplasms

Perhaps the most promising advances in genitourinary pathology have been in the development of tissue-specific antibodies, eg, those reacting only with prostatic epithelium or only with kidney tissue. By the use of polyclonal antibodies to prostatic acid phosphatase and prostate-specific antigen under well-controlled test conditions, the prostatic origin of a metastatic neoplasm can be documented with nearly absolute certainty (**FIGURES 8–12** through **8–18**). Prostatic acid phosphatase is sometimes not expressed by poorly differentiated or metastatic prostate carcinomas; but we have found prostate-specific antigen invariably present, although it may be focally distributed within the tumor. The only tissue cross-reacting with the antibody to prostate-specific antigen is salivary duct epithelium.

Adenocarcinoma of salivary gland origin may, on a rare occasion, present as a metastatic lesion; and a false-positive result would be obtained with a prostate-specific antibody, although we have not encountered this particular situation. For all practical purposes, the prostate immunohistochemical screen system is extremely useful in diagnostic surgical pathology.

Renal Cell Carcinoma

When confronted with a poorly differentiated carcinoma containing a clear cell component, the surgical pathologist has been forced to rely on nonspecific histochemical features such as glycogen and lipid content to document renal cell origin of such a neoplasm. Several monoclonal antibodies (Uro-1 through 10) have been developed that, in conjunction with other monoclonal antibodies, recognize various components of the nephron and urothelium (**FIGURES 8–19** and **8–20**), as summarized in Table 8–2.

Experience with these monoclonal antibodies has been most promising. Nonrenal cell carcinomas, large cell lymphomas, and malignant melanoma have not expressed antigens recognized by Uro-2. These reagents will undoubtedly be very helpful in confirming that metastatic, poorly differentiated carcinoma is of renal cell or urothelial origin.

Other Kidney Diseases

Although applications for detection of the Tamm-Horsfall protein (urinary uromucoid) are limited (**FIGURE 8–21**), it may be useful for detecting some kidney problems. Maldistribution of this substance can provide evidence for rupture of the

TABLE 8–2. Intrarenal Distribution of Antigens Defined by Monoclonal Antibodies, AE1/3, and Uro Series

Antibody	Glomerular Epithelium	Proximal Tubules	Henle's Loop	Distal Tubules	Collecting Duct	Urothelium	Vascular Endothelium	Renal Cell Carcinoma	Bladder Carcinoma
Uro-1	+	−	−	−	−	+	−	+	+
Uro-2	+	+	−	−	−	−	+	+	−
Uro-3	−	+	−	−	−	−	−	+	−
Uro-4	−	+	+	−	−	+	−	+	−
Uro-5	−	−	+	+	+	+	−	−	+
Uro-7[a]	+	−	−	−	−	−	−	+	−
Uro-8	−	−	+	−	−	−	−	?	?
Uro-9	−	−	−	−	−	+	−	−	+
Uro-10	−	+	−	−	−	−	−	(+)	+
AE1/3[b]	−	−	−	+	+	+	−	(+)	+

ABBREVIATIONS: + indicates present, − indicates absent, ? indicates not established, (+) indicates variably present.

[a]Uro-6 was not available at the time of the study.

[b]Monoclonal antibody to cytokeratins.

distal nephron, collecting ducts, and renal pelvis, as is occasionally found with massive hematuria requiring nephrectomy.

Bladder Carcinoma

Bladder epithelial cells express blood group antigens in concert with ABO erythrocyte phenotype. Because of the immunoadherence of red blood cells coated with natural isohemagglutinins, these red cells can be used to determine the phenotypic expression of blood group antigens by noninvasive bladder tumors. An immunoadherence technique using these red blood cells has been advocated for predicting the biologic potential of these tumors. Thus, in several large series in which this technique was used, stage 0 papillary bladder tumors that expressed the blood group antigenic phenotype tended to have a more benign course without invasive recurrences. Conversely, stage 0 papillary tumors that did not express the blood group antigenic phenotype had a more aggressive biologic course with more frequent recurrences of invasive tumor.

Phenotypic blood group antigen expression can be profiled using immunohistochemical techniques as well as passive erythrocyte immunoadherence procedures (**FIGURES 8–22** through **8–24**). However, the large body of literature on red cell immunoadherence may not necessarily be applicable to results derived immunohistochemically. Available procedures include indirect, PAP, and ABC immunoperoxidase techniques using human isoagglutinins; indirect and ABC methods using lectins as primary reagents; and indirect, PAP, and ABC methods using monoclonal primary antibodies. Results vary with the procedure used and the type of tissue fixation. Furthermore, immunostaining patterns are not uniform. Diffuse staining of epithelial cells, staining of basal cells only, and focal 4+ staining in predominantly negative tumor have been observed; and the clinical relevance of each pattern remains undefined. In our experience, the optimal system uses paraffin sections fixed in absolute ethanol and immunostained with the ABC-PO technique and monoclonal antibodies to blood groups A, B, and O.

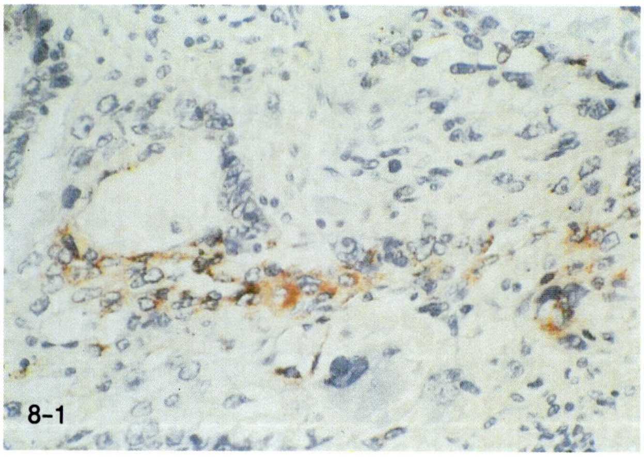

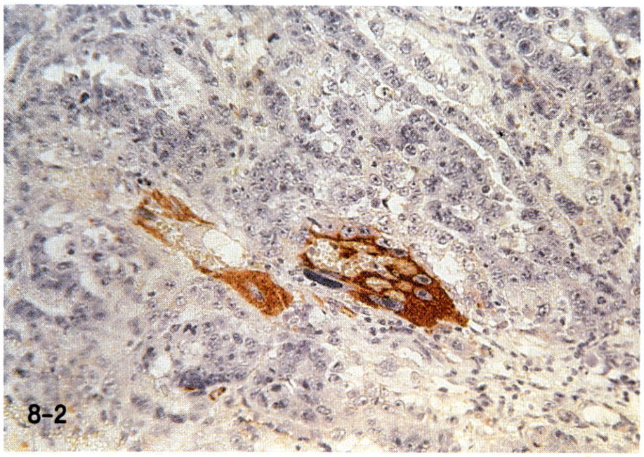

FIGURE 8–1. Endodermal sinus tumor of the testis immunostained for α-fetoprotein (ABC-PO with AEC, hematoxylin counterstain). *Slide 82.*

FIGURE 8–2. Mixed germ cell tumor of the testis immunostained for β subunit of human chorionic gonadotropin (β-HCG; ABC-PO with AEC, hematoxylin counterstain). *Slide 83.*

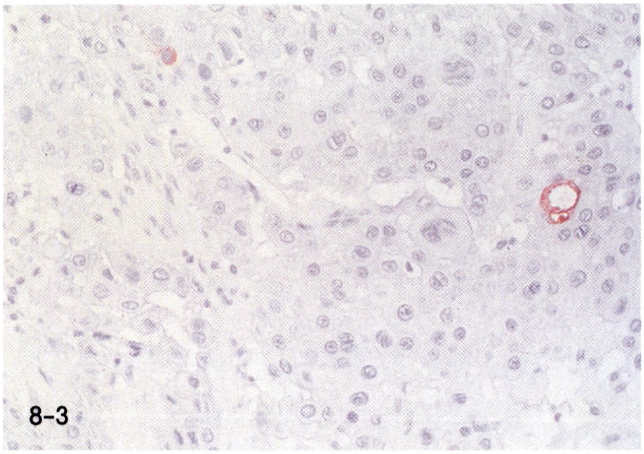

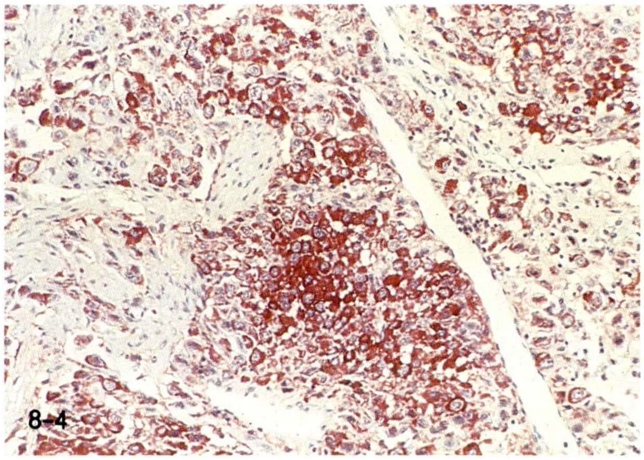

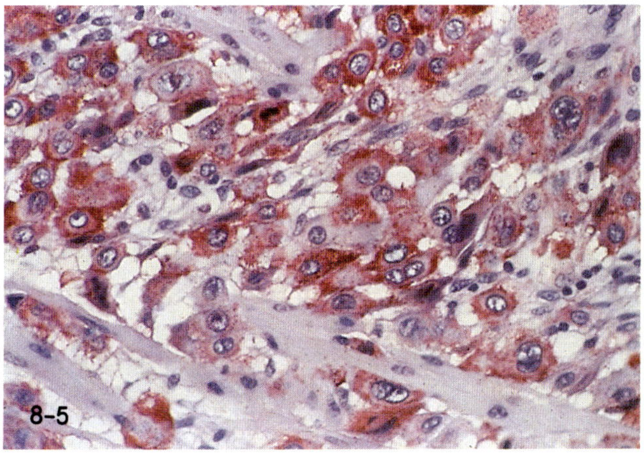

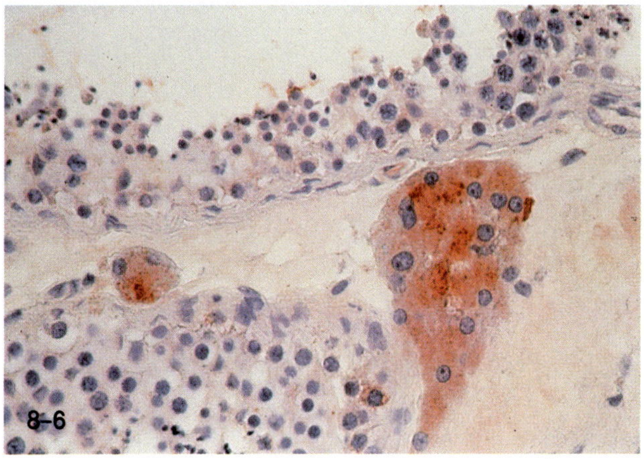

FIGURE 8–3. Placental site trophoblastic tumor. Figures 8–3 through 8–5 are from the same case. Only occasional cells contain immunoreactive β-HCG (ABC-PO with AEC, hematoxylin counterstain).

FIGURE 8–4. Same case as 8–3. Numerous "intermediate trophoblastic" cells contain placental lactogen (ABC-PO with AEC, hematoxylin counterstain).

FIGURE 8–5. Same case as 8–3, higher magnification of Figure 8–4. Numerous "intermediate trophoblastic" cells contain abundant placental lactogen (ABC-PO with AEC, hematoxylin counterstain).

FIGURE 8–6. Normal testis immunostained for testosterone (red; ABC-PO with AEC, hematoxylin counterstain).

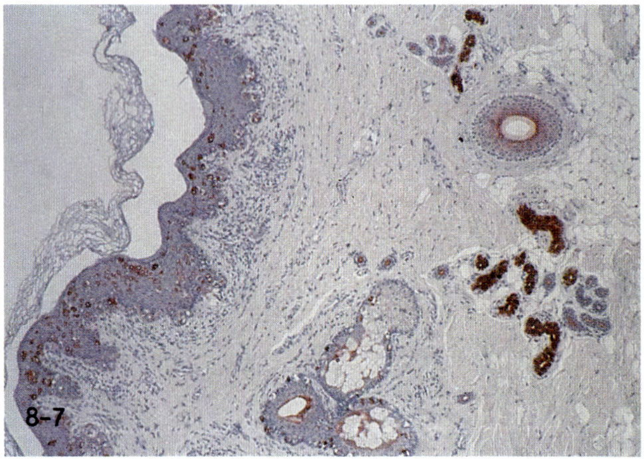

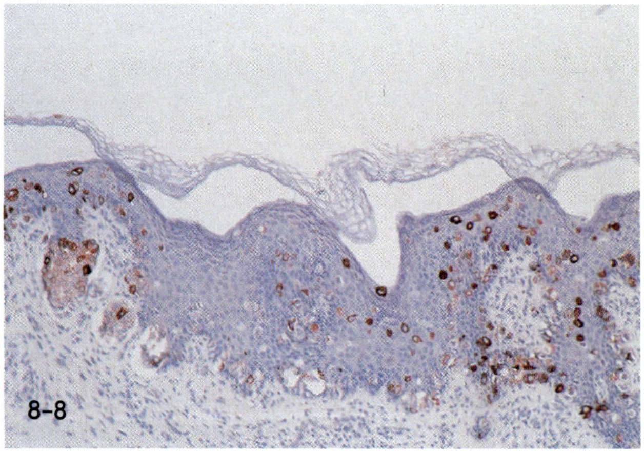

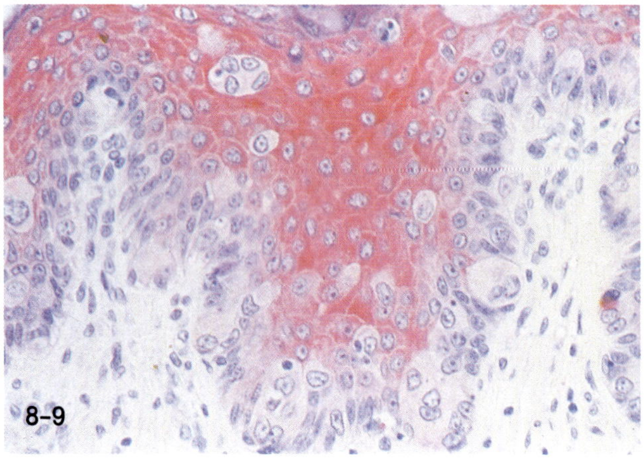

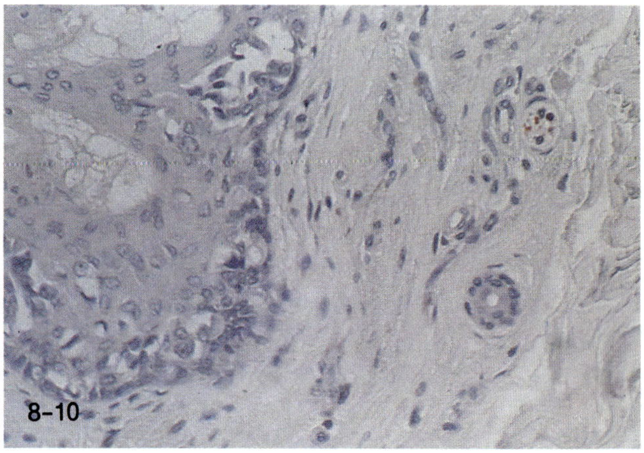

FIGURE 8–7. Paget's disease of the vulva. Figures 8–7 through 8–11 are from the same case. The neoplastic cells invading the epidermis contain cytokeratins defined by AE1/3 (ABC-PO with AEC, hematoxylin counterstain).

FIGURE 8–8. Same case as 8–7. Higher magnification showing neoplastic cells containing cytokeratins defined by AE1/3 (ABC-PO with AEC, hematoxylin counterstain). *Slide 84.*

FIGURE 8–9. Same case as 8–7. The neoplastic cells do not contain keratins of relatively high molecular weight defined by a polyclonal rabbit antibody (Dako). The normal epidermal cells are positive (ABC-PO with AEC, hematoxylin counterstain).

FIGURE 8–10. Same case as 8–7. The neoplastic cells lack S-100 protein; Schwann cells of a small nerve are positive (upper right; ABC-PO with AEC, hematoxylin counterstain).

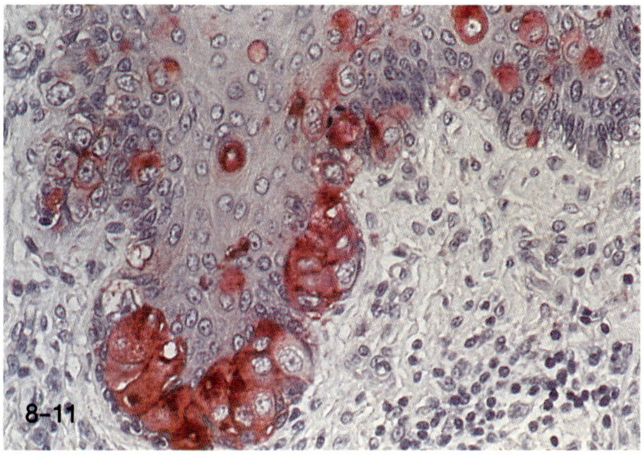

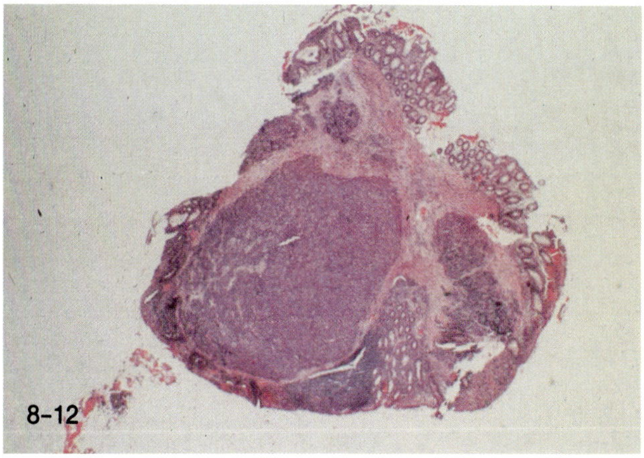

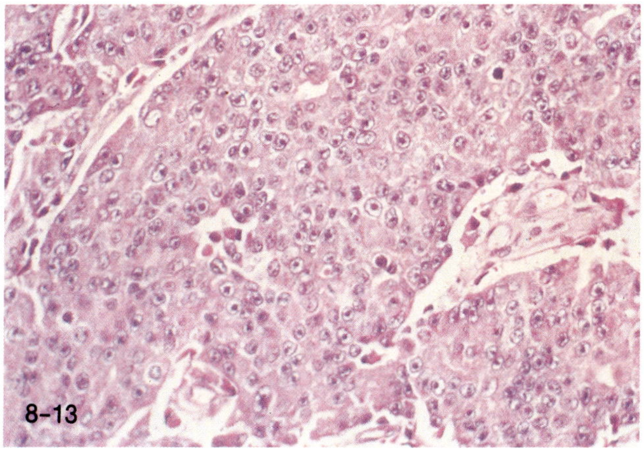

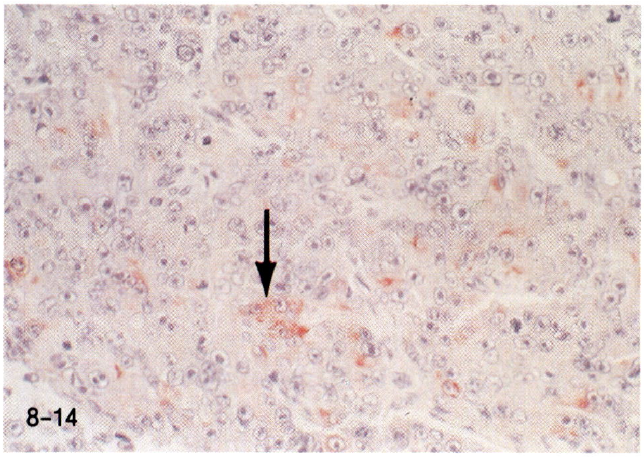

FIGURE 8–11. Same case as 8–7. The neoplastic cells also contain carcinoembryonic antigen (red; ABC-PO with AEC, hematoxylin counterstain).

FIGURE 8–12. Metastatic adenocarcinoma involving the rectal wall. Figures 8–12 through 8–14 are from the same case. There was no history of neoplasm, and tests for serum prostatic acid phosphatase were negative. This tissue section is stained with H & E.

FIGURE 8–13. Same case as 8–12. Higher magnification of the tissue section shows cells with prominent nucleoli suggestive of prostatic carcinoma (H & E).

FIGURE 8–14. Same case as 8–12. The neoplasm demonstrates cytoplasmic prostate-specific antigen in a few cells (arrow). Prostatic acid phosphatase was not demonstrable (ABC-PO with AEC, hematoxylin counterstain).

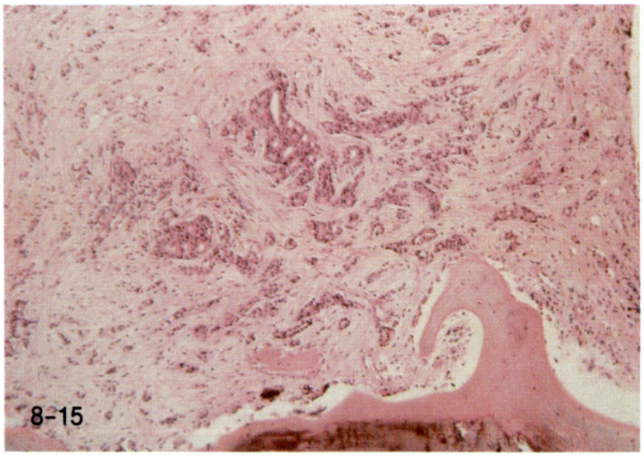

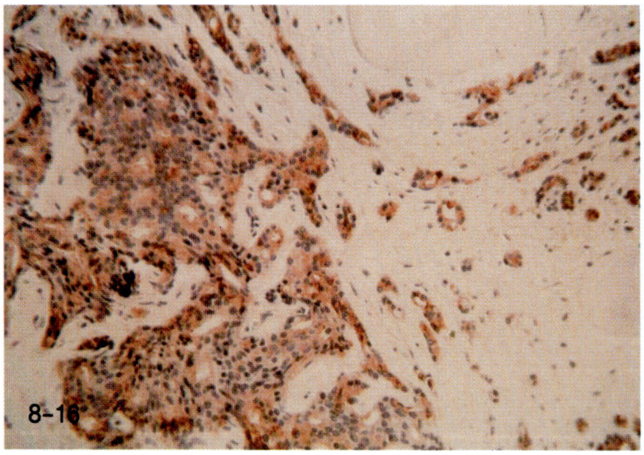

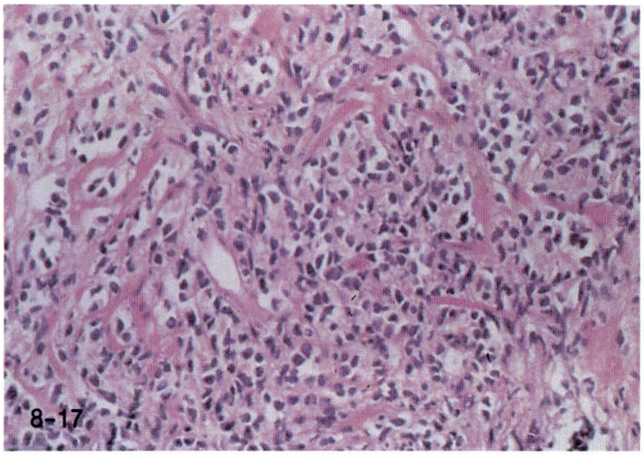

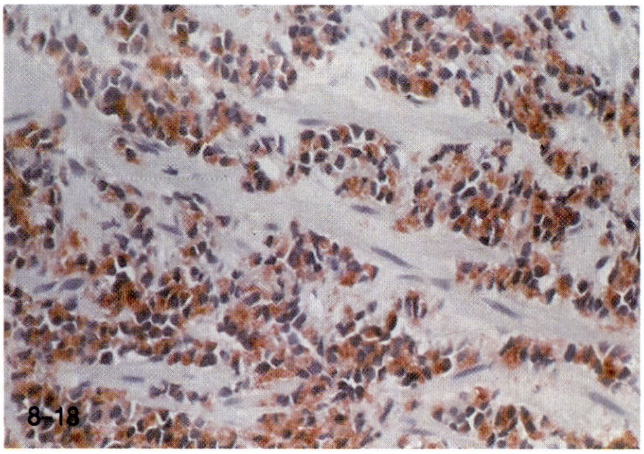

FIGURE 8–15. Metastatic carcinoma in bone marrow from a patient without elevation of serum prostatic acid phosphatase. Figures 8–15 and 8–16 are from the same case. Subsequent study of a needle biopsy specimen of the prostate showed adenocarcinoma. This tissue section is stained with H & E.

FIGURE 8–16. Same case as 8–15. Prostate-specific antigen is expressed by metastatic carcinoma in bone marrow (ABC-PO with AEC, hematoxylin counterstain). *Slide 85.*

FIGURE 8–17. Poorly differentiated invasive malignant neoplasm in the prostate gland. Figures 8–17 and 8–18 are from the same case. The tissue was unclassifiable by light microscopy; and serum and tissue were negative for prostatic acid phosphatase. This tissue section is stained with H & E.

FIGURE 8–18. Same case as 8–17. Despite the absence of architectural differentiation, phenotypic expression of prostate-specific antigen is documented (ABC-PO with AEC, hematoxylin counterstain). *Slide 86.*

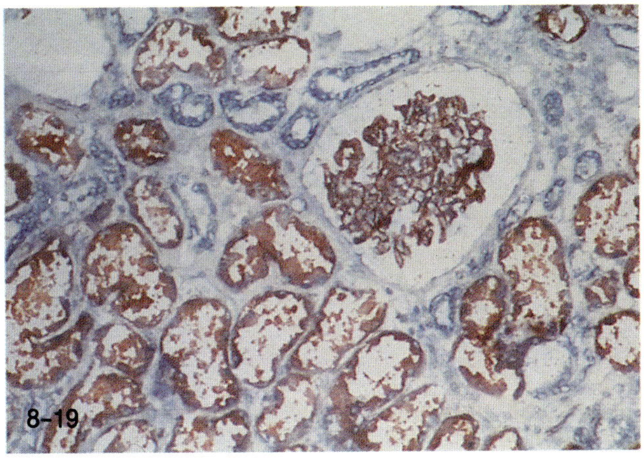

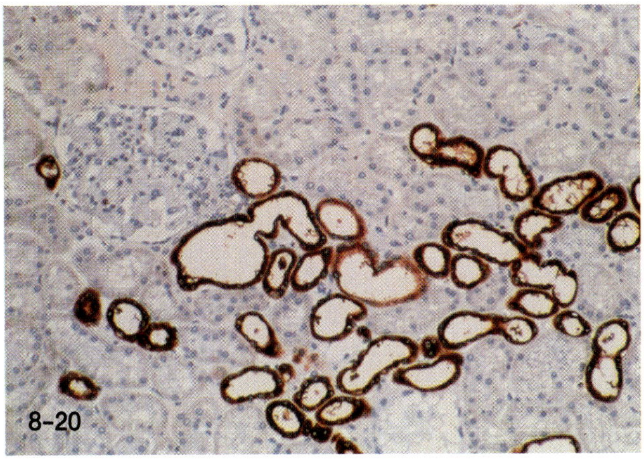

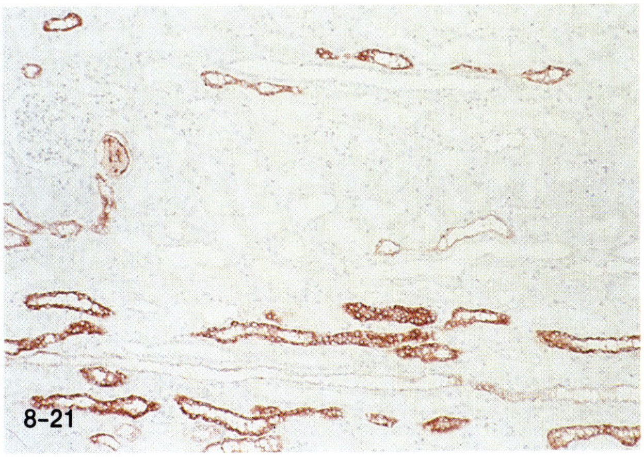

FIGURE 8–19. Normal kidney, distribution of Uro-2, an antigen defined by monoclonal antibody. The antibody delineates the glomerulus and proximal tubules (ABC-PO with AEC, hematoxylin counterstain).

FIGURE 8–20. Normal kidney, distribution of epithelial membrane antigen, an antigen defined by monoclonal antibody. The distal nephron is immunostained (ABC-PO with AEC, hematoxylin counterstain).

FIGURE 8–21. Normal kidney immunostained for urinary uromucoid (Tamm-Horsfall protein). The antigen is present primarily in tubular epithelium and casts (ABC-PO with AEC, hematoxylin counterstain).

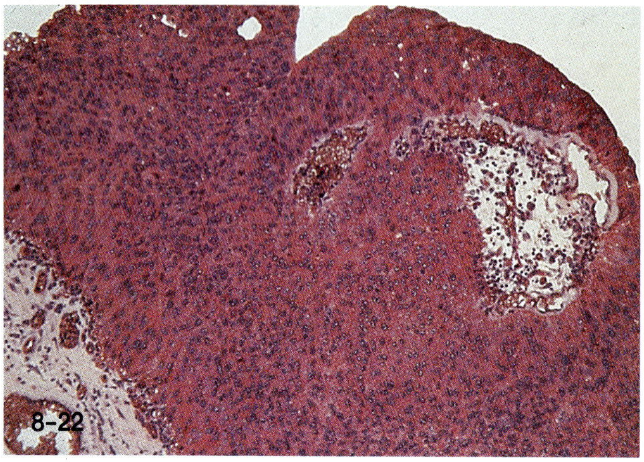

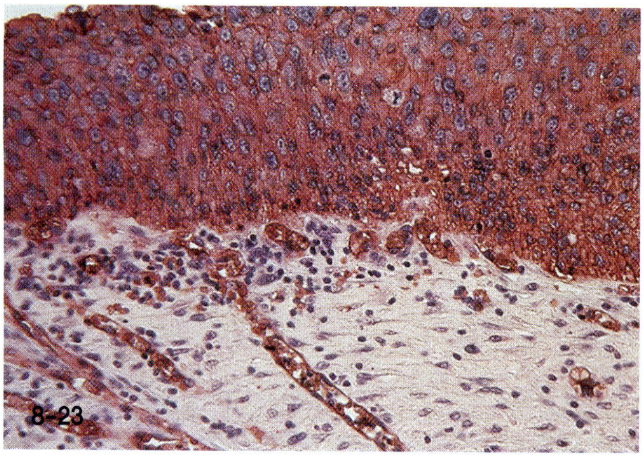

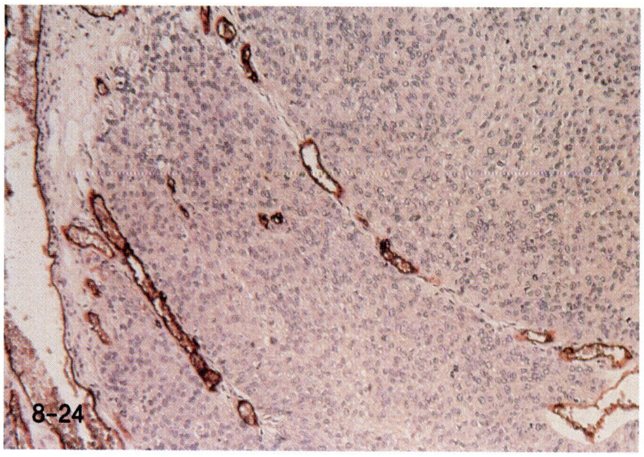

FIGURE 8–22. Stage 0 transitional cell carcinoma of the urinary bladder. Figures 8–22 and 8–23 are from the same case. This section was immunostained for monoclonal antibody to blood group O (H substance; ABC-PO with AEC, biotinylated antibody modification [biotinylated anti-*Ulex*], hematoxylin counterstain).

FIGURE 8–23. Same case as 8–22. The neoplastic urothelium expresses H substance in concert with the patient's blood type. Note the positive red blood cells and endothelium (ABC-PO with AEC, biotinylated antibody modification [biotinylated anti-*Ulex*], hematoxylin counterstain). *Slide 87.*

FIGURE 8–24. Another stage 0 transitional cell carcinoma of the urinary bladder immunostained for monoclonal antibody to blood group O (H substance). This case shows deletion of H substance. The endothelium and red blood cells remain positive (red), an internal positive control (ABC-PO with AEC, biotinylated antibody modification [biotinylated anti-*Ulex*], hematoxylin counterstain). *Slide 88.*

9 Soft Tissue Tumors

Immunohistochemical detection of antigens expressed by mesenchymal neoplasms is in an embryonic phase. Currently, except for detection of factor VIII–related antigen in angiosarcomas, myoglobin in some rhabdomyosarcomas, and S-100 protein in granular cell tumors and Schwannomas, immunohistochemistry has little to offer the surgical pathologist that is of any more value than conventional histopathology and electron microscopy. For the most part, available systems depend on the detection of secreted cell products or functional molecules such as contractile protein. Consequently, they are sometimes undetectable in poorly differentiated tumors, for which additional information is needed. Furthermore, the inadequate specificity of many commercial reagents, the tendency for intermediate filament antibodies to bind nonspecifically to fixed embedded tissue, and antigen absorption from contiguous normal tissues to tumor cells and phagocytosis of normal antigen by tumor cells (eg, myoglobin in normal muscle by malignant histiocytes) greatly limit the utility of diagnostic immunohistochemistry for soft tissue tumors.

FIGURES 9–1 through **9–9** illustrate immunostained spindle cell tumors. Antigens described in normal mesenchymal tissue and their respective differentiated tumors may not be expressed in less differentiated neoplasms. For example, in our experience myoglobin is sometimes not present in spindle cell tumors that have been classified as rhabdomyosarcoma by histopathology and are devoid of cross-striations. Also, some angiosarcomas do not contain immunoreactive factor VIII in the tumor cells. However, some additional information can be obtained with immunohistochemistry, using a battery of antibodies to intermediate filaments, combinations of which may be characteristic of a particular sarcoma (see Chapter 12, Table 12–1). In particular, desmin may be detectable in the small, primitive cells of embryonal rhabdomyosarcoma (**FIGURES 9–8** and **9–9**). These latter immunotypes are only tentative, and much immunohistochemical screening still needs to be done in this area.

On rare occasions, epithelial tumors and malignant melanoma may resemble sarcomas, consisting principally of neoplastic spindle cells. Immunohistochemistry may be helpful to document the expression of cytoplasmic keratin in epithelial tumors and antigens detected by melanoma-specific monoclonal antibodies in malignant melanoma.

In addition to an array of antigenic markers, the most significant advances in the classification of sarcomas may come with the development of tumor-specific antigens detected by monoclonal antibodies. Panels of monoclonal antibodies have been developed with selective reactivity for different small, round cell tumors. Such antibodies can potentially be helpful in differentiating between rhabdomyosarcoma, neuroblastoma, and Ewing's sarcoma.

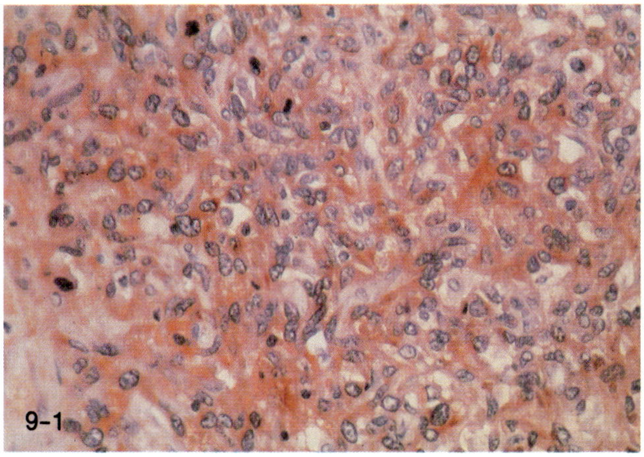

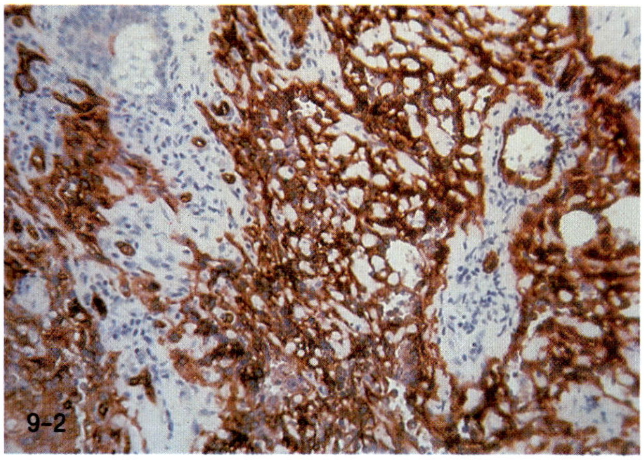

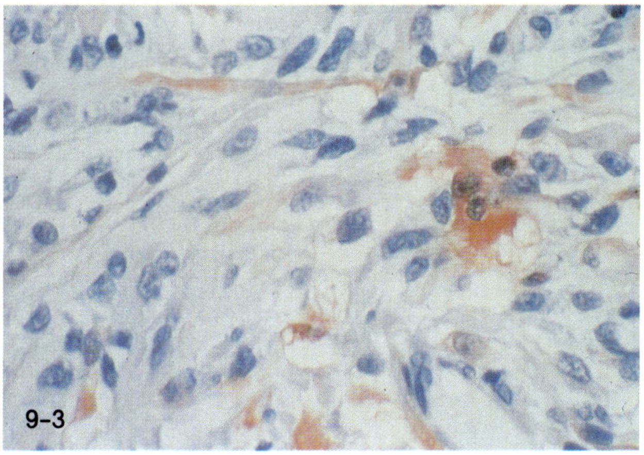

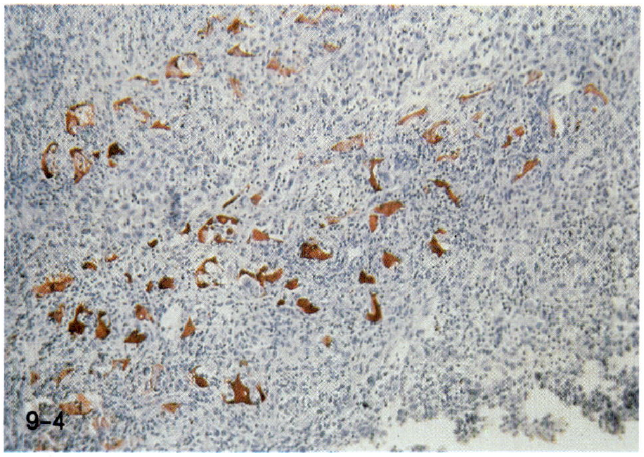

FIGURE 9–1. Angiosarcoma. Figures 9–1 and 9–2 are from the same case. This photomicrograph shows factor VIII–related antigen in the tumor cells (ABC-PO with AEC, hematoxylin counterstain).

FIGURE 9–2. Same case as 9–1. When *Ulex europaeus* lectin is used as the primary reagent, the *Ulex* reagent binds to blood group O cells expressing blood group H substance and endothelium (ABC-PO with AEC, hematoxylin counterstain).

FIGURE 9–3. Rhabdomyosarcoma immunostained for myoglobin. Occasional tumor cells are positive (ABC-PO with AEC, hematoxylin counterstain). *Slide 89.*

FIGURE 9–4. Leiomyosarcoma infiltrating skeletal muscle. Residual skeletal muscle cells are myoglobin-positive (red), but tumor cells are negative (ABC-PO with AEC, hematoxylin counterstain).

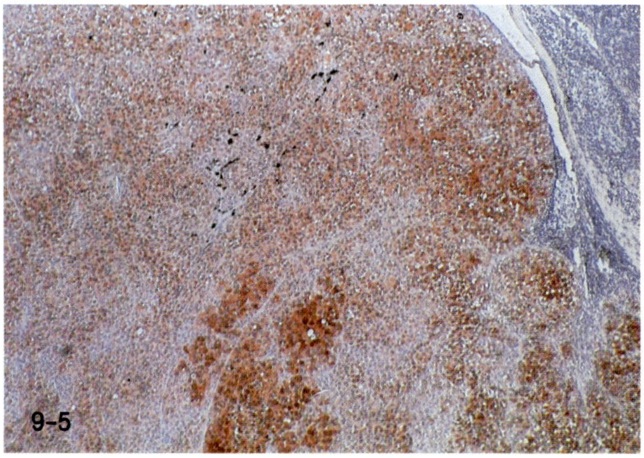

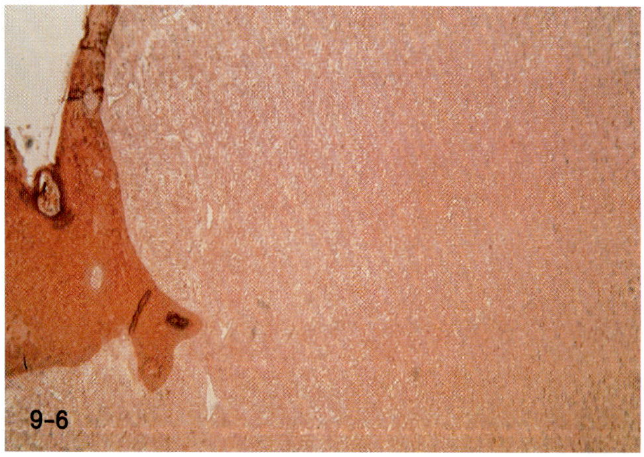

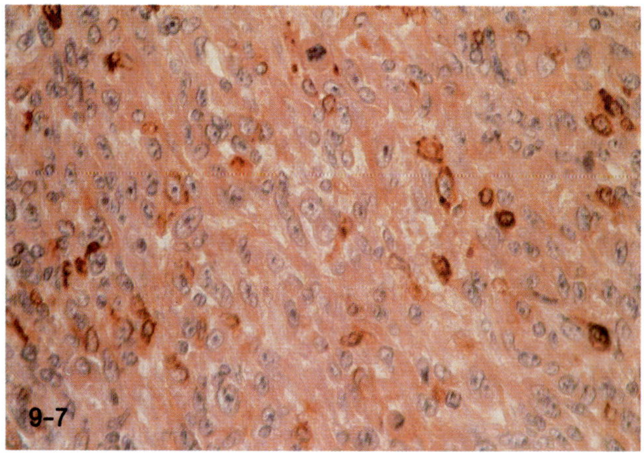

FIGURE 9–5. Metastatic spindle cell and epithelioid amelanotic melanoma presenting as idiopathic lymphadenopathy immunostained for S-100 protein. A small portion of noneffaced lymph node is present in the upper right (ABC-PO with AEC, hematoxylin counterstain). *Slide 90.*

FIGURE 9–6. Spindle cell dermal and subcutaneous neoplasm suggestive of spindle cell squamous carcinoma. Figures 9–6 and 9–7 are from the same case. This section is immunostained for cytokeratins (Dako rabbit antibody and ABC-PO with AEC, hematoxylin counterstain).

FIGURE 9–7. Same case as 9–6. Higher magnification shows positive staining of tumor cells for cytokeratins (ABC-PO with AEC, hematoxylin counterstain). *Slide 91.*

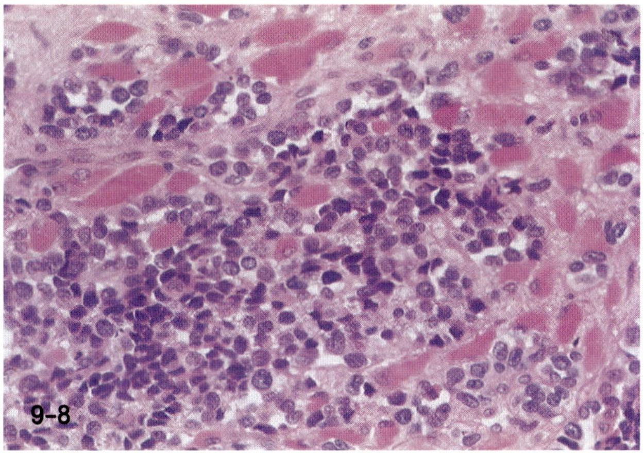

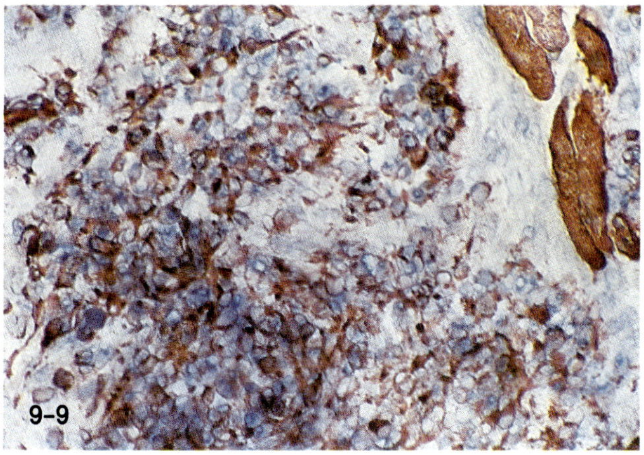

FIGURE 9–8. Embryonal rhabdomyosarcoma invading skeletal muscle. Figures 9–8 and 9–9 are from the same case. This tissue section is stained with H & E.

FIGURE 9–9. Same case as 9–8. Immunostained with monoclonal antibody to desmin. Despite the primitive appearance of this small cell tumor, desmin is readily detected in the small rim of cytoplasm in malignant cells. Note the staining of skeletal muscle contiguous to the tumor at upper right (ABC-PO with AEC, in a frozen tissue section, hematoxylin counterstain).

10 Gastrointestinal and Hepatic Pathology

Gastrointestinal Tract

There appear to be several areas of current practical application for immunohistochemical techniques in the gastrointestinal (GI) tract: (1) study of the distribution and immunomorphology of neuroendocrine cells in the normal and diseased GI tract, (2) classification of gut lymphomas and their distinction from reactive lymphoid hyperplasias (pseudolymphomas), and (3) use of tumor markers in the differential diagnosis of unusual or metastic neoplasia involving the GI tract.

Neuroendocrine Cells and Corresponding Neoplasms

Immunohistochemistry has played a significant role in the study of the gastrointestinal tract neuroendocrine system and associated pathology. Techniques are now available to identify a large number of common and uncommon gut-associated hormones found in these neuroendocrine cells, although some of these antigenic determinants are destroyed by routine fixation and embedding and thus require frozen section material.

The identification of many of these antigens is now considered experimental, but there are several practical applications. In general, neoplasms of neuroendocrine cells, despite their variable morphologic appearance, distribution, and biologic potential, express common antigens. Thus, although a particular tumor may not contain an individual polypeptide such as serotonin, in many (but not all) cases the neoplasm can be confirmed as neuroendocrine with a panreactive antibody such as "neuron-specific" enolase. Such a stain can be used in conjunction with conventional hemotoxylin and eosin preparations and the Grimelius or some other histochemical stain.

Immunohistochemistry can be used to classify neuroendocrine tumors throughout the GI tract and thereby aid in making clinicopathologic correlations. The technique can also be used to document primary G-cell hyperplasia in the stomach. **FIGURE 10–1** illustrates immunoreactive gastrin in a duodenal gastrinoma from a patient with the Zollinger-Ellison syndrome. As in the pancreas, neuroendocrine tumors in the gut have been shown to be multihormonal and may contain ectopic hormones such as adrenocorticotropic hormone. It remains to be seen whether immunohistochemical classification of neuroendocrine tumors of the GI tract will help in predicting clinical behavior.

Lymphoid Lesions

The immunohistochemical techniques, interpretation, and theory used in the study of lymphoid proliferations in the GI tract are virtually identical to those used for the node-based lesions outlined in Chapter 5. Although many studies of gut lymphomas based on paraffin-embedded material appear in the literature, our experience has shown that frozen-section immunohistochemistry, ideally coupled with parallel cell suspension correlates, is the only reliable method for demonstrating lymphocyte differentiation antigens. A major pitfall involves obtaining frozen-section material in the first place. We advocate working closely with clinical colleagues, paying close attention to previous biopsy diagnoses in handling resection specimens, and frequent use of frozen-section histology in directing the subsequent immunologic workup of unusual-appearing lesions in GI resections.

As in the lymph node and other extranodal sites, the majority of GI lymphomas are of B-cell origin and manifest monoclonal light chain surface immunoglobulins, whereas pseudolymphoma and reactive lymphoid proliferations are polyclonal for light chains (**FIGURES 10–2** through **10–5**). We have now seen several cases of monoclonal lymphoma arising focally in polyclonal pseudolymphoma or associated with polyclonal reactive lymphoid proliferations. To minimize the chance of sampling error, we recommend the routine immunologic study of several frozen-section blocks in this situation.

True histiocytic lymphomas (THL) of the bowel are probably more rare than originally thought (see Grody et al). Cell markers in THL show either negative or polyclonal light chain staining (presumably from internalized light chains), negative results of B- and T-cell marker studies (B1, B2, T11, and T3), and positive immunohistologic demonstration of muramidase, α-1-antitrypsin, and α-1-antichymotrypsin (**FIGURES 5–49** through **5–52** in Chapter 5).

Some non-Hodgkin's lymphomas of the GI tract are of cytotoxic-suppressor T-cell origin and have been referred to as "epitheliotropic lymphoma of small bowel." Frozen material is required for accurate immunotyping of such tumors. It is sometimes difficult to distinguish between reactive and neoplastic T-cell proliferations immunologically because true "clonal" markers are not available. However, anomalous deletions of individual T-cell antigens are common in T-cell lymphomas.

Other Primary and Metastatic Tumors

Classification of unusual or metastatic tumors involving the GI tract is a difficult area of differential diagnosis. In such cases, immunohistochemistry can be invaluable. Chapter 8 illustrated the usefulness of prostatic acid phosphatase and prostate-specific antigen to distinguish prostatic adenocarcinoma that secondarily involves the colon from primary colonic adenocarcinoma. Similarly, S-100 protein can be used to help confirm the diagnosis of malignant melanoma (**FIGURES 10–6** and **10–7**). Use of epithelial antigens (keratin, epithelial membrane antigen) and common leukocyte antigens can aid in distinguishing lymphoma from undifferentiated carcinoma. With advances in monoclonal technology and the identification of tumor-specific antigens, one can expect many more aids to be developed in differential diagnostic staining.

In summary, immunohistochemistry can be extremely useful in the classification and differential diagnosis of gut lymphoid proliferations and unusual or metastatic epithelial malignancies involving the gut. In addition, it can be used as documentation or diagnosis of primary G-cell hyperplasia and for classification and clinicopathologic correlation of gut neuroendocrine tumors.

Hepatic Pathology

In hepatic pathology, immunohistochemistry can be used in the investigation of hepatitis and cirrhosis and as a differential diagnostic aid in distinguishing primary from metastatic neoplasm involving the liver.

It has been stated that the most specific indicator of the carrier state for the P_1Z gene in α-1-antitrypsin deficiency is the demonstration of immunoreactive α-1-antitrypsin within diastase-resistant PAS-positive globules **(FIGURES 10–8** and **10–9)**.

Immunohistochemical localization of hepatitis-B surface and core antigens in acute and chronic hepatitis has been well documented in the literature. Hepatitis-B surface antigen (HBsAg) can easily be demonstrated by immunohistochemical techniques and usually appears as diffuse staining within the cytoplasm **(FIGURE 10–10)**. On certain occasions, it can appear as staining associated with the liver cell membrane. Positive staining correlates well with both orcein-positivity and serum assays positive for HBsAg. Hepatitis-B core antigen (HBcAg) can also easily be demonstrated in nuclei and occasionally in the cytoplasm of infected hepatocytes **(FIGURE 10–11)**. Clinicopathologic correlates of the patterns of core and surface antigen immunostaining are well described in the literature and are beyond the scope of this manual.

Although most liver biopsy specimens containing carcinoma are from patients with a well-established history of a primary tumor, some specimens present a diagnostic challenge. Thus, in the absence of a history of a primary neoplasm, a needle biopsy specimen may be useful for diagnosing cases of poorly differentiated epithelioid neoplasm. Differential diagnosis may include tumors such as melanoma or tumors of neuroendocrine origin in which specific immunohistochemical markers may be obtained to corroborate light microscopic findings (see Chapter 4).

More common is the diagnostic dilemma of differentiating primary hepatocellular carcinoma from metastatic poorly differentiated carcinoma. In this setting, immunostaining for carcinoembryonic antigen (CEA) may be helpful in making the distinction. Hepatocellular carcinoma usually demonstrates striking canalicular immunostaining with the CEA antibody **(FIGURE 10–12)**. Conversely, metastatic carcinoma usually demonstrates cytoplasmic staining of individual tumor cells in variable numbers **(FIGURES 10–13** and **10–14)**.

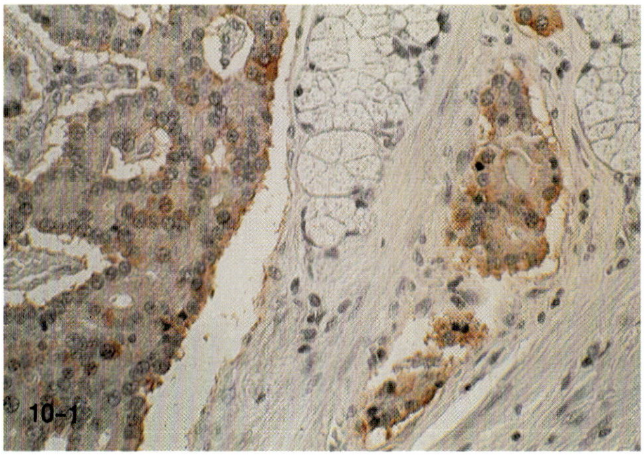

FIGURE 10–1. Gastrinoma of the duodenal wall immunostained for gastrin (red) from patient with Zollinger-Ellison syndrome (ABC-PO with AEC, hematoxylin counterstain). *Slide 92.*

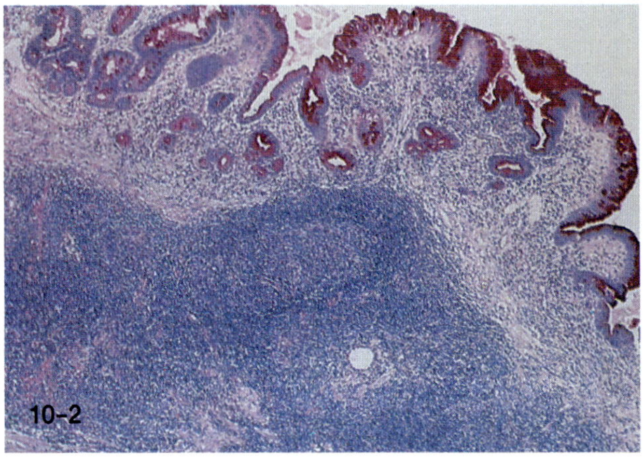

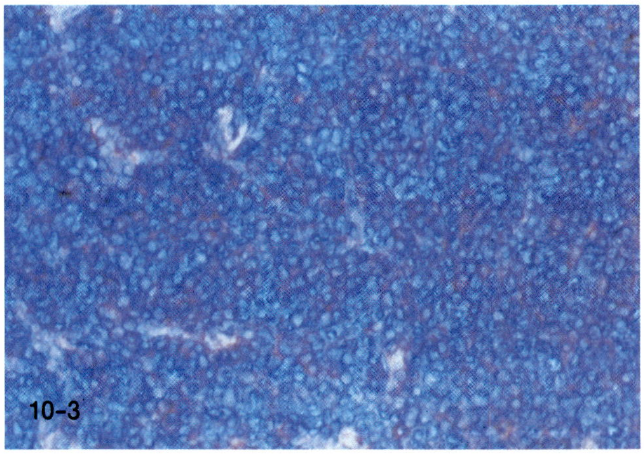

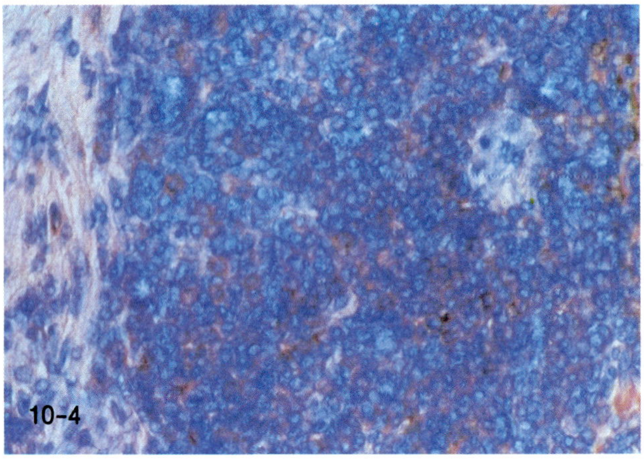

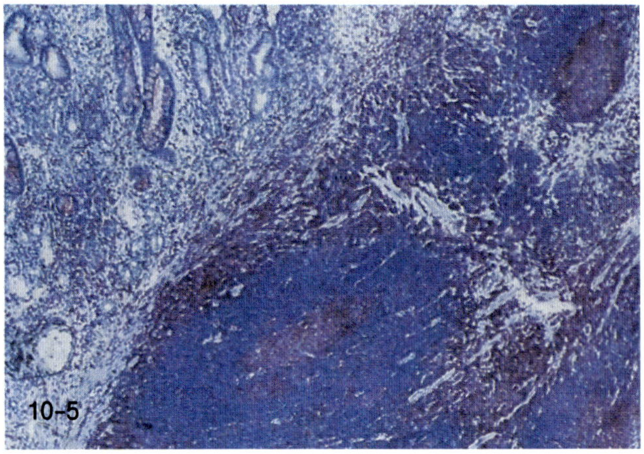

FIGURE 10–2. Gastric pseudolymphoma. Figures 10–2 through 10–5 are from the same case. Germinal center formation is present (PAS with hematoxylin counterstain).

FIGURE 10–3. Same case as 10–2. κ light chains are present (direct IMP with AEC, hematoxylin counterstain).

FIGURE 10–4. Same case as 10–2. λ light chains are also present (direct IMP with AEC, hematoxylin counterstain).

FIGURE 10–5. Same case as 10–2. T-cells as identified by antibody directed against T11 antigen are also part of the lymphoid proliferation (ABC-PO with AEC, hematoxylin counterstain).

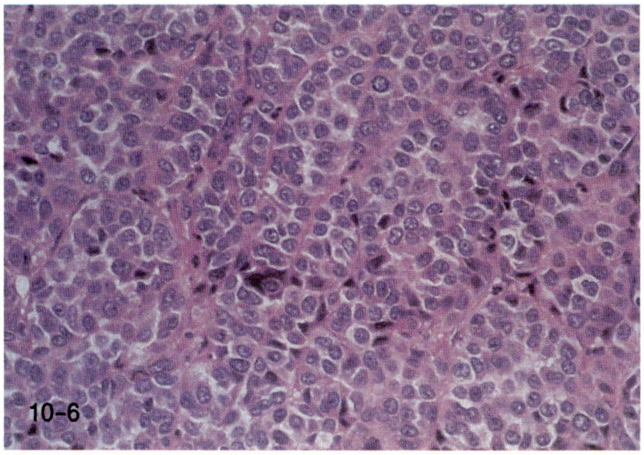

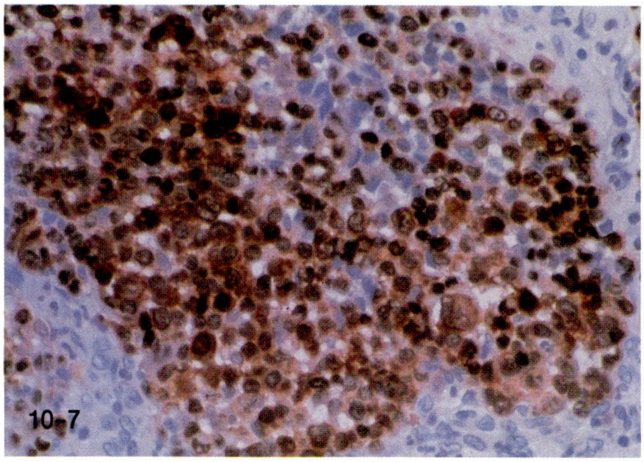

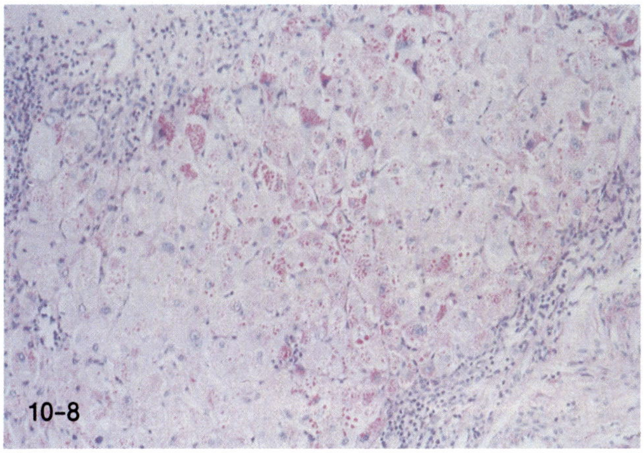

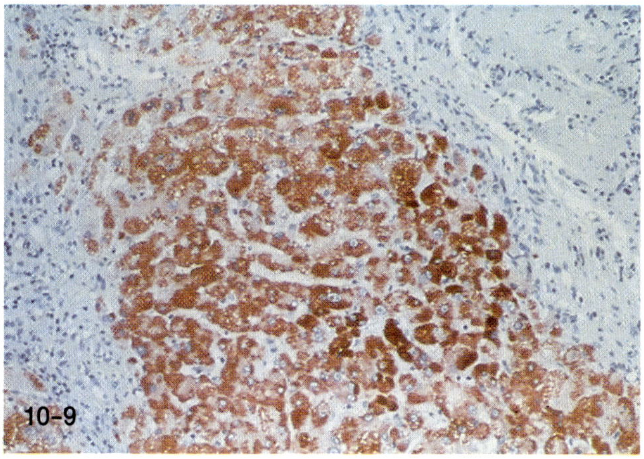

FIGURE 10–6. Rectal melanoma. Figures 10–6 and 10–7 are from the same case. This tissue section is stained with H & E.

FIGURE 10–7. Same case as 10–6. Intense S-100 protein immunoreactivity is present (ABC-PO with AEC, hematoxylin counterstain).

FIGURE 10–8. Liver from a patient with α-1-antitrypsin deficiency. Figures 10–8 and 10–9 are from the same case. This photomicrograph shows cytoplasmic PAS-positive globules (PAS with hematoxylin counterstain).

FIGURE 10–9. Same case as 10–8. Immunoreactive α-1-antitrypsin is present in many hepatocytes (ABC-PO with AEC, hematoxylin counterstain).

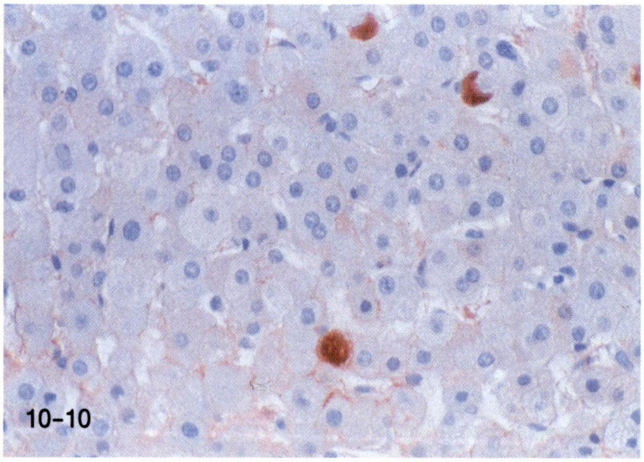

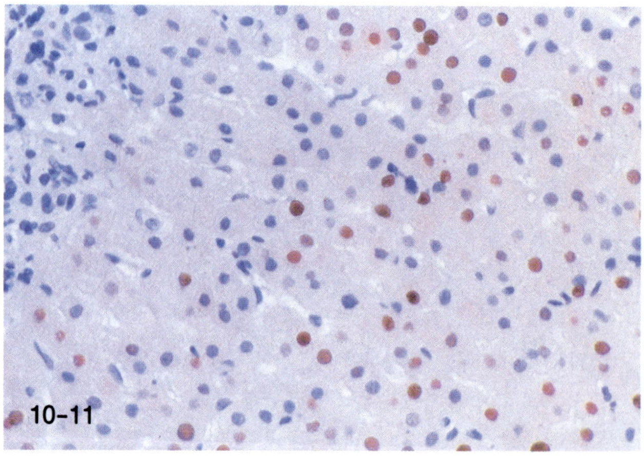

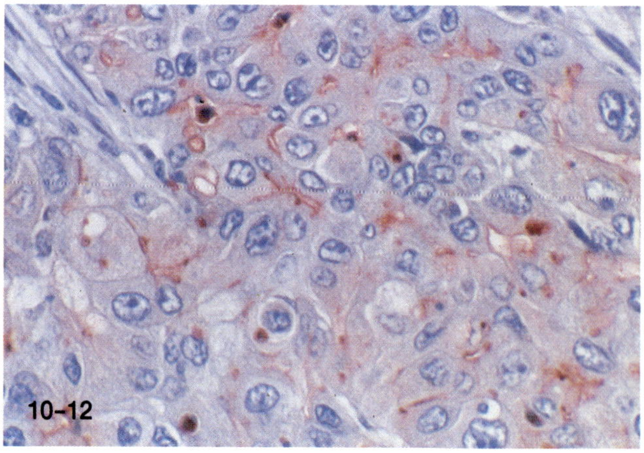

FIGURE 10–10. Chronic hepatitis. Figures 10–10 and 10–11 are from the same case. Diffuse cytoplasmic immunostaining in hepatocytes for HBsAg is present in this figure. Focal membrane-associated immunostaining is also demonstrated (ABC-PO with AEC, hematoxylin counterstain). *Slide 93.*

FIGURE 10–11. Same case as 10–10. Many nuclei illustrated are positive for immunoreactive HBcAg. Note the color distinction between true-red positive nuclei and negative blue nuclei (ABC-PO with AEC, hematoxylin counterstain). *Slide 94.*

FIGURE 10–12. Hepatocellular carcinoma immunostained for carcinoembryonic antigen (CEA). Note the striking canalicular positivity (ABC-PO with AEC, hematoxylin counterstain). Figure courtesy of Thomas Bauer, MD, PhD. *Slide 95.*

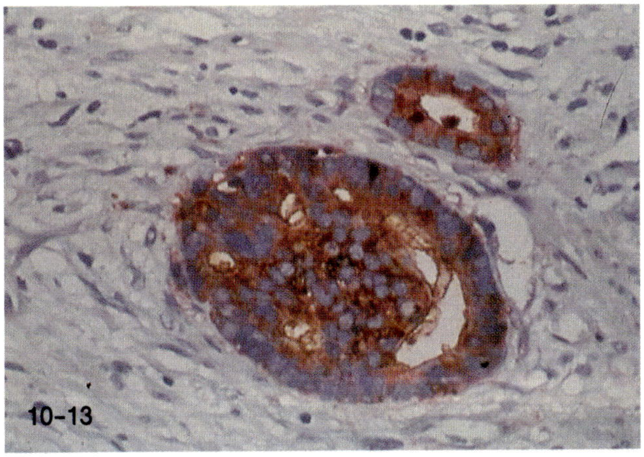

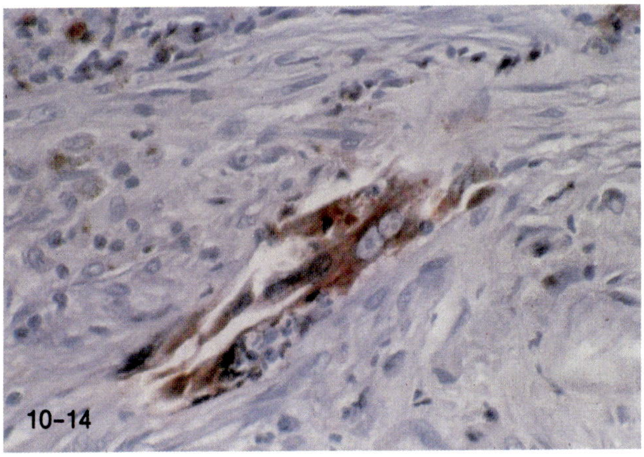

FIGURE 10–13. Adenocarcinoma metastatic to liver. In contrast to Figure 10–12, this tumor shows cytoplasmic rather than canalicular CEA within the tumor cells (ABC-PO with AEC, hematoxylin counterstain). *Slide 96.*

FIGURE 10–14. Another focus from another case of metastatic carcinoma in liver shows cytoplasmic CEA (ABC-PO with AEC, hematoxylin counterstain).

11 Other Applications

Immunohistochemistry is an evolving technology, and eventually its application will pervade all disciplines of pathology. For some disease processes, immunohistochemistry is only beginning to be used; for others, immunohistochemistry has limited diagnostic applications.

Although immunohistochemical procedures have been used to study autoimmune renal disease, only a few investigators have used these techniques in evaluating cutaneous autoimmune illness. Current immunofluorescence procedures are very reliable. Immunohistochemistry presents the potential for technically superior evaluation of bullous diseases and deserves further study. Techniques for profiling immunoglobulin and differentiation antigen markers in lymphoid tissue are equally applicable to cutaneous and other extranodal mononuclear cell infiltrates. These procedures can be helpful in confirming the benign reactive nature of mononuclear cell infiltrates and for immunotyping malignant cutaneous lymphoid infiltration.

Antigens expressed by viruses may also be detected with immunohistochemistry. Antibodies to hepatitis-B surface antigen (HBsAg) have been used to study cirrhosis and hepatocellular carcinoma occurring in the posthepatitic setting. The ability to correlate the expression of hepatitis-B surface and core antigens in liver biopsy specimens with histopathologic features may be of value in understanding the evolution of hepatitis-B infections and may yield prognostic information (Chapter 10). Other antibodies available include those directed against herpes simplex virus, papillomavirus, cytomegalovirus, and Epstein-Barr virus (capsid, nuclear, and other antigens). Biotinylated probes of complementary DNA may be a superior approach to identifying specific viruses in tissue (see Chapter 12).

A few immunohistochemical applications for diagnostic neuropathology have been developed. Glial fibrillary acidic protein (GFAP) is expressed in central nervous system tumors of glial origin (**FIGURE 11–1**). However, there is an inverse relationship between degree of differentiation (and consequently diagnostic challenge) and expression of GFAP. Other applications include the documentation of metastatic carcinoma by the use of oncodevelopmental and cytoskeletal antigens described earlier and the use of specific monoclonal antibodies for melanoma (**FIGURES 11–2** through **11–4**), renal cell carcinoma, and possibly other neoplasms. In addition, cerebellar-pontine angle tumors may occasionally present a difficulty in distinguishing between Schwannoma and meningioma. In this setting, S-100 protein and Leu-7 may be helpful in recognizing Schwannian derivation to corroborate the light microscopic impression.

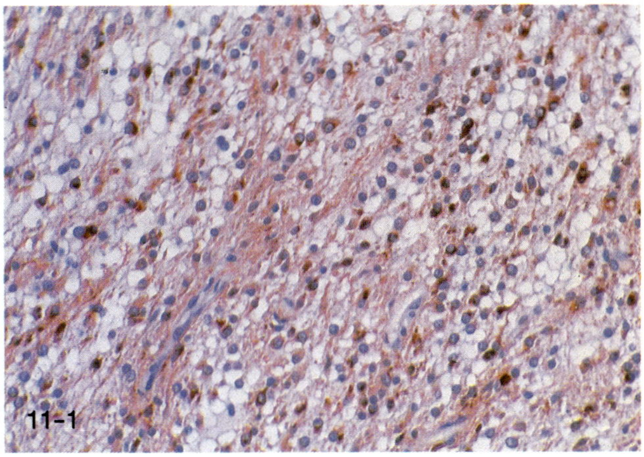

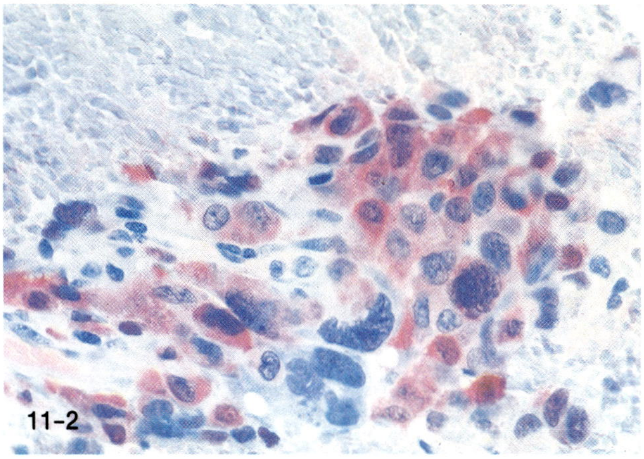

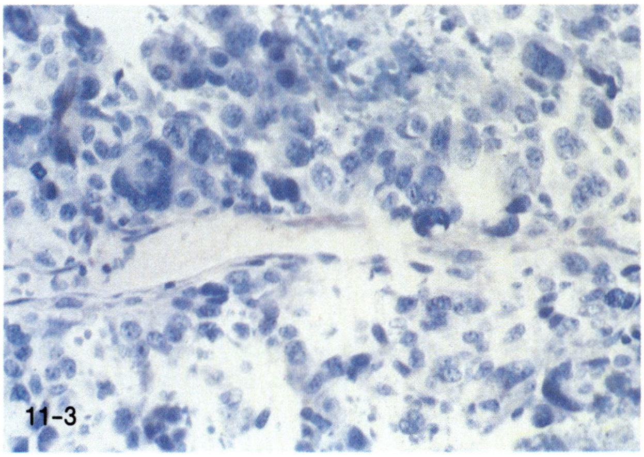

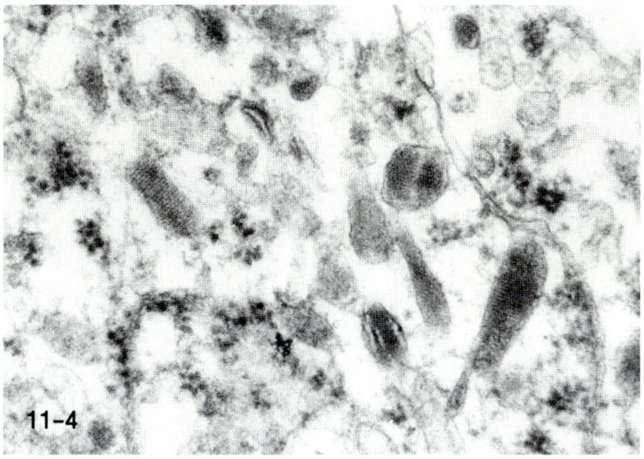

FIGURE 11–1. Cerebellar astrocytoma immunostained for glial fibrillar acidic protein. Tumor cells contain the antigen (ABC-PO with AEC, hematoxylin counterstain).

FIGURE 11–2. Metastatic amelanotic malignant melanoma in the brain. Figures 11–2 through 11–4 are from the same case. This figure shows tumor cells that contain S-100 protein (ABC-PO with AEC, hematoxylin counterstain). *Slide 97.*

FIGURE 11–3. Same case as 11–2. The tumor cells show a lack of cytokeratins as defined by AE1/3 (ABC-PO with AEC, hematoxylin counterstain).

FIGURE 11–4. Same case as 11–2. Premelanosomes are identified by electron microscopy (lead citrate and uranyl acetate).

12 Future Directions

Applications of immunohistochemistry are now firmly established as corroborative techniques in surgical pathology. Integration of this technology into all disciplines of diagnostic pathology will continue and, we hope, flourish. Advances during the next decade will appear on several levels.

One of the more common problems confronting the pathologist is that of a metastatic neoplasm of unknown origin presenting in a lymph node or other site. As outlined in Tables 12–1 and 12–2 and **FIGURES 12–1** and **12–2**, immunohistochemistry may help clarify the tissue of origin and, consequently, the classification of the tumor by means of a combination of monoclonal and polyclonal antibodies to tissue-specific antigens and intermediate filaments. These antigenic distributions are only tentative, and additional screening still will need to be done. In particular, "cytokeratins" must be more precisely identified and corresponding antibodies characterized and standardized. We agree wholeheartedly with the timely cautionary comments of Erlandson in this regard.

After Kohler and Milstein's development of hybridoma technology, the detection of monospecific tumor-associated antibodies by means of monoclonal antibodies seemed imminent. The development of tissue-specific, as opposed to tumor-specific, reagents is probably possible but still requires laborious and time-consuming screening of cell fusions and realistic, controlled study design to assess diagnostic efficiency and predictive value. This kind of effort has made available reagents like Uro-2, which will be very helpful in confirming the renal origin of metastatic carcinoma. The development of other tissue-specific monoclonal antibodies will require a similar commitment to the screening of cell fusions to identify the desired clones. For practical purposes, monoclonal antibodies will need to be available for many tissues and their corresponding neoplasms (eg, lung, stomach, colon, breast, pancreas).

The importance of freezing aliquots of tissue, in addition to processing in the conventional manner, cannot be overstressed. In our view, every diagnostic pathology laboratory should be both freezing aliquots and doing the conventional tissue processing. Most of the tissue-specific monoclonal antibodies that are currently available or are being developed are active only in frozen tissue sections. The frozen tissue need not be stored indefinitely.

As knowledge regarding immunohistochemistry is accumulated, tumors will eventually be

TABLE 12–1. Tentative Differential Distribution of Cellular Antigens in Spindle Cell Neoplasms

	AE 1/3	Vimentin	Desmin	Fibronectin	S-100 Protein	NAE	Myoglobin	VIII R:Ag	*Ulex*	Muramidase	α-1-Antitrypsin/ α-1-Chymotrypsin
Spindle cell carcinoma	+	–	–	–	–	–	–	–	(+)	–	–
Spindle cell melanoma	–	+	–	–	+	–	–	–	–	–	–
Fibrosarcoma	–	+	–	+	–	–	–	–	–	–	–
Malignant fibrous histiocytoma	–	+	(+)	+[a]	–	–	–	–	–	(+)	+
Leiomyosarcoma	–	+	+	–	–	–	–	–	–	–	–
Rhabdomyosarcoma	–	+	+	–	–	–	(+)	–	–	–	–
Liposarcoma	–	+	–	(+)	–	–	–	–	–	–	–
Granular cell tumor	–	+	–	–	+	?	–	–	–	–	–
Schwannoma	–	+	–	–	+	+	–	–	–	–	–
Synovial sarcoma	+[b]	+	–	–	–	–	–	–	–	–	–
Angiosarcoma	–	+	–	–	–	–	–	+	+	–	–

ABBREVIATIONS: NAE = neuron-associated enolase, VIII R:Ag = factor VIII–related antigen, + indicates present, – indicates absent, (+) indicates variably present, ? indicates not well established.

NOTE: Distributions are only tentative. Much specificity screening still needs to be done to verify these patterns.

[a]Fibrous component.

[b]Epithelial component.

identified that cannot be classified by either light microscopy or electron microscopy. Information is accumulating regarding the immunohistologic findings in spindle cell tumors (Table 12–1). In some instances, immunohistochemistry may provide the only means for classifying a neoplasm. Such situations currently arise with poorly differentiated adenocarcinoma of the prostate, and immunohistochemistry is very helpful in this setting.

However, in a neoplasm such as the tumor illustrated in **FIGURES 12–3** through **12–5**, interpretation is much more difficult. This spindle cell and epithelioid neoplasm presented as widespread peritoneal and mesenteric implants. It was ultimately classified as a probable amelanotic malignant melanoma because of its intense expression of S-100 antigen and because of cytoplasmic expression of three antigens defined by monoclonal antibodies thought to be specific for melanoma. Preliminary screening suggested that these antibodies react only with melanocytic

TABLE 12–2. Differential Distribution of Antigens in Undifferentiated Large Cell Neoplasms

Neoplasms	Cytokeratins (AE1/3, PKK-1)	Common Leukocyte Antigen	LN1	LN2	S-100 Protein	Mel-5/ BMA	Uro-2[b]
Amelanotic melanoma	−	−	−	−[a]	+	+	−
Large cell lymphoma	−	+	+	+	−	−	−
Renal cell carcinoma	(−)	−	−	−	−	−	+
Other carcinomas	+	−	+	(−)	(−)	−	−

ABBREVIATIONS: BMA = Biogenix melanoma antibody, + indicates positive, − indicates negative, (−) indicates usually negative, but some are focally positive.

NOTE: Generalizations are based on current literature and our experience; further tissue specificity screening is needed to corroborate these observations.

[a]Although a rare LN2-positive melanoma has been observed, most are negative.

[b]Uro-2 also labels endothelium in all tissues; superficial review of richly vascularized nonrenal tumors can result in erroneous interpretation.

cells and neoplasms derived from them, and other markers for poorly differentiated carcinomas were negative. However, premelanosomes could not be identified by transmission electron microscopy. It will take several more years and much immunohistochemical screening to identify the tissue- and tumor-specific monoclonal antibodies that would permit precise classification in the absence of architectural or ultrastructural differentiation, as in the tumor illustrated in **FIGURES 12–3** through **12–5**.

Furthermore, classification should be clinically relevant, and for many widely metastatic poorly differentiated neoplasms, there are really no effective treatments. Some encouraging results have been obtained using immunotherapy, including monoclonal antibodies labeled with cell toxins. In this setting, immunohistochemistry may facilitate not only the classification but also the profiling of tumor antigen expression before immunotherapy with the corresponding specific monoclonal antibody labeled with a cell toxin.

Significant strides can still be made in the refinement of techniques. Biotinylation of antibodies does not appear to affect immunoreactivity to a detectable degree, so that two-step or even one-step ABC procedures using biotinylated primary antibodies and preformed complexes for all systems could be developed. Two areas of great need are the development of alternative enzymes to peroxidase with favorable enzyme-substrate-chromogen kinetics and the development of monoclonal antibodies that recognize fixed antigens, particularly differentiation antigen immunotypes. The optimal system for lymphoid cells would be one using 1 μm thick plastic sections of tissue fixed in B-5 in conjunction with monoclonal antibodies recognizing fixed antigens in tissue sections.

Most of the literature on immunoperoxidase describes work done on tissue sections. Cytologic preparations can also be used for immunomicroscopy (**FIGURES 12–6** and **12–7**). However, great care must be taken in interpreting the results. In our experience, best results have been achieved using air-dried cytocentrifuge preparations. However, some artifact is induced during the preparation of the specimen. Overstaining of Papanicolaou's stain can be done, but there is a significant problem with nonspecific adherence of preimmune serum in such preparations. Thus, great caution must be exercised in performing and interpreting the preparations.

Molecular probes for complementary DNA material are gaining increasing importance in identifying virus in tissue-cultured cells and other preparations. Because nucleotide probes can be biotinylated, a biotinylated peroxidase-avidin complex or other biotin-avidin system can be used to detect in situ hybridization with the biotinylated probe. Such an application has already been devised for detection of cytomegalovirus and other viruses in tissue (**FIGURES 12–8** through **12–11**).

Because estrogen receptor activity is regulated by specific molecules, it is possible to isolate the protein responsible for the receptor activity. Rat monoclonal antibodies have been successfully developed against the estrogen receptor protein and may ultimately have great usefulness in evaluation of breast carcinoma and in the therapeutic approach to the management of such patients (**FIGURE 12–12**).

Rat monoclonal antibodies have been developed that recognize the encoded proteins of the v-H-*ras* and other oncogene products detected by immunohistology (**FIGURE 12–13**). Such reagents offer great potential in understanding neoplastic transformation at the level of cellular DNA.

Most of the immunohistologic literature has depended on qualitative and semiquantitative assessment. Cell-by-cell differential counting can be done, but it is laborious and currently adds little useful information. Gray-level morphometry may play a role in time-efficient quantitation for immunohistochemical preparations.

The future of immunohistochemistry greatly depends on the way these techniques are used now. Advances must be based on realistic expectations for the techniques, clear understanding of their complexity and limitations, and strict adherence to quality assurance programs in the diagnostic pathology laboratory. The appropriate role for immunohistochemistry in the pathologist's consultative practice should always be complementary and integrated with conventional histopathologic interpretation as tempered by experience and consultation.

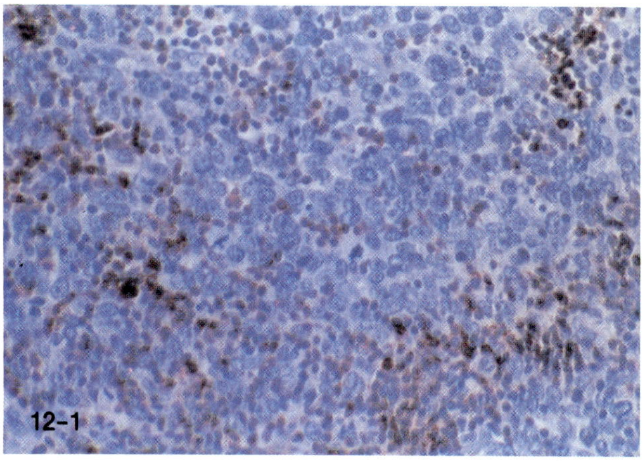

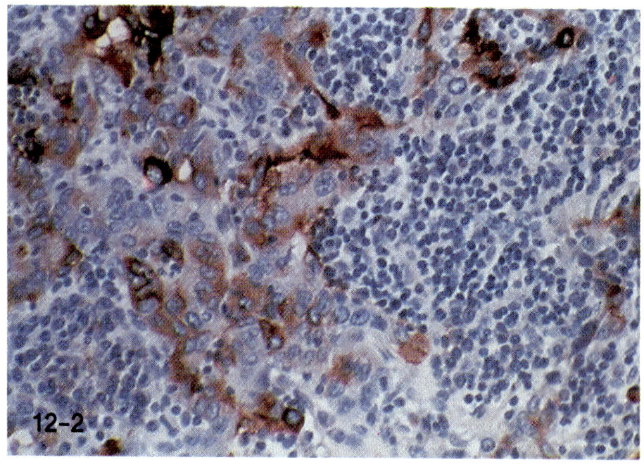

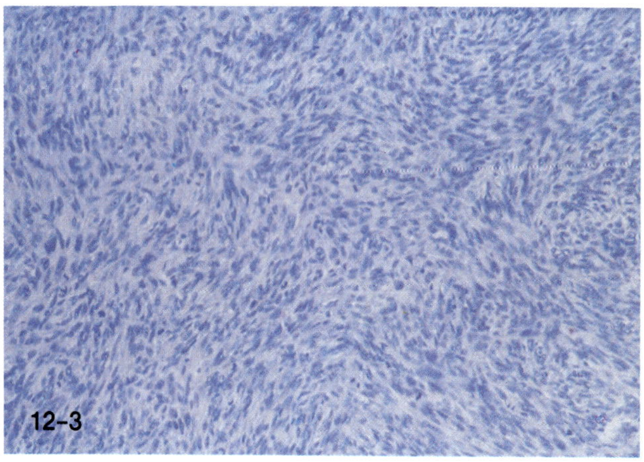

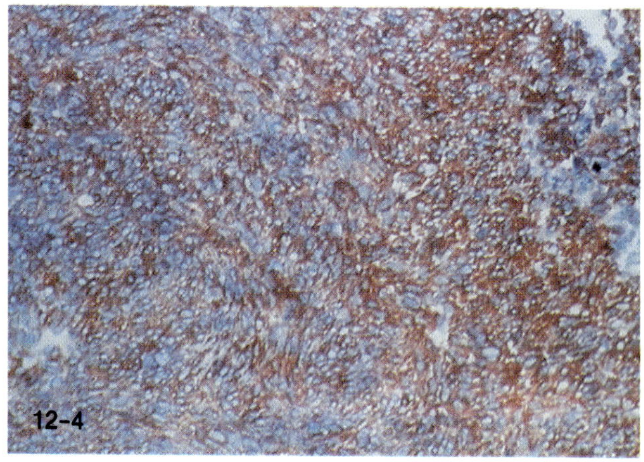

FIGURE 12–1. Undifferentiated malignant neoplasm presenting as a large neck mass. Figures 12–1 and 12–2 are from the same case. While large tumor cells do not express common leukocyte antigen, the latter is identified in small contiguous lymphocytes (ABC-PO with AEC, hematoxylin counterstain). *Slide 98.*

FIGURE 12–2. Same case as 12–1. Cytokeratins (AE1/3) are expressed by large tumor cells. Lymphocytes are negative for AE1/3 (ABC-PO with AEC, hematoxylin counterstain). *Slide 99.*

FIGURE 12–3. Spindle cell and epithelioid neoplasm presenting as multiple peritoneal implants in a patient with no history of primary tumor. Figures 12–3 through 12–5 are from the same case. This figure shows that no staining is present in the negative control for S-100 protein (IgG fraction of preimmune rabbit serum; ABC-PO with AEC, hematoxylin counterstain).

FIGURE 12–4. Same case as 12–3. The neoplasm contains tumor antigen identified with monoclonal antibody Mel-5 (ABC-PO with AEC, in a frozen tissue section, hematoxylin counterstain).

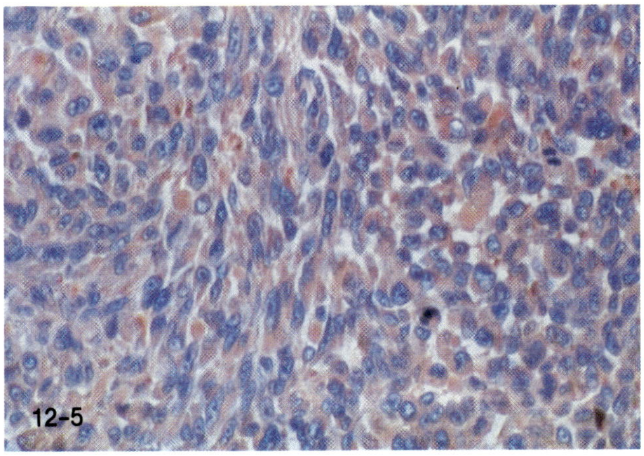

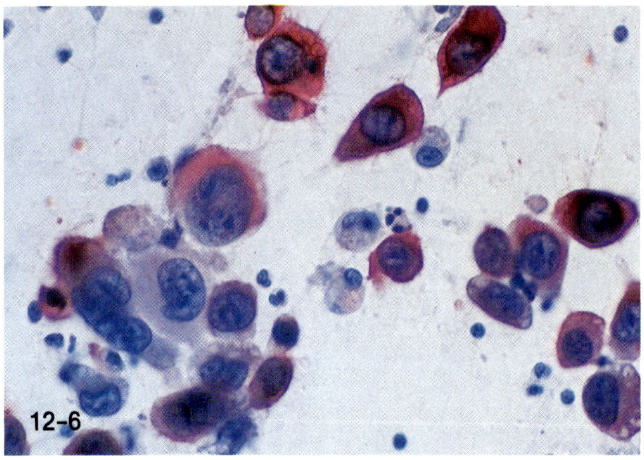

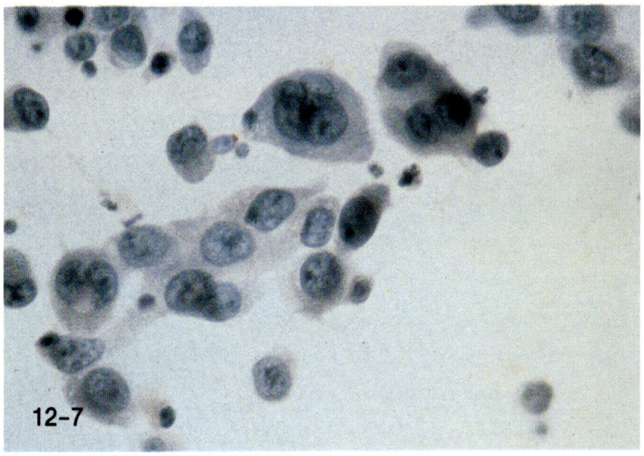

FIGURE 12–5. Same case as 12–3. Cytoplasmic expression of S-100 protein is present (ABC-PO with AEC, hematoxylin counterstain).

FIGURE 12–6. Undifferentiated large cell carcinoma, lung aspiration specimen. Figures 12–6 and 12–7 are from the same case. A Papanicolaou cytologic preparation overstained with antibody to epithelial membrane antigen shows positive staining in nucleolated tumor cells (ABC-PO with AEC, Papanicolaou counterstain). Preparation courtesy of Steven Becker, MD. *Slide 100.*

FIGURE 12–7. Same case as 12–6. No staining is present in the negative control using nonimmune mouse IgG as a substitute for the primary reagent (ABC-PO with AEC, Papanicolaou counterstain). Preparation courtesy of Steven Becker, MD.

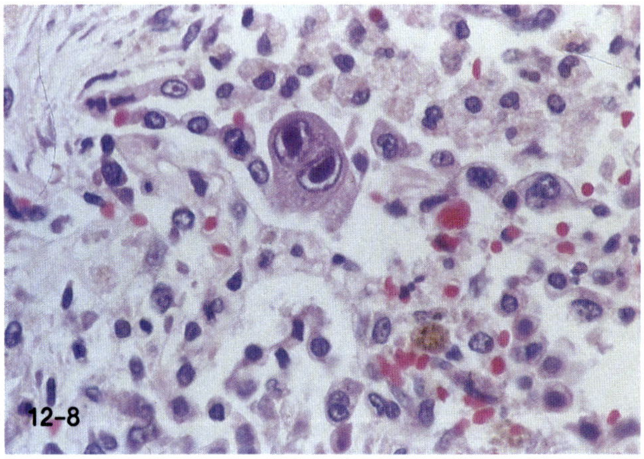

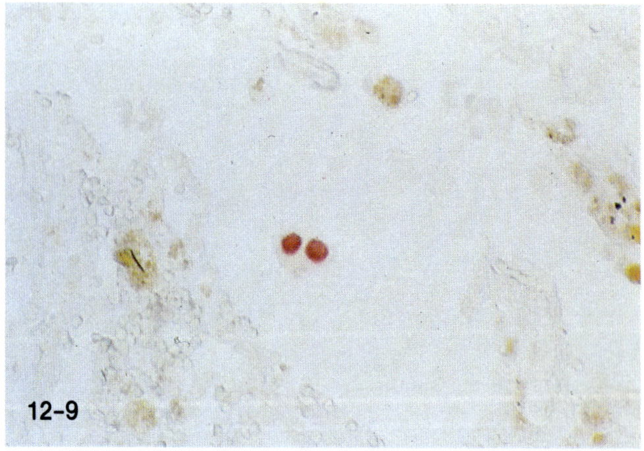

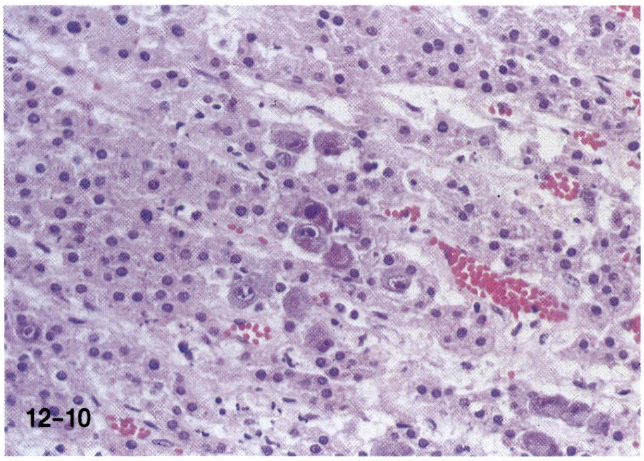

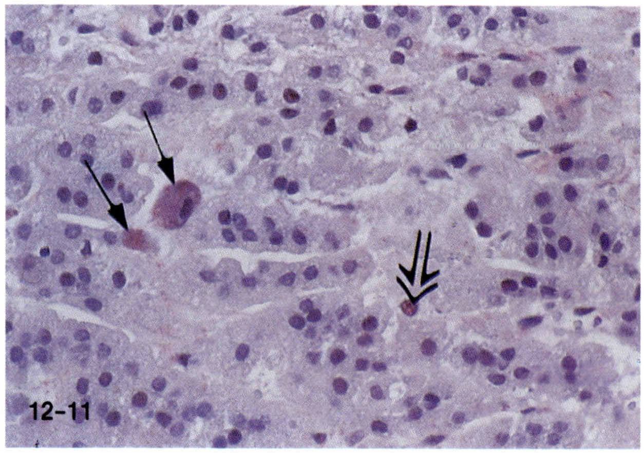

FIGURE 12–8. Cytomegalovirus pneumonia. Figures 12–8 and 12–9 are from the same case. This tissue section is stained with H & E.

FIGURE 12–9. Same case as 12–8. In situ hybridization (red) of cytomegalovirus using a biotinylated complementary probe. Note contrast with hemosiderin (biotinylated primary modification of ABC-PO with AEC, no counterstain).

FIGURE 12–10. Cytomegalovirus adrenalitis. Figures 12–10 and 12–11 are from the same case. This tissue section is stained with H & E.

FIGURE 12–11. Same case as 12–10. In situ hybridization. Viral DNA is identified in the obvious nuclear inclusion, in cytoplasmic inclusions (arrows), and in a nucleus without an obvious inclusion (double arrow; ABC-PO, biotinylated primary modification, with AEC, hematoxylin counterstain). *Slide 101.*

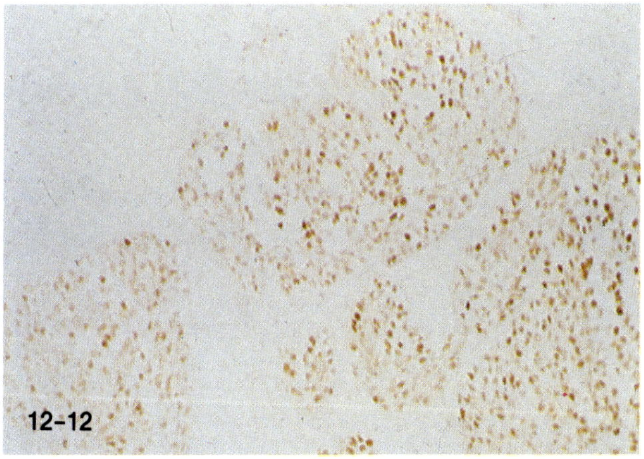

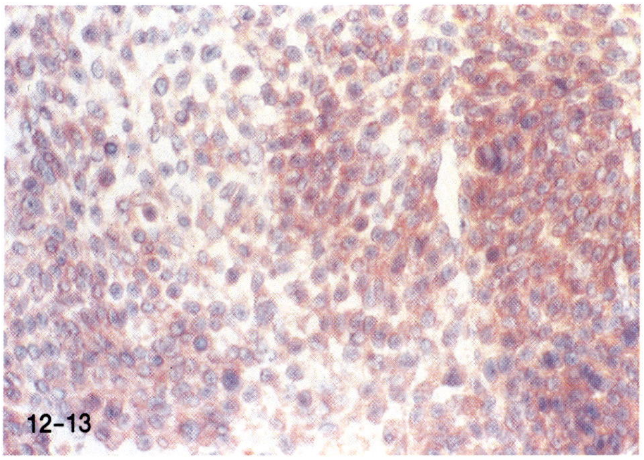

FIGURE 12–12. Breast carcinoma demonstrating positive nuclear staining with rat monoclonal antibody to estrogen receptor protein (rat peroxidase-antiperoxidase with DAB, no counterstain; materials to perform estrogen receptor immunocytochemical assay—ERICA—provided by Abbott Diagnostics).

FIGURE 12–13. Transitional cell carcinoma of bladder immunostained with rat monoclonal antibody to the oncogene encoded protein v-H-*ras* (ABC-PO with AEC, hematoxylin counterstain).

A Buffers

A–1. Phosphate-Buffered Saline, pH 7.2

BACKGROUND

Phosphate-buffered saline (PBS) is the principal working buffer for immunohistochemistry. It serves as a diluent for antibodies and as a washing buffer to remove excess reagent from tissue sections.

MATERIALS

1. FTA hemagglutination buffer (BBL Laboratories, No. 11248)
2. Distilled water

PROCEDURE

1. Dissolve 9.23 g FTA hemagglutination buffer (which consists of 7.65 mg NaCl, 1.2688 g Na_2HPO_4, 0.1 g NaH_2PO_4, and 0.2113 g KH_2PO_4) in 1 L distilled water.
2. The pH should be 7.2.

A–2. Modified Phosphate-Buffered Saline

BACKGROUND

Modified PBS is used as a diluent for some monoclonal antibody systems, in which its use yields reaction products of relatively greater intensity.

MATERIALS

1. K_2HPO_4
2. Distilled water
3. NaCl
4. NaH_2PO_4
5. Thimerosal (Sigma, No. T5125)

PROCEDURE

1. To make the stock solution, dissolve 188.0 g K_2HPO_4 in 100 mL distilled water (use heat if necessary); then add 180.0 g NaCl and 33.0 g NaH_2PO_4 and dilute with distilled water to 1 L.
2. To make the working solution, dilute 40 mL of the stock solution with 960 mL distilled water. Then dissolve 20 mg thimerosal in the liter of buffer.

REFERENCE

Wood GS, Warnke RA: The immunologic phenotyping of bone marrow biopsies and aspirates: Frozen section techniques. *Blood* 1982;59:913–922.

A–3. Acetate Buffer, 0.02 M, pH 5.2

BACKGROUND

Acetate buffer is used as a buffer for aminoethylcarbazole, a peroxidase/hydrogen peroxide chromogen.

MATERIALS

1. Sodium acetate, 0.2 M (16.4 g/L)
2. Acetic acid, 0.2 M (11.4 mL glacial acetic acid/L)

PROCEDURE

1. To 730 mL of 0.2 M sodium acetate, add 270 mL of 0.2 M acetic acid.

A–4. Tris HCl, 0.1 M, pH 7.6

BACKGROUND

Tris HCl is used as the principal buffer for the Hanker-Yates peroxidase chromogen system.

MATERIALS

1. Tris HCl, molecular weight 149.0, reagent grade (Sigma, No. T4253)
2. Distilled water

PROCEDURE

1. Dissolve 7.45 g Tris HCl in 1 L distilled water.
2. The pH should be 7.6.

A–5. Tris Buffer, pH 8.2

BACKGROUND

This buffer is used for the alkaline phosphatase chromogenic substrate.

MATERIALS

1. Tris, 0.1 M
2. Concentrated HCl
3. Distilled water

PROCEDURE

1. Dissolve 12.1 g Tris in 950 mL distilled water.
2. Adjust pH to 8.2 with concentrated HCl; add distilled water to make final volume of 1,000 mL.

B Chromogens and Substrates

B–1. Aminoethylcarbazole

BACKGROUND

Aminoethylcarbazole (AEC) is a chromogen used with immunoperoxidase systems. In the presence of hydrogen peroxide and peroxidase, AEC yields a red reaction product that is soluble in organic solvents.

MATERIALS

1. 3-Amino-9-ethylcarbazole (Sigma IsoPac, No. A5754)
2. Acetate buffer, 0.02 M, pH 5.2 (Appendix A–3)
3. *N,N*-dimethylformamide (Baker, No. 9221-1)
4. 30% Hydrogen peroxide (Fisher, No. H325)

PROCEDURE

1. Dissolve 25 mg AEC with 10 mL dimethylformamide.
2. Add 100 mL acetate buffer.
3. Add 40 μL of 30% hydrogen peroxide just before immersing slides.

NOTE

1. AEC is a potentially hazardous substance.
2. Use gloves and do all AEC reactions under a hood.
3. Discard the AEC solution and the first wash with PBS into a special, appropriate container.

B–2. Hanker-Yates Reagent

BACKGROUND

Hanker-Yates reagent (HYR; *p*-phenylenediamine and pyrocatechol) is a chromogen used with immunoperoxidase systems. In the presence of hydrogen peroxide and peroxidase, HYR yields a brown-black reaction product that is insoluble in organic solvents. It is preferred for renal immunohistochemistry.

MATERIALS

1. Hanker-Yates reagent (HYR; Polysciences, No. 8661)
2. Tris buffer, pH 8.2 (Appendix A–5)
3. 30% Hydrogen peroxide (Fisher, No. H325)

PROCEDURE

1. Place 75 mg of HYR into each of 4 to 6 Coplin jars.
2. Add 50 mL of Tris buffer to each jar.
3. Place slides in the HYR solution, then add 20 μL of 30% hydrogen peroxide to each jar.
4. Incubate slides at room temperature for 3 to 4 minutes (best results are achieved when incubation jars are mechanically shaken).
5. Monitor controls; usually 3 to 5 changes of chromogen are required to adequately develop reaction product.

NOTE

1. Do *not* make up HYR ahead of time. Prepare just before immersing slides.

B–3. Alkaline Phosphatase (Fast Red) Chromogenic Substrate

BACKGROUND

Alkaline phosphatase chromogenic substrate is used in alkaline phosphatase immunohistochemical systems, especially for analysis of tissues rich in endogenous peroxidases and pseudoperoxidases. The reaction product is red and is not soluble in organic solvents.

MATERIALS

1. Naphthol ASTR (Sigma, No. 6125)
2. *N,N*-dimethylformamide (Baker, No. 9221-1)
3. Fast red K salt (Sigma, No. 8379)
4. Levamisole (Sigma, No. L-9756), optional
5. Tris buffer, pH 8.2 (Appendix A–5)

PROCEDURE

1. Dissolve 10 mg naphthol ASTR in 2 mL dimethylformamide.
2. Dissolve 50 mg fast red K salt and 12 mg levamisole in 50 mL Tris buffer.
3. Add the Tris buffer solution to the dimethylformamide solution.
4. Incubate slides for 10 to 15 minutes at room temperature.

NOTE

1. The addition of levamisole is optional; it inhibits endogenous alkaline phosphatase (excluding the intestinal form). It reduces the intensity of staining to some extent. Do not use routinely.
2. For a blue reaction product, use fast blue BBN (50 mg) in place of fast red.

C Techniques

For the best results, each antigen-antibody system should be adjusted for optimal reactivity with respect to both dilutions of primary antibodies and to tissue processing. Approximate recommended dilutions appear in the tables in Appendix D. Recommendations for optimal tissue processing appear in Table 3–1 (page 18).

C–1. Avidin-Biotin Flush

BACKGROUND

Biotin-avidin systems are particularly useful in immunohistochemistry because of their increased sensitivity. However, some tissues may have endogenous biotin activity (eg, liver, kidneys) and require biotin suppression for reliable interpretation of the specific stain. Endogenous biotin is usually not detectable in paraffin sections, only in frozen tissue sections.

MATERIALS

1. Avidin D (Vector, No. A2000)
2. PBS and modified PBS (Appendixes A–1, A–2)
3. Biotin (Sigma, No. B4501)
4. Avidin D solution, 0.01% in modified PBS
   a. Make stock solution by reconstituting 10 mg avidin D with 1 mL PBS.
   b. Make working solution by diluting 0.1 mL of stock solution in 10 mL modified PBS.
5. Biotin solution, 0.005%
   a. Dissolve 0.015 g biotin in 500 mL modified PBS solution.

PROCEDURE

1. Fix tissue appropriately as specified for antigen to be tested (usually acetone).
2. Rinse tissues in modified PBS.
3. Incubate slides for 20 minutes in avidin D working solution.
4. Wash and then incubate in modified PBS for 5 minutes.
5. Incubate tissue in biotin solution for 20 minutes.
6. Wash in modified PBS for 5 minutes.
7. Proceed with primary antibody and immunoperoxidase procedure.

REFERENCE

Wood GS, Warnke R: Suppression of endogenous avidin-binding activity in tissues and its relevance to biotin-avidin detection systems. *J Histochem Cytochem* 1981;29:1196–1204.

C–2. Direct Immunoperoxidase: Entrapped Immune Complexes and Autoantibody Detection

BACKGROUND

Entrapment of autoantibody or immune complexes is the hallmark of many disease processes mediated by immune mechanisms. The direct immunoperoxidase procedure profiles the tissue deposition of these components of the immune response as an adjunct to the pathologic classification of disease.

MATERIALS

1. Modified PBS (Appendix A–2)
2. Antibody conjugates
   a. PO-anti-IgG Fc (Cappell, $F(ab')_2$ fragment), diluted 1:80 in modified PBS (see step 6)
   b. PO-anti-IgA Fc (Cappell, $F(ab')_2$ fragment), diluted 1:20 in modified PBS (see step 6)
   c. PO-anti-IgM Fc (Dako), diluted 1:15 in modified PBS (see step 6)
   d. PO-anti-C3 (Dako), diluted 1:20 in modified PBS (see step 6)
3. Hanker-Yates reagent (HYR; Polysciences, No. 8661)
4. 30% Hydrogen peroxide (Fisher, No. H325)
5. Tris buffer (Appendix A–5)
6. Periodic acid
7. Schiff's reagent
8. Hematoxylin
9. Gum tragacanth (Kodak, No. 15409)

PROCEDURE

1. Place 75 mg HYR in each of 4 to 6 Coplin jars. Set aside until needed.
2. Freeze fresh tissue (attached to a chuck by gum tragacanth) by immersing it in a container of isopentane, which has been cooled to −120 °C by immersion in liquid nitrogen. Store tissue at −70 °C or colder.
3. Using a cryostat, cut frozen tissue into sections 4 μm thick. Place 4 sections per slide on 2 slides.
4. Allow sections to air-dry completely.
5. Allow slides to reach room temperature for 5 minutes.
6. Dilute antibodies with modified PBS as specified in materials list.
7. Pipette monospecific conjugated antibodies onto tissue sections. Each antibody is applied to one section on each slide. Incubate sections in humidified chamber for 30 minutes at ambient temperature.
8. Remove adherent antibody from tissue surface as follows: Hold slide flat, then flood with modified PBS by pouring on one edge of slide. Tilt the slide while continuing to flood sections with modified PBS. *Do not pour buffer directly onto tissue.*
9. Wash sections rapidly in three additional changes of modified PBS.
10. Wash sections briefly in Tris buffer.

C–2. Direct Immunoperoxidase: Entrapped Immune Complexes and Autoantibody Detection/*continued*

11. Develop the colored reaction product in 3 to 6 consecutive changes of HYR as follows.
    a. Add 50 mL Tris buffer to the HYR in each Coplin jar to be used.
    b. Place slides in the solution.
    c. Add 20 μL of 30% hydrogen peroxide to each Coplin jar.
    d. Best results are achieved with a mechanical shaker or continuous agitation. Monitor positive control staining if desired.
    e. Wash slides briefly in Tris buffer between changes of HYR solution.
    f. When HYR solution turns dark, transfer slides to fresh HYR solution.
12. Wash both slides in Tris buffer briefly.
13. Counterstain one of the 2 slides with periodic acid for 5 minutes; wash in Tris buffer; stain with Schiff's reagent for 45 minutes. Wash with hot water for 30 minutes. Counterstain with hematoxylin; dehydrate, clear, and mount.
14. Dehydrate the noncounterstained slide in graded alcohols and xylene; dehydrate, clear, and mount.

REFERENCE

Sheibani K, Tubbs RR, Gephardt GN, et al: Comparison of alternative chromogens for renal immunohistochemistry. *Hum Pathol* 1981;12:349–354.

C–3. Direct Immunoperoxidase: Cellular Immunoglobulin Immunotypes

BACKGROUND

The direct immunoperoxidase procedure is used to identify cell-associated immunoglobulins. The antigens are altered by most fixatives, and paraffin sections of such material are not acceptable. Thus, frozen tissue sections and cytocentrifuge preparations are used. A monolayer of cells ideal for immunostaining of cytocentrifuge preparations is obtained with cell suspensions containing approximately 2×10^6 cells/mL.

MATERIALS

1. 3-Amino-9-ethylcarbazole (AEC; Sigma IsoPac, No. A5754)
2. Acetate buffer, 0.02 M, pH 5.2 (Appendix A–3)
3. *N,N*-dimethylformamide (Baker, No. 9221-1)
4. 30% Hydrogen peroxide (Fisher, No. H325)
5. Modified PBS (Appendix A–2)
6. Poly-L-lysine, MW >300,000 (Sigma No. P1524), 0.1% in distilled water
7. Acetone, reagent grade
8. Affinity-purified immunoglobulin conjugates
   a. Peroxidase-conjugated anti-κ Fab (HPO-aκ, Tago, No. 2396), diluted 1:100 and 1:300 in modified PBS
   b. Peroxidase-conjugated anti-λ Fab (HPO-aλ; Tago, No. 2398), diluted 1:100 and 1:300 in modified PBS
   c. Peroxidase-conjugated chrompure goat IgG (negative control, HPO-C; Jackson, No. 005-3004), diluted 1:100 and 1:300 in modified PBS
9. Hematoxylin
10. Aquamount (Lerner through American Scientific Products, No. M7644-1)

PROCEDURE

1. Precoat slides with poly-L-lysine (0.1% in distilled water) and allow to air-dry.
2. Using a cryostat, cut frozen tissue into 8 μm thick sections.
3. Place 3 sections per slide on each of 3 poly-L-lysine-coated slides. On each slide, 2 sections (left and right) will be immunostained; the third (the middle section) will serve as a negative control.
4. Air-dry slides overnight at room temperature.
5. Make a control slide with frozen sections of tonsil tissue.
6. Make 3 slides with specimens from a cytocentrifuge preparation.
7. Fix "frozen" sections, tonsil control, and cytocentrifuge preparations for 10 minutes in fresh, reagent-grade acetone. Air-dry.
8. Wash slides with modified PBS for 5 minutes and wipe around sections.
9. Apply the 1:300 dilutions of the immunoglobulin conjugates to the first slide and the tonsil control in the following manner: HPO-aκ to the section on the left, HPO-aλ to the section on the right, and HPO-C to the section in the middle.
10. Apply the 1:100 dilutions of the immunoglobulin conjugates to the second and third slides in the same manner.
11. Apply the 1:100 dilutions of HPO-aκ to one cytocentrifuge preparation, of HPO-aλ to the second cytocentrifuge preparation, and of HPO-C to the third cytocentrifuge preparation.
12. Incubate all the slides for *only* 10 minutes at room temperature in a humidified chamber.

C–3. Direct Immunoperoxidase: Cellular Immunoglobulin Immunotypes/*continued*

13. Wash with modified PBS, making several changes over 5 minutes.
14. Develop the colored reaction product with AEC as follows.
    a. Observe precautions for AEC (Appendix B–1).
    b. Dissolve 25 mg AEC in 10 mL of dimethylformamide.
    c. Add 100 mL of 0.02 M acetate buffer (pH 5.2).
    d. Add 40 μL of 30% hydrogen peroxide.
    e. Incubate slides for 10 minutes.
15. Wash with PBS, making several changes over 5 minutes.
16. Counterstain all the cytocentrifuge preparations, the third frozen section slide, and the tonsil control with fresh hematoxylin (no alcohol).
17. Do *not* dehydrate in alcohols.
18. Apply a coverslip with Aquamount.
19. Seal edges of the coverslip with nail polish and label the slides.

REFERENCES

Huang WM, Gibson SJ, Facer P, et al: Improved section adhesion for immunocytochemistry using high molecular weight polymers of L-lysine as a slide coating. *Histochemistry* 1983;77:275–279.

Tubbs RR, Fishleder A, Weiss RA, et al: Immunohistologic cellular phenotypes of lymphoproliferative disorders: Comprehensive evaluation of 564 cases including 257 non-Hodgkin's lymphomas classified by the International Working Formulation. *Am J Pathol* 1983;113:207–221.

C–4. Mouse Avidin-Biotinylated Peroxidase Complex (ABC-PO) for Frozen Sections

BACKGROUND

The mouse ABC procedure is used for identifying cellular antigens with monoclonal antibodies. Some antigens are preserved in paraffin sections of fixed tissue. Most are destroyed in the processing; therefore, frozen tissue sections or cytocentrifuge preparations are usually required for good antigen preservation. See Table 3–1 for details of optimal specimen processing.

MATERIALS

1. 3-Amino-9-ethylcarbazole (AEC; Sigma IsoPac, No. A5754)
2. Modified PBS (Appendix A–2)
3. Acetate buffer, 0.02 M, pH 5.2 (Appendix A–3)
4. 30% Hydrogen peroxide (Fisher, No. H325)
5. *N,N*-dimethylformamide (Baker, No. 9221-1)
6. Absolute acetone, reagent grade
7. Poly-L-lysine, MW > 300,000 (Sigma No. P1524), 0.1% in distilled water
8. Mouse ABC kit (Vector, No. PK-4002), consists of the following:
   a. Biotinylated horse anti-mouse IgG
   b. Avidin DH
   c. Biotinylated peroxidase
9. Appropriately diluted mouse monoclonal antibodies (Table D–2)
10. HPO anti-mouse IgG (Dako, No. P-260), diluted 1:60 in modified PBS
11. Aquamount (Lerner through American Scientific Products, No. M7644-1)

PROCEDURE

1. Cut frozen tissue in a cryostat into 8 μm thick sections.
2. Place on poly-L-lysine-coated slides and allow to air-dry overnight at room temperature.
3. Fix "frozen" sections in reagent-grade acetone for 10 minutes. Air-dry.
4. Preform ABC-PO reagent from kit.
   a. Combine 20 μL avidin DH (reagent A), 20 μL biotinylated peroxidase (reagent B), and 1.6 mL modified PBS.
   b. Allow to stand at room temperature for at least 30 minutes before use.
5. Wash sections in modified PBS, 3 changes over 5 minutes.
6. Apply mouse monoclonal antibodies and mouse IgG control to the sections and incubate in a humidified chamber at room temperature for 15 minutes.
7. Wash in modified PBS, 3 changes over 5 minutes.
8. Apply biotinylated affinity-purified horse anti-mouse Ig (diluted 1:200 in modified PBS) for 15 minutes at room temperature. For those tissues rich in indirect biotin, a simple, indirect immunoperoxidase procedure can be used instead of the ABC-PO method. See "Indirect Option" on page 143.
9. Wash in modified PBS, 3 changes over 5 minutes.

C–4. Mouse Avidin-Biotinylated Peroxidase Complex (ABC-PO) for Frozen Sections/ *continued*

10. Apply preformed ABC reagent for 15 minutes in humidified chamber at room temperature.
11. Wash in modified PBS, 3 changes over 5 minutes.
12. Develop the colored reaction product with AEC as follows.
    a. Observe precautions for AEC (Appendix B–1).
    b. Dissolve 25 mg AEC in 10 mL of dimethylformamide.
    c. Add 100 mL of 0.02 M acetate buffer (pH 5.2).
    d. Add 40 μL of 30% hydrogen peroxide.
    e. Incubate slides for 10 minutes.
13. Wash in PBS for 5 minutes, making several changes.
14. Counterstain with fresh hematoxylin (no alcohol).
15. Do *not* dehydrate in alcohols.
16. Apply a coverslip with Aquamount.
17. Seal edges of the coverslip with nail polish and label the slides.

INDIRECT OPTION

1. Follow steps 1 through 7.
2. Apply HPO anti-mouse IgG (diluted 1:60 in modified PBS) for 15 minutes at room temperature.
3. Wash in modified PBS, 3 changes over 5 minutes.
4. Then proceed with step 11 and resume procedure sequence.

REFERENCE

Hsu SM, Cossman J, Jaffe S: A comparison of ABC, unlabeled antibody and conjugated immunohistochemical methods with monoclonal and polyclonal antibodies: An examination of germinal center of tonsils. *Am J Clin Pathol* 1983;80:429–435.

C–5. Mouse ABC-PO: Lymphocyte Differentiation Antigens for Paraffin Sections

BACKGROUND

The mouse ABC-PO procedure is used for identifying cellular antigens with monoclonal antibodies. Although most antigens are destroyed during processing for paraffin sectioning, some are preserved. See Table 3–1 for details of optimal specimen processing.

MATERIALS

1. 3-Amino-9-ethylcarbazole (AEC; Sigma IsoPac, No. A5754)
2. Modified PBS (Appendix A–2)
3. Acetate buffer, 0.02 M, pH 5.2 (Appendix A–3)
4. 30% Hydrogen peroxide (Fisher, No. H325)
5. *N,N*-dimethylformamide (Baker, No. 9221-1)
6. Acetone, reagent grade
7. Mouse ABC kit (Vector, No. PK-4002), consists of the following:
   a. Biotinylated horse anti-mouse IgG
   b. Avidin DH
   c. Biotinylated peroxidase
8. Appropriately diluted mouse monoclonal antibodies (Table D–2)
9. HPO anti-mouse IgG (Dako, No. P-260), diluted 1:20 in modified PBS
10. Normal horse serum (Vector, special order)
11. Aquamount (Lerner through American Scientific Products, No. M7644-1)

PROCEDURE

1. Fix tissue 1 to 2 mm in thickness in ample volumes of the fixative chosen for the antigen. Pronase digestion (Appendix C–7) is usually helpful only for keratins and S-100 protein but is useless or deleterious for other antigens.
2. Cut paraffin sections 4 to 6 μm thick. Place 2 sections per slide on each of 2 slides. Dry in 60 °C oven until immunostaining is to be performed (a few hours or less).
3. Deparaffinize slides in 2 changes of xylene and 2 changes of absolute alcohol.
4. Block endogenous peroxidase by immersing slides for 30 minutes in a solution consisting of 6 mL of 30% hydrogen peroxide and 94 mL absolute methanol.
5. Wash briefly in distilled water and in modified PBS, 3 changes over 5 minutes.
6. Apply blocking 5% normal horse serum, diluted in modified PBS, for 30 to 60 minutes to all sections, using either flat slide incubation or immersion.
7. Preform ABC-PO reagent from kit.
   a. Combine 20 μL avidin DH (reagent A), 20 μL biotinylated peroxidase (reagent B), and 1.6 mL modified PBS.
   b. Allow to stand at room temperature for at least 30 minutes before use.
8. Wash in modified PBS, 3 changes over 5 minutes.
9. Apply mouse monoclonal antibodies and mouse IgG control to sections and incubate in a humidified chamber at room temperature for 15 minutes.

C–5. Mouse ABC-PO: Lymphocyte Differentiation Antigens for Paraffin Sections/ *continued*

10. Wash in modified PBS, 3 changes over 5 minutes.
11. Apply biotinylated affinity-purified horse anti-mouse Ig (diluted 1:200 in modified PBS) for 15 minutes at room temperature. For those tissues rich in endogenous biotin, a simple indirect immunoperoxidase procedure can be used instead of the ABC-PO method. See "Indirect Option."
12. Wash in modified PBS, 3 changes over 5 minutes.
13. Apply preformed ABC reagent for 15 minutes in a humidified chamber at room temperature.
14. Wash in modified PBS, 3 changes over 5 minutes.
15. Develop the colored reaction product with AEC as follows.
    a. Observe precautions for AEC (Appendix B–1).
    b. Dissolve 25 mg AEC in 10 mL of dimethylformamide.
    c. Add 100 mL of 0.02 M acetate buffer (pH 5.2).
    d. Add 40 μL of 30% hydrogen peroxide.
    e. Stain slides for 10 minutes.
16. Wash in PBS for 5 minutes, making several changes.
17. Counterstain with hematoxylin (no alcohol).
18. Do *not* dehydrate in alcohols.
19. Apply a coverslip with Aquamount.
20. Seal edges of coverslip with nail polish and label the slides.

INDIRECT OPTION

1. Follow steps 1 through 10.
2. Apply HPO anti-mouse IgG (diluted 1:60 in modified PBS) for 15 minutes.
3. Wash in modified PBS, 3 changes over 5 minutes.
4. Then proceed with development of AEC colored reaction product (step 15).

REFERENCES

Hsu SM, Cossman J, Jaffe S: A comparison of ABC, unlabeled antibody and conjugated immunohistochemical methods with monoclonal and polyclonal antibodies: An examination of germinal center of tonsils. *Am J Clin Pathol* 1983;80:429–435.

Huang WM, Gibson SJ, Facer P, et al: Improved section adhesion for immunocytochemistry using high molecular weight polymers of L-lysine as a slide coating. *Histochemistry* 1983;77:275–279.

C–6. Biotinylated Primary Antibody Modification of ABC-PO

BACKGROUND

The avidin-biotinylated peroxidase complex can be directly linked to a biotinylated nucleotide probe or to a biotinylated primary antibody. The use of the biotinylated primary antibody eliminates one step in the ABC-PO procedure with essentially no loss in reaction intensity.

Tissue DNA must be heat- or formamide-denatured before incubation with the biotinylated probe for in situ hybridization. (The in situ hybridization technique is still in the preliminary stages of development.)

MATERIALS

1. 3-Amino-9-ethylcarbazole (AEC; Sigma IsoPac, No. A5754)
2. Modified PBS (Appendix A–2)
3. Acetate buffer, 0.02 M, pH 5.2 (Appendix A–3)
4. 30% Hydrogen peroxide (Fisher, No. H325)
5. *N,N*-dimethylformamide (Baker, No. 9221-1)
6. Acetone, reagent grade
7. Biotinylated nucleotide probe or antibody, dilutions must be empirically optimized
8. Vectastain standard ABC kit (Vector, No. PK-4000)
9. Aquamount (Lerner through American Scientific Products, No. M7644-1)

PROCEDURE

1. Preform ABC-PO reagent from kit.
   a. Combine 20 μL avidin DH (reagent A), 20 μL biotinylated peroxidase (reagent B), and 1.6 mL modified PBS.
   b. Allow to stand at room temperature for at least 30 minutes before use.
2. Cut frozen tissue in a cryostat into 8 μm thick sections. Place 3 sections on one slide. If paraffin sections are used, follow the procedure in C–8, steps 1 through 7, then proceed to step 4 below.
3. Fix in reagent-grade acetone for 10 minutes and allow to air-dry.
4. Wash in modified PBS, 3 changes over 5 minutes.
5. Apply biotinylated nucleotide probe or appropriately diluted biotinylated antibody. (Dilutions must be empirically determined, but usually approximate the immunoglobulin concentration of nonbiotinylated antibody.)
6. Incubate in humidified chamber at room temperature for 15 minutes.
7. Wash in modified PBS, 3 changes over 5 minutes.
8. Apply preformed ABC reagent and incubate for 15 minutes in a humidified chamber at room temperature.

C–6. Biotinylated Primary Antibody Modification of ABC-PO/*continued*

9. Wash in modified PBS, 3 changes over 5 minutes.
10. Develop the colored reaction product with AEC as follows.
    a. Observe precautions for AEC (Appendix B–1).
    b. Dissolve 25 mg AEC in 10 mL of dimethylformamide.
    c. Add 100 mL of 0.02 M acetate buffer (pH 5.2).
    d. Add 40 μL of 30% hydrogen peroxide.
    e. Incubate slides for 10 minutes.
11. Wash in modified PBS for 5 minutes, making several changes.
12. Counterstain with fresh hematoxylin *(no alcohol)*.
13. Do *not* dehydrate in alcohols.
14. Apply a coverslip with Aquamount.
15. Seal the edges of the coverslip with nail polish and label the slides.

REFERENCE

Hsu SM, Cossman J, Jaffe S: A comparison of ABC, unlabeled antibody and conjugated immunohistochemical methods with monoclonal and polyclonal antibodies: An examination of germinal center of tonsils. *Am J Clin Pathol* 1983;80:429–435.

C–7. Pronase Digestion

BACKGROUND

Enzyme pretreatment is used in selected cases to enhance specific staining of certain antigens. Pronase digestion enhances keratin and S-100 protein immunostaining but has a negligible or deleterious effect on other antigens.

MATERIALS

1. Poly-L-lysine, MW > 300,000 (Sigma, No. P1524), 0.1% in distilled water
2. Protease VIII (Sigma, No. P5255)
3. Pentyl acetate (Eastman Kodak, No. EKC2360), optional *(Be sure to use under the hood.)*
4. Parlodion, 0.5% (Mallinckrodt, No. 6552), 0.5 g in 100 mL pentyl acetate, optional
5. PBS (Appendix A–1)
6. 30% Hydrogen peroxide (Fisher, No. H325)
7. Normal goat serum (Dako, No. X907)

PROCEDURE

1. Precoat slides with poly-L-lysine (0.1% in distilled water) and allow to air-dry.
2. Cut paraffin-embedded tissue into 6 μm thick sections and place on poly-L-lysine-coated slides.
3. Place slides in 60 °C oven for at least one hour to cause sections to adhere to slides.
4. Rehydrate sections in xylene and graded alcohols to water.
5. Rinse in PBS.
6. Prepare 0.1% protease solution.
   a. Dissolve 0.05 g protease in 50 mL PBS.
   b. Heat to 37 °C.
7. Incubate slides in 0.1% protease at 37 °C for one minute.
8. Wash sections in distilled water.
9. Dehydrate in graded alcohols.
10. Block endogenous peroxidase by immersing slides for 30 minutes in a solution consisting of 6 mL of 30% hydrogen peroxide and 94 mL absolute methanol.
11. Wash briefly in distilled water and in modified PBS, 3 changes over 5 minutes.
12. Apply antibody, normal goat serum, diluted 1:20 in modified PBS for 30 to 60 minutes.

C–7. Pronase Digestion/*continued*

OPTION FOR NONADHERENT TISSUE OR RUSH CASES

1. Dilute 0.5% Parlodion solution in pentyl acetate to make a 0.05% solution. (Be sure to use pentyl acetate under the hood. Do *not* use ether alcohol.)
2. Dip slides into 0.05% Parlodion and allow to dry overnight (preferably for 3 days).
3. Cut unstained paraffin sections and float onto Parlodion-coated slides and allow to dry for 30 minutes at 56 °C before immunostaining.
4. If unstained sections are already cut, the section on the slide can be dipped into the 0.5% Parlodion and allowed to dry for 30 minutes at 56 °C before immunostaining.

C–8. ABC-PO: Rabbit Primary Antibodies

BACKGROUND

In our experience, the avidin-biotinylated peroxidase complex (ABC-PO) procedure has been the most reliable system for routine detection of most tissue antigens in paraffin sections.

MATERIALS

1. Primary rabbit antibodies at optimized dilutions (Table D–1)
2. Vectastain rabbit IgG ABC kit (Vector, No. PK 4001), consists of the following
   a. Biotinylated goat anti-rabbit IgG
   b. Avidin DH
   c. Biotinylated peroxidase
3. Modified PBS (Appendix A–2)
4. Acetate buffer, 0.02 M, pH 5.2 (Appendix A–3)
5. 3-Amino-9-ethylcarbazole (AEC; Sigma IsoPac, No. A5754)
6. *N,N*-dimethylformamide (Baker, No. 9221-1)
7. 30% Hydrogen peroxide (Fisher, No. H325)
8. Normal goat serum (Dako, No. X907)
9. Preimmune or normal rabbit serum, preferably IgG purified fraction (Dako, No. X903)
10. Aquamount (Lerner through American Scientific Products, No. M7644-1)

PROCEDURE

1. Fix tissue 1 to 2 mm thick in ample volumes of the fixative chosen for the antigen (see Table 3–1 for recommended fixatives).
2. Cut paraffin sections 4 to 6 μm thick.
3. Place 2 sections per slide on each slide and dry in a 60 °C oven until immunostaining is to be performed.
4. Deparaffinize slides in 2 changes of xylene and 2 changes of absolute alcohol.
5. Block endogenous peroxidase by immersing slides for 30 minutes in a solution consisting of 6 mL of 30% hydrogen peroxide and 94 mL absolute methanol.
6. Wash briefly in distilled water and in modified PBS, 3 changes over 5 minutes.
7. Apply blocking normal goat serum, diluted 1:20 in modified PBS, for 30 to 60 minutes to all sections, using either flat slide incubation or immersion.
8. Preform ABC-PO reagent from kit.
   a. Combine 20 μL avidin DH (reagent A), 20 μL biotinylated peroxidase (reagent B), and 1.6 mL modified PBS.
   b. Allow to stand at room temperature for at least 30 minutes before use.
9. Apply primary rabbit antibody to the left tissue section and normal control rabbit IgG to the right tissue section.
   a. Immunoglobulin concentration should approximate the concentration of the primary antibody.
   b. If several primary antibodies are used, the protein concentration of normal control rabbit IgG should be the same as that of the antibody used in the *highest* concentration.
10. Incubate for 30 minutes in a humidified chamber at room temperature.
11. Wash in modified PBS, 3 changes over 5 minutes.
12. Apply biotinylated affinity-purified goat anti-rabbit IgG (diluted 1:400 in modified PBS) to both tissue sections on each slide, and incubate for 30 minutes.
13. Wash in modified PBS, 3 changes over 5 minutes.

C–8. ABC-PO: Rabbit Primary Antibodies/*continued*

14. Incubate in preformed ABC reagent for 30 minutes.
15. Wash in modified PBS, 3 changes over 5 minutes.
16. Develop the colored reaction product with AEC as follows.
    a. Observe precautions for AEC (Appendix B–1).
    b. Dissolve 25 mg AEC in 10 mL dimethylformamide.
    c. Add 100 mL of 0.02 M acetate buffer (pH 5.2).
    d. Add 40 μL of 30% hydrogen peroxide.
    e. Incubate slides for 10 minutes.
17. Wash in modified PBS for 5 minutes.
18. Wash with tap water.
19. Counterstain in Mayer's hematoxylin for 10 minutes. For antibody systems directed against nuclear antibodies (such as HBcAg), stain one slide with hematoxylin and do not counterstain the other slide.
20. Wash in tap water for 5 minutes.
21. Do *not* dehydrate in alcohols.
22. Apply a coverslip with Aquamount.
23. Seal the edges of the coverslip with nail polish and label the slides.

REFERENCE

Hsu SM, Raine L, Fanger H: A comparative study of the PAP method and avidin-biotin-complex method for studying polypeptide hormones with radioimmunoassay antibodies. *Am J Clin Pathol* 1981;75:734–738.

C–9. ABC-PO: Goat Primary Antibodies

BACKGROUND

Although most of the primary antibodies used for diagnostic immunohistochemistry are produced in rabbits or mice, a few are derived from goats (eg, HBsAg). The procedure is essentially the same as that for rabbit primary antibodies (Appendix C–8) with a few changes in reagents.

MATERIALS

1. Goat antibodies at optimized dilutions (Table 3–1)
2. Vectastain goat IgG ABC kit (Vector, No. PK 4005), consists of the following
   a. Biotinylated rabbit anti-goat IgG
   b. Avidin DH
   c. Biotinylated peroxidase
3. Modified PBS (Appendix A–2)
4. Acetate buffer, 0.02 M, pH 5.2 (Appendix A–3)
5. 3-Amino-9-ethylcarbazole (AEC; Sigma IsoPak, No. A5754)
6. *N,N*-dimethylformamide (Baker, No. 9221-1)
7. 30% Hydrogen peroxide (Fisher, No. H325)
8. Normal rabbit serum (Dako, No. X902)
9. IgG fraction of preimmune or normal goat serum (Jackson, No. 005-0004)
10. Aquamount (Lerner through American Scientific Products, No. M7644-1)

PROCEDURE

1. Fix tissue 1 to 2 mm thick in ample volumes of the fixative chosen for the antigen (see Table 3–1 for recommended fixatives).
2. Cut paraffin sections 4 to 6 μm thick.
3. Place 2 sections per slide on each slide and dry in a 60 °C oven until immunostaining is to be performed.
4. Deparaffinize slides in 2 changes of xylene and 2 changes of absolute alcohol.
5. Block endogenous peroxidase by immersing slides for 30 minutes in a solution consisting of 6 mL of 30% hydrogen peroxide and 94 mL absolute methanol.
6. Wash briefly in distilled water and in modified PBS, 3 changes over 5 minutes.
7. Apply blocking normal rabbit serum, diluted 1:20 in modified PBS, for 30 to 60 minutes using either flat slide or immersion method.
8. Preform ABC-PO reagent from kit.
   a. Combine 20 μL avidin DH (reagent A), 20 μL biotinylated peroxidase (reagent B), and 1.6 mL modified PBS.
   b. Allow to stand at room temperature for at least 30 minutes before use.
9. Apply goat primary antibody to the left tissue section and equivalently diluted normal goat IgG to the right tissue section.
   a. Immunoglobulin concentration of normal goat IgG should approximate the concentration of the primary goat antibody.
   b. If several primary antibodies are used, the protein concentration of normal goat IgG should be the same as that of the antibody used in the *highest* concentration.
10. Incubate for 30 minutes in a humidified chamber at room temperature.
11. Wash in modified PBS, 3 changes over 5 minutes.
12. Apply biotinylated affinity-purified rabbit anti-goat IgG (diluted 1:400 in modified PBS) to both tissue sections on each slide and incubate for 30 minutes in a humidified chamber room temperature.
13. Wash in modified PBS, 3 changes over 5 minutes.
14. Incubate in preformed ABC reagent for 30 minutes.
15. Wash in modified PBS, 3 changes over 5 minutes.

C–9. ABC-PO: Goat Primary Antibodies/*continued*

16. Develop the colored reaction product with AEC as follows.
    a. Observe precautions for AEC (Appendix B–1).
    b. Dissolve 25 mg AEC in 10 mL dimethylformamide.
    c. Add 100 mL of 0.02 M acetate buffer (pH 5.2).
    d. Add 40 μL of 30% hydrogen peroxide.
    e. Incubate slides for 20 minutes.
17. Wash in modified PBS for 5 minutes.
18. Wash with tap water.
19. Counterstain in Lerner's hematoxylin for 2 to 5 minutes.
20. Wash in tap water for 5 minutes.
21. Do *not* dehydrate in alcohols.
22. Apply a coverslip with Aquamount.
23. Seal the edges of the coverslip with nail polish and label the slides.

REFERENCE

Hsu SM, Raine L, Fanger H: A comparative study of the PAP method and avidin-biotin-complex method for studying polypeptide hormones with radioimmunoassay antibodies. *Am J Clin Pathol* 1981;75:734–738.

C–10. Avidin-Biotinylated Alkaline Phosphatase Complex (ABC-AP)

BACKGROUND

The avidin-biotinylated alkaline phosphatase (ABC-AP) procedure can be used to evaluate antigens expressed in tissues containing large amounts of endogenous peroxidase or pseudoperoxidases, especially in tissues such as peripheral blood, where pretreatment with methanolic hydrogen peroxide destroys morphologic detail. The use of levamisole inhibits all the isoenzymes of alkaline phosphatase except for the intestinal form. In addition to the ABC-AP procedure, an indirect option is provided. An enzyme-antienzyme alkaline phosphatase–antialkaline phosphatase (APAAP) method has also been described (Erber et al).

MATERIALS

1. Primary mouse antibodies at optimized dilutions (Table D–2)
2. ABC-AP kit (Vector, special order)
   a. Alternative 1: Alkaline phosphatase–avidin D (Vector, No. A-2100)
   b. Alternative 2: Streptavidin–alkaline phosphatase (Enzo, No. EBP-822-2)
3. Tris buffer, pH 8.2 (Appendix A–5)
4. Alkaline phosphatase–conjugated rabbit anti-mouse IgG (Dako, No. D314), diluted 1:20, for indirect procedure
5. Modified PBS (Appendix A–2)
6. Alkaline phosphatase chromogenic substrate (Appendix B–3)
   a. Alternative: substrates from Vector kit
7. Biotinylated affinity-purified horse anti-mouse IgG (from Vector kit), diluted 1:200
8. Levamisole (Sigma, No. L-9756)
9. Acetone, reagent grade
10. Aquamount (Lerner through American Scientific Products, No. M7644-1)

PROCEDURE

1. Fix frozen tissue sections in reagent-grade acetone for 10 minutes and allow to air-dry.
2. Cut paraffin sections 4 to 6 μm thick.
3. Place 2 sections per slide on each of 2 slides and dry in a 60 °C oven until immunostaining is to be performed.
4. Deparaffinize slides in 2 changes of xylene and 2 changes of absolute alcohol.
5. Wash in modified PBS.
6. Incubate with appropriately diluted mouse monoclonal antibody for 30 minutes in a humidified chamber at room temperature.
7. Preform the ABC-AP reagent from kit.
   a. Combine 20 μL avidin DH, 20 μL biotinylated alkaline phosphatase, and 1.6 mL Tris buffer (pH 8.2).
   b. Allow to stand at room temperature for at least 30 minutes.
8. Wash in modified PBS, 3 changes over 5 minutes.
9. Apply biotinylated horse anti-mouse IgG (diluted 1:200 in modified PBS), and incubate for 30 minutes in a humidified chamber at room temperature. The indirect option can be used at this point. See "Indirect Option" on page 155.
10. Wash in PBS, 3 changes over 5 minutes.
11. Apply preformed ABC-AP reagent or streptavidin-alkaline phosphatase (10 μL per section, undiluted), and incubate for 30 minutes in a humidified chamber at room temperature.
12. Wash in modified PBS, 3 changes over 5 minutes.

C–10. Avidin-Biotinylated Alkaline Phosphatase Complex (ABC-AP)/*continued*

13. Develop the alkaline phosphatase substrate-chromogen colored reaction product as follows.
    a. Warm the alkaline phosphatase chromogenic substrate to 37 °C.
    b. Immerse slides.
    c. Incubate slides for 5 to 15 minutes at 37 °C (monitor positive control slide for optimum result).
14. Wash briefly in modified PBS.
15. Counterstain with hematoxylin (no alcohol).
16. Do *not* dehydrate in alcohols.
17. Apply a coverslip with Aquamount.
18. Seal the edges of the coverslip with nail polish and label the slides.

INDIRECT OPTION

1. Follow steps 1 through 8.
2. Add alkaline phosphatase–conjugated rabbit anti-mouse IgG (diluted 1:20 in Tris buffer [pH 8.2]) to the slide surface.
3. Incubate for 30 minutes in a humidified chamber at room temperature.
4. Wash with modified PBS.
5. Proceed with the development of the alkaline phosphatase chromogenic substrate (step 13).

REFERENCES

Erber WN, Pinching AJ, Mason DY: Immunocytochemical detection of T and B cell populations in routine blood smears. *Lancet* 1984;1:1042–1046.

Hsu SM, Raine L, Fanger H: A comparative study of the PAP method and avidin-biotin-complex method for studying polypeptide hormones with radioimmunoassay antibodies. *Am J Clin Pathol* 1981;75:734–738.

C–11. Multilabel Immunohistology

BACKGROUND

On rare occasions, it may be desirable to perform double-label or triple-label immunohistologic staining. In theory, more than three labels could be used simultaneously, but practical applications for such procedures are quite limited. It is very difficult to generalize about a multilabel procedure. Thus, a specific example is used. Obviously, by interchanging primary antibodies and enzyme labels, other multilabeled preparations can be made.

In multilabeling, it is important to shorten the time intervals involved, and this requires changing reagent dilutions. This protocol outlines one specific multilabel application. Other applications can be developed based on this example.

MATERIALS

1. Primary antibodies
   a. Rabbit antiglucagon, diluted 1:100
   b. Rabbit antisomatostatin, diluted 1:500
   c. Guinea pig anti-insulin, diluted 1:1,000
2. Vectastain rabbit IgG ABC-PO kit (Vector, No. PK 4001)
3. Alkaline phosphatase–avidin D (Vector, No. A-2100)
   a. Alternative: Streptavidin–alkaline phosphatase (Enzo, No. EBP-822-2)
4. Modified PBS (Appendix A–2)
5. Hanker-Yates reagent (HYR; Polysciences, No. 8661)
6. Tris HCl, pH 7.6 (Appendix A–4)
7. 30% Hydrogen peroxide (Fisher, No. H325)
8. Tris buffer, pH 8.2 (Appendix A–5)
9. Hydrochloric acid, 1 N
10. Normal goat serum (Dako, No. X501)
11. IgG fraction of normal rabbit serum (Dako, No. X903)
12. IgG fraction of guinea pig serum (Cappel, No. 6007-0080)
13. Normal rabbit serum (Dako, No. X902)
14. Naphthol ASTR (Sigma, No. 6125)
15. *N,N*-dimethylformamide (Baker, No. 9221-1)
16. Fast red K salt (Sigma, No. 8379)
17. Fast blue (substrate III from ABC-AP kit, Vector, special order)
18. Aquamount (Lerner through American Scientific Products, No. M7644-1)

PROCEDURE

1. Fix tissue 1 to 2 mm thick in ample volumes of the fixative chosen for the antigens (in this instance, Bouin's or Hollande's).
2. Cut paraffin sections 4 μm thick.
3. Place 2 sections per slide on each of 2 slides and dry in a 60 °C oven until immunostaining is to be performed.
4. Deparaffinize slides in 2 changes of xylene and 2 changes of absolute alcohol.
5. Block endogenous peroxidase by immersing slides for 30 minutes in a solution consisting of 6 mL of 30% hydrogen peroxide and 94 mL absolute methanol.
6. Wash briefly in distilled water and in modified PBS, 3 changes over 5 minutes.
7. Apply antibody, normal goat serum, diluted 1:20 in modified PBS, for 15 minutes.
8. Preform ABC-PO reagent from kit.
   a. Combine 20 μL avidin D (reagent A), 20 μL biotinylated peroxidase (reagent B), and 1.6 mL modified PBS.
   b. Allow to stand at room temperature for at least 30 minutes before use.

C–11. Multilabel Immunohistology/*continued*

9. Apply rabbit anti-glucagon (diluted 1:100 in modified PBS) to the left tissue section and equivalently diluted IgG fraction of normal rabbit serum to the right tissue section.
10. Incubate for 15 minutes in a humidified chamber at room temperature.
11. Wash in modified PBS, 3 changes over 5 minutes.
12. Apply biotinylated affinity-purified goat anti-rabbit IgG (diluted 1:200; notice that this is more concentrated than in the single label ABC-PO procedure) to both sections of tissue and incubate for 15 minutes.
13. Wash in modified PBS, 3 changes over 5 minutes.
14. Incubate in preformed ABC-PO reagent for 15 minutes.
15. Wash in modified PBS, 3 changes over 5 minutes.
16. Develop brown reaction product with HYR as in Appendix B–2.
17. Wash in modified PBS.
18. Incubate for 10 minutes in 1 N hydrochloric acid followed by washing in hot tap water.
19. Apply normal goat serum (diluted 1:20 in modified PBS), and incubate for 15 minutes.
20. Apply rabbit antisomatostatin (diluted 1:500 in modified PBS) to left tissue section and equivalently diluted IgG fraction of normal rabbit serum to the right tissue section.
21. Incubate for 15 minutes in a humidified chamber at room temperature.
22. Wash in modified PBS, 3 changes over 5 minutes.
23. Apply biotinylated affinity-purified goat anti-rabbit IgG (diluted 1:200).
24. Incubate in a humidified chamber at room temperature for 15 minutes.
25. Wash in modified PBS, 3 changes over 5 minutes.
26. Apply 10 μL of undiluted alkaline phosphatase–avidin D or of undiluted streptavidin–alkaline phosphatase to each section.
27. Incubate for 15 minutes.
28. Wash in modified PBS, 3 changes over 5 minutes.
29. Develop blue reaction product with fast blue as follows.
    a. Incubate slides in fast blue for 5 minutes.
30. Wash several times in modified PBS.
31. Incubate for 10 minutes in 1 N hydrochloric acid.
32. Wash in hot tap water, then wash several times in modified PBS.
33. Apply normal rabbit serum (diluted 1:20 in modified PBS), and incubate for 15 minutes.
34. Apply guinea pig anti-insulin (diluted 1:2,000 in modified PBS) to the left tissue section and equivalently diluted IgG fraction of normal guinea pig IgG to the right tissue section.
35. Incubate for 15 minutes at room temperature in a humidified chamber.
36. Wash in modified PBS, 3 changes over 5 minutes.
37. Apply biotinylated affinity-purified rabbit anti-guinea pig IgG (diluted 1:200 in modified PBS).
38. Incubate for 15 minutes in a humidified chamber at room temperature.
39. Wash in modified PBS, 3 changes over 5 minutes.
40. Apply 10 μL of undiluted alkaline phosphatase–avidin D or of undiluted streptavidin–alkaline phosphatase to each section.
41. Incubate for 15 minutes in a humidified chamber at room temperature.
42. Wash briefly in Tris buffer (pH 8.2).

(Continues on next page)

C–11. Multilabel Immunohistology/*continued*

43. Develop red reaction product with fast red as follows.
    a. Dissolve 10 mg naphthol ASTR and 50 mg fast red K salt in 2 mL dimethylformamide.
    b. Add 50 mL Tris buffer (pH 8.2).
    c. Incubate for 5 minutes at room temperature.
44. Wash briefly in PBS.
45. Do *not* counterstain with hematoxylin.
46. Apply a coverslip with Aquamount.
47. Seal the edges of the coverslip with nail polish and label the slides.

REFERENCES

Erber WN, Pinching AJ, Mason DY: Immunocytochemical detection of T and B cell populations in routine blood smears. *Lancet* 1984;1:1042–1046.

Hsu SM, Raine L, Fanger H: A comparative study of the PAP method and avidin-biotin-complex method for studying polypeptide hormones with radioimmunoassay antibodies. *Am J Clin Pathol* 1981;75:734–738.

Moir DJ, Ghosh AK, Abdulaziz Z, et al: Immunoenzymatic staining of haematological samples with monoclonal antibodies. *Br J Haematol* 1983;55:395–410.

C–12. Rapid ABC-PO

BACKGROUND

The extraordinary sensitivity of the ABC-PO method permits the use of a rapid modification of the procedure. This modification depends on the formation of all of the antibody and the enzyme-lectin complex components into a large macromolecular complex in fluid phase, while the tissue section is being prepared.

Sensitivity in this system is reduced. Primary antibodies must be used at much higher concentrations than are required for the conventional three-step ABC-PO procedure. However, since 5 μL from primary antibody stock are used for either the conventional or rapid method, the net effect on antibody consumption is unchanged.

Not all systems are amenable to the use of a rapid ABC-PO procedure. Each must be evaluated independently. For this reason, only an example is provided.

MATERIALS

1. Primary rabbit anti-human growth hormone (Dako, No. A570), final dilution will be 1:100 in the preformed complex in step 3b.
2. Vectastain rabbit ABC-PO kit (Vector, No. PK 4001)
3. Modified PBS (Appendix A–2)
4. 3-Amino-9-ethylcarbazole (AEC; Sigma IsoPac, No. A5754)
5. *N,N*-dimethylformamide (Baker, No. 9221-1)
6. Acetate buffer, 0.02 M, pH 5.2 (Appendix A–3)
7. 30% Hydrogen peroxide (Fisher, No. H325)
8. Aquamount (Lerner through American Scientific Products No. M7644-1)

PROCEDURE

1. Cut paraffin sections 4 to 6 μm thick.
2. Place 2 sections on each of 2 slides and dry in a 60 °C oven until immunostaining is to be performed.
3. Preform macromolecular staining complex as follows:
   a. Preform ABC-PO reagent by adding 10 μL of avidin DH (reagent A) and 10 μL of biotinylated peroxidase (reagent B) to 1,000 μL of modified PBS. Incubate for 5 minutes at room temperature.
   b. Add 5 μL biotinylated anti-rabbit IgG and 10 μL of rabbit anti-growth hormone to the ABC-PO reagent. Incubate at room temperature for 15 minutes. Steps 4 and 5 below can be done during this 15-minute incubation.
4. Deparaffinize slides in 2 changes of xylene and 2 changes of absolute alcohol.
5. Wash in modified PBS.
6. Incubate with macromolecular complex (formed in step 3b) for 15 minutes in a humidified chamber at room temperature.
7. Wash in modified PBS, 3 changes over 5 minutes.
8. Develop the colored reaction product with AEC as follows.
   a. Observe precautions for AEC (Appendix B–1).
   b. Dissolve 25 mg AEC in 10 mL of dimethylformamide.
   c. Add 100 mL of 0.02 M acetate buffer (pH 5.2).
   d. Add 40 μl of 30% hydrogen peroxide.
   e. Incubate slides for 10 minutes at room temperature.

(Continues on next page)

C–12. Rapid ABC-PO/*continued*

9. Wash in modified PBS for 5 minutes, making several changes.
10. Counterstain with fresh hematoxylin (no alcohol).
11. Do *not* dehydrate in alcohols.
12. Apply a coverslip with Aquamount.
13. Seal edges of the coverslip with nail polish and label the slides.

REFERENCE

Lloyd RV, Schmidt K, Blaivas L, et al: A rapid immunostaining method utilizing preformed antibody-avidin-biotin-peroxidase complexes. *Am J Clin Pathol* 1985;83:636-639.

D Antibody Dilutions and Detection Systems

In Appendix D, dilutions of rabbit, goat, and mouse primary antibodies are summarized in Tables D–1, D–2, and D–3, with the commercial source and order numbers supplied for each antigen. Table D–4 summarizes the available detection systems that have been referred to in the previous chapters, their commercial sources, and their order numbers. Additional information on the suppliers appears in Appendix E.

Upon receipt, primary antibodies should be dated with a one-year expiration date. However, shelf life is best determined by antibody performance in immunostaining control tissues.

Dilutions of primary antibodies can best be made by removing 5 μL aliquots from the primary antibody stock solution. Then dilute the 5 μL aliquot in the diluent buffer to the appropriate final concentration.

TABLE D–1. Rabbit Polyclonal Primary Antibodies

Antigen	Approximate Working Dilution[a]	Commercial Source	Order No.
Serotonin	1:1,200	Immunonuclear	43H2T
Glucagon	1:4,500	Dako	A565
Somatostatin	1:1,000	Dako	A566
Gastrin	1:2,500	Dako	A568
Vasoactive intestinal polypeptide (VIP)	1:1,000	Immunonuclear	39H2T
Enolase	1:1,000	Dako	A589
Growth hormone (GH)	1:1,200	Dako	A570
Prolactin	1:1,200	Dako	A569
Luteinizing hormone	1:1,500	Dako	A572
Follicle-stimulating hormone (FSH)	1:1,200	Dako	A573
Thyroid-stimulating hormone (TSH)	1:2,000	Dako	A574
Adrenocorticotropic hormone (ACTH)	1:2,000	Dako	A571
Thyroglobulin	1:4,500	Dako	A251
Calcitonin	1:2,500	Dako	A576
Cytokeratins	1:800	Dako	
Carcinoembryonic antigen (CEA)	1:2,000	Dako	A115
α-Fetoprotein	1:800	Dako	A008
β-Subunit of human chorionic gonadotropin (β-HCG)	1:1,200	Dako	A231
Placental lactogen (HPL)	1:1,000	Dako	A137
Hepatitis-B core antigen (HBcAg)	1:800	Dako	B586
Factor VIII	1:800	Dako	A082
Muramidase (lysozyme)	1:1,000	Dako	A099
Myoglobin	1:2,000	Dako	A578
α-1-Antitrypsin	1:2,000	Dako	A012
α-1-Chymotrypsin	1:1,200	Dako	A022
Glial fibrillary acidic protein (GFAP)	1:400	Dako	A561
S-100 protein	1:1,000	Dako	Z311
Prostate-specific antigen (PSA)	1:3,000	Dako	A562
Prostatic acid phosphatase	1:5[b]	Immulok	583015
IgG fraction, normal rabbit serum	Variable	Dako	X903

[a]These are approximate dilutions for the rabbit ABC-PO and indirect immunoperoxidase systems. Each lot should be tested and optimized.

[b]1:5 dilution of prediluted commercial stock.

TABLE D–2. Mouse Monoclonal Primary Antibodies for Frozen Tissue Sections

Antigen	Approximate Working Dilution[a]	Commercial Source	Order No.
Hematopoietic			
T1	No dilution	Dako	M705
Leu-1	1:15	Becton-Dickinson	6300
T3	No dilution	Coulter	6602331
Leu-4	1:10	Becton-Dickinson	7340
Leu-9	1:15	Becton-Dickinson	7480
T4/OKT4	1:10[b]	Coulter or Ortho	6602309 or 7042
Leu-3a/Leu-3b	1:5[b]	Becton-Dickinson	6320
T8	1:50	Coulter	6602310
Leu-2a/Leu-2b	1:10[b]	Becton-Dickinson	2G7350
Leu-15	1:10	Becton-Dickinson	7557
T6	1:50	Coulter	6602323
T9	1:40	Ortho	7092
T10	1:50	Ortho	7102
Leu-8	1:10	Becton-Dickinson	7440
T11	1:40	Coulter	6602308
Leu-10	1:15	Becton-Dickinson	7450
Leu-14	No dilution	Becton-Dickinson	7570
B1	1:5	Coulter	6602311
B2	1:5	Coulter	6602324
J5	1:30	Coulter	6602314
CALLA	1:15	Becton-Dickinson	7500
LN1, LN2, LN3	No dilution	Diamedex	LN1, LN2, LN3
I2	1:20	Coulter	6602313
CLA	1:10	Dako	M701
Leu-7	1:15	Becton-Dickinson	7390
Leu-11a	1:15	Becton-Dickinson	7530
Leu-M1	1:5	Becton-Dickinson	7420
Other			
Blood group A	1:3	Dako	A581
Blood group B	1:3	Dako	A582
Blood group H	1:3	Dako	A583
AE1/3	1:80	Hybritech (Boehringer Mannheim)	0702
Desmin	1:100	Oncogene Science	Desmin Ab-1
PKK-1	1:30	Labsystems	6400 200
Uro-2 through Uro-5	1:10	Cambridge Research	Uro-2 through Uro-5
Melanoma antibody	1:10	Biogenex	HPO 1-20

NOTE: Frozen tissue sections are preferred, except in the following cases: for blood group antibodies, fixation in absolute alcohol is preferred; for LN1, LN2, LN3, fixation in B-5 or Bouin's fixative is preferred; for AE1/3, frozen sections or pronase-digested paraffin sections of formalin-fixed tissue are preferred.

[a]These are approximate dilutions for the ABC-PO (mouse IgG Vectastain) and indirect immunoperoxidase systems. Each lot should be tested and optimized.

[b]Use a multiclonal preparation, both antibodies in the same volume, eg, 5 μL Coulter T4, 5 μL OKT4, and 40 μL buffer.

TABLE D–3. Other Primary Antibodies and Biotinylated Reagents

Reagent	Approximate Working Dilution[a]	Commercial Source	Order No.
Biotinylated viral nucleotide probes (in situ hybridization)	No dilution	Enzo	Various
Hepatitis-B surface antigen (goat)	1:20	Immulok (Ortho)	587015
Insulin (guinea pig)	1:1,000	Dako	A564
IgG fraction, normal goat serum	Variable[b]	Jackson	005-0004
IgG fraction, normal guinea pig serum	Variable[b]	Jackson	006-0003
Estrogen receptor protein (rat monoclonal)	None	Abbott Diagnostics	PAP kit, special order
Oncogene encoded proteins (rat monoclonal)	Varies	Oncogene Science	OPO1, OPO2, others

[a]These are approximate dilutions for the ABC-PO (Vectastain) systems. Dilutions must be optimized for each primary antibody lot.

[b]Concentration of nonimmune (preimmune IgG) for negative control should be equivalent to the highest concentration of primary antibody used.

TABLE D–4. Detection Systems

Detection System	Commercial Source	Order No.
Biotin-avidin systems		
Peroxidase		
Vectastain rabbit IgG	Vector	PK4001
Vectastain mouse IgG	Vector	PK4002
Vectastain goat IgG	Vector	PK4005
Vectastain guinea pig IgG	Vector	PK4007
Vectastain rat IgG	Vector	PK4004
Alkaline phosphatase–avidin D	Vector	A2100
Streptavidin–alkaline phosphatase	Enzo	EBP-822-2
Glucose oxidase (standard kit)	Vector	OK3000
Enzyme-antienzyme systems		
Rabbit peroxidase–antiperoxidase	Dako	Z113
Goat peroxidase–antiperoxidase	Dako	B157
Mouse peroxidase–antiperoxidase	Dako	B650
Mouse alkaline phosphatase–antialkaline phosphatase	Dako	Z651
Labeled secondary antibodies		
Peroxidase rabbit anti-mouse Ig (1:60)[a]	Dako	P161
Alkaline phosphatase rabbit anti-mouse Ig (1:20)[a]	Dako	D314
Chromogens/substrates/solubilizers		
Aminoethylcarbazole	Sigma IsoPac	A5754
Hanker-Yates reagent	Polysciences	8661
30% Hydrogen peroxide	Fisher	H325
N,N-dimethylformamide	Baker	9221-1
Fast red K salt	Sigma	8379
Fast blue BBN	Sigma	F0125
Naphthol ASTR	Sigma	6125
Levamisole	Sigma	L-9756

NOTE: The detection systems listed in this table are for procedures used in this atlas.

[a]Approximate dilution; test each lot.

E Sources for Reagents

Abbott Laboratories
Diagnostics Division
Abbott Park, Dept 49B
North Chicago, IL 60064
(312) 937-2163

American Scientific Products
1430 Waukegan Road
McGaw Park, IL 60085
(312) 689-8410

JT Baker Chemical Company
222 Red School Lane
Phillipsburg, NJ 08865
See American Scientific Products

BBL Microbiology Systems
PO Box 243
Cockeysville, Maryland
See American Scientific Products

Becton-Dickinson
PO Box 7375
Mountain View, CA 94039
(800) 223-8226

Biogenex
6529 Sierra Lane
Dublin, CA 94568
(800) 421-4149

Cambridge Research Labsystems
195 Albany Street
Cambridge, MA 02139
(617) 491-2300

Cappel-Worthington
(Cooper Biomedical, Inc)
One Technology Court
Malvern, PA 19355
(800) 523-7620

Coulter Electronics, Inc
Immunology Division
440 West 20 Street
Hialeah, FL 33010
(800) 327-3778

Dako Corporation
22 North Milpas Street
Santa Barbara, CA 93101
(800) 235-5743

Diamedex
3301 South Harbor Boulevard
Santa Ana, CA 92704
(714) 241-9854

Eastman Kodak Company
343 State Street
Rochester, NY 14650
(716) 724-4000

Enzo Biochem, Inc
325 Hudson Street
New York, NY 10013
(800) 221-7705

Fisher Scientific Company
585 Alpha Drive
Pittsburgh, PA 15238
(412) 784-2600

Hybritech, Inc
(Boehringer Mannheim Diagnostics)
7941 Castleway Drive
Indianapolis, IN 46250
(800) 428-5433

Immulok
(800) 235-6963
See Ortho Diagnostic Systems

Immunonuclear Corporation
PO Box 285
Stillwater, MN 55082
(800) 328-1482

Jackson Immuno Research
PO Box 683
Avondale, PA 19311
(215) 268-3601

Labsystems
PO Box 48723
Chicago, IL 60648
(312) 967-5220

Lerner Laboratories
17 James Street
New Haven, CT 06513
See American Scientific Products

Linscott's Directory
(a comprehensive compendium of commercially available reagents)
40 Glen Drive
Mill Valley, CA 94941
(415) 681-3344

Mallinckrodt, Inc
675 McDonnell Boulevard
St Louis, MO 63134
(314) 895-2402

Oncogene Science, Inc
222 Station Plaza North
Mineola, NY 11501
(800) ONC-2616, or
(516) 877-2882

Ortho Diagnostic Systems
Route 202
Raritan, NJ 08869
(800) 631-5807

Polysciences, Inc
PO Box 697
Warrington, PA 18976
(800) 523-2575

Sigma Chemical Company
PO Box 14508
St Louis, MO 63178
(800) 325-3010

Tago, Inc
PO Box 4463
887 Mitten Road
Burlingame, CA 94010
(415) 692-4015

Vector Laboratories
1429 Rollins Road
Burlingame, CA 94010
(415) 348-3737

Guide to Optional Slide Set

SLIDE 1
Anti–glomerular basement membrane disease. Diffuse generalized deposits of IgG (brown) in the glomerular basement membrane can be simultaneously correlated with a cellular extracapillary crescent occupying the urinary space (IMPAS with DAB, hematoxylin counterstain). *Figure 2–1.*

SLIDE 2
Systemic lupus erythematosus nephritis with cellular crescents. Generalized deposits of C3 (HYR, brown) in a glomerulus and a tubular epithelial cell containing cytokeratins (AEC, red) are visible. The glomerular crescent is negative for AE1/3 (for C3: direct IMP with HYR; for AE1/3: ABC-PO with AEC, hematoxylin counterstain). *Figure 2–4.*

SLIDE 3
Pancreatic islet cells with triple-label. Glucagon (brown; ABC-PO with DAB), somatostatin (blue; ABC-AP with fast blue), and insulin (red; ABC-AP with fast red) are simultaneously visible (no counterstain). *Figure 2–13.*

SLIDE 4
Indirect immunoperoxidase technique. *Figure 2–16.*

SLIDE 5
Unlabeled peroxidase-antiperoxidase (PAP) technique. *Figure 2–18.*

SLIDE 6
Avidin-biotinylated peroxidase complex (ABC-PO) immunoperoxidase technique. *Figure 2–21.*

SLIDE 7
Avidin-biotin flush technique. This flush technique is used to mask endogenous biotin. The tissue section is first exposed to excess avidin and then to biotin, a process that renders the endogenous biotin unavailable for binding to the ABC. *Figure 3–2.*

SLIDE 8
Working controls: tissue control slide. *Table 3–2.*

SLIDE 9
Working controls: test slide from patient's tissue. *Table 3–3.*

SLIDE 10
Pancreatic islet cells show immunoreactive insulin (red) in the beta cells (ABC-PO with AEC, hematoxylin counterstain). *Figure 4–1.*

SLIDE 11
Pancreatic islet cells show two antigens simultaneously, insulin and glucagon, by use of two chromogens. In the more numerous and centrally located beta cells, the insulin stains red (ABC-PO with AEC). In the less numerous and peripherally located alpha cells, the glucagon stains brown-black (ABC-PO with DAB, hematoxylin counterstain). Reproduced with permission from *Cleve Clin Q* 1981;48:258. *Figure 4–2.*

SLIDE 12
Pancreatic islet. Alpha cells, which contain immunoreactive glucagon (red), are present in lesser numbers than the beta cells (ABC-PO with AEC, hematoxylin counterstain). *Figure 4–3.*

SLIDE 13
Pancreatic islet. Somatostatin (red) is visible in the delta cells (ABC-PO with AEC, hematoxylin counterstain). *Figure 4–4.*

SLIDE 14
Gastric antrum control for gastrin. Occasional G-cells stain red (ABC-PO with AEC, hematoxylin counterstain). *Figure 4–5.*

SLIDE 15
Islet cell tumor. Immunoreactive vasoactive intestinal polypeptide (red) is visible in almost all the cells (ABC-PO with AEC, hematoxylin counterstain). *Figure 4–7.*

SLIDE 16
Normal pituitary gland used as a control for ACTH (red-brown; ABC-PO with AEC, hematoxylin counterstain). *Figure 4–11.*

SLIDE 17
Thyroid C-cell hyperplasia used as a positive (red) calcitonin control (ABC-PO with AEC, hematoxylin counterstain). *Figure 4–16.*

SLIDE 18
Metastatic papillary carcinoma in a lymph node stained for thyroglobulin. The positive reaction (red) establishes that this tumor originated from the thyroid. As with other endocrine neoplasia, not all cells stain positively (ABC-PO with AEC, hematoxylin counterstain). *Figure 4–18.*

SLIDE 19
Medullary thyroid carcinoma metastatic to liver. Staining the tumor tissue for immunoreactive calcitonin (red) establishes this tumor as metastatic medullary thyroid carcinoma (ABC-PO with AEC, hematoxylin counterstain). *Figure 4–20.*

SLIDE 20
Carcinoid tumor arising in an immature coccygeal teratoma. The tumor cells contain serotonin (red; ABC-PO with AEC, hematoxylin counterstain). *Figure 4–23.*

SLIDE 21
Processing protocol for lymph node biopsy specimens. Source: *Semin Diagn Pathol* 1984;1:273, used with permission. Note: Frozen tissue can also be used for gene rearrangement studies. *Figure 5–3.*

SLIDE 22
Tonsil immunostained for IgM (red). Both follicle center cells and the mantle zone lymphocytes are positive (direct IMP with AEC, no counterstain). *Figure 5–4.*

SLIDE 23
Tonsil immunostained for IgD (red). Positive cells are confined to the follicle mantle zones (direct IMP with AEC, no counterstain). *Figure 5–5.*

SLIDE 24
Tonsil immunostained for κ light chains (direct IMP in a frozen section, hematoxylin counterstain). *Figure 5–8.*

SLIDE 25
Tonsil immunostained for λ light chains (direct IMP in a frozen section, hematoxylin counterstain). *Figure 5–9.*

SLIDE 26
Follicular hyperplasia of lymph node. Distribution of a broadly expressed T-cell antigen, Leu-1 (red), is illustrated (ABC-PO with AEC, hematoxylin counterstain). *Figure 5–11.*

SLIDE 27
Tonsil immunostained for the T-cell differentiation antigen, T6. Lymphoid cells are not stained, but Langerhan's cells associated with tonsillar epithelium (arrow) are positive (red; ABC-PO with AEC in a frozen section, hematoxylin counterstain). *Figure 5–14.*

SLIDE 28
Tonsil immunostained for the T-cell differentiation antigen, T4. The T-cell germinal center subpopulation is predominantly $T4^+$ (red). Compare this figure with Slides 26 and 29 (ABC-PO with AEC in a frozen section, hematoxylin counterstain). *Figure 5–15.*

SLIDE 29
Tonsil immunostained for the T-cell differentiation antigen, T8. Positive cells (red) are essentially restricted to interfollicular zones (ABC-PO with AEC in a frozen section, hematoxylin counterstain). *Figure 5–16.*

SLIDE 30
Spleen immunostained for the T-cell differentiation antigen, T8. The sinusoidal endothelium is positive (ABC-PO with AEC, hematoxylin counterstain). *Figure 5–17.*

SLIDE 31
Follicular hyperplasia of lymph node immunostained for the B-cell differentiation antigen, Leu-14 (red). Both germinal centers and mantle zones are positive (ABC-PO with AEC, hematoxylin counterstain). *Figure 5–19.*

SLIDE 32
Spleen immunostained for the B-cell differentiation antigen, LN2. The germinal center and mantle zone lymphocytes stain positively, but the periarteriolar sheaths are negative (ABC-PO with AEC in a paraffin section of tissue fixed in B-5, hematoxylin counterstain). *Figure 5–21.*

SLIDE 33
Follicular large cell lymphoma. Slides 33 and 34 are from the same case. Here, the κ light chains are immunostained in the large atypical cells (direct IMP with AEC in a cytocentrifuge preparation, hematoxylin counterstain). *Figure 5–23.*

SLIDE 34
Follicular large cell lymphoma. This figure shows that the atypical large cell population is negative for λ light chains (direct IMP with AEC in a cytocentrifuge preparation, hematoxylin counterstain). *Figure 5–24.*

SLIDE 35
Follicular predominantly small cleaved cell lymphoma, with the immunotype $\kappa^+ \lambda^-$. Slides 35 through 38 are from the same case. Here, the neoplastic follicles stain positively for κ light chains (direct IMP with AEC in a frozen section, no counterstain). *Figure 5–28.*

SLIDE 36
Follicular predominantly small cleaved cell lymphoma. Neoplastic follicles do not stain for λ light chains (direct IMP with AEC in a frozen section, no counterstain). *Figure 5–29.*

SLIDE 37
Follicular predominantly small cleaved cell lymphoma. Use of Leu-1 shows T-cells concentrated at the periphery of the neoplastic nodules and in interfollicular areas. Some T-cells infiltrate the neoplastic follicles, but most lie outside, as in this figure (ABC-PO with AEC, hematoxylin counterstain). *Figure 5–30.*

SLIDE 38
Follicular predominantly small cleaved cell lymphoma. Neoplastic follicles are positive for the differentiation antigen, B1 (ABC-PO with AEC, biotinylated primary modification, in a frozen section, hematoxylin counterstain). *Figure 5–32.*

SLIDE 39
Small noncleaved cell lymphoma. Slides 39 through 41 are from the same case. This section is stained for κ light chains. The nonspecific adherence to capillary walls (arrows) is apparent. Similar adherence to collagen occurs in other sites, eg, skin, desmoplastic large cell lymphomas (direct IMP with AEC in a frozen section, no counterstain). *Figure 5–34.*

SLIDE 40
Small noncleaved cell lymphoma. This section is stained for λ light chains. Each individual cell stained positively (direct IMP with AEC in a frozen section, no counterstain). *Figure 5–35.*

SLIDE 41
Small noncleaved cell lymphoma. When stained with B1 differentiation antigen, the cells are diffusely positive (ABC-PO with AEC, biotinylated primary modification, in a frozen section, hematoxylin counterstain). *Figure 5–37.*

SLIDE 42
Small noncleaved cell lymphoma. Slides 42 and 43 are from the same case. Here, the rare, nonnucleolated small lymphocytes are positive (red) for κ light chains. The nucleolated tumor cells are negative (direct IMP with AEC in a cytocentrifuge preparation, hematoxylin counterstain). *Figure 5–38.*

SLIDE 43
Small noncleaved cell lymphoma. This section is stained for λ light chains (red). The nucleolated tumor cells are positive (direct IMP with AEC, hematoxylin counterstain). *Figure 5–39.*

SLIDE 44
Lymphoblastic (convoluted cell) lymphoma. Slides 44 through 47 are from the same case. When immunostained for the T-cell antigen, Leu-1, the atypical convoluted cells are positive (ABC-PO with AEC in a cytocentrifuge preparation, hematoxylin counterstain). *Figure 5–41.*

SLIDE 45
Lymphoblastic (convoluted cell) lymphoma. When immunostained for the B-cell differentiation antigen, Leu-14, a few residual B-cells are positive (lower right), but most of the cells are negative (ABC-PO with AEC in a frozen section, hematoxylin counterstain). *Figure 5–43.*

SLIDE 46
Lymphoblastic (convoluted cell) lymphoma. When immunostained for the T-cell differentiation antigen, T11, most of the cells are positive, but the intensity varies (ABC-PO with AEC in a frozen section, hematoxylin counterstain). *Figure 5–44.*

SLIDE 47
Lymphoblastic (convoluted cell) lymphoma. When stained for the differentiation antigen, LN2, the macrophages are positive, but the tumor cells are negative (ABC-PO with AEC in a paraffin section of tissue fixed in B-5, hematoxylin counterstain). *Figure 5–45.*

SLIDE 48
Acute leukemia. Slides 48 and 49 are from the same case. When immunostained for the T-cell differentiation antigen, T11, the small lymphocytes are $T11^+$ and the large blasts are $T11^-$ (ABC-PO with AEC in a cytocentrifuge preparation, hematoxylin counterstain). Figure courtesy of Andrew Fishleder, MD, and Richard A. Savage, MD. *Figure 5–46.*

SLIDE 49
Acute leukemia. When stained for the differentiation antigen, J5 (CALLA), the blasts are $J5^+$ and the small lymphocytes are $J5^-$ (ABC-PO with AEC in a cytocentrifuge preparation, hematoxylin counterstain). Figure courtesy of Andrew Fishleder, MD, and Richard A. Savage, MD. *Figure 5–47.*

SLIDE 50
Hodgkin's disease. When immunostained for the differentiation antigen, LN2, the neoplastic cells are positive. A positive Reed-Sternberg cell (red) is visible in the upper left corner (ABC-PO with AEC in a paraffin section of tissue fixed in B-5, hematoxylin counterstain). *Figure 5–55.*

SLIDE 51
Mixed cell thymoma. When immunostained with AE1/3 for cytokeratins (red), the epithelial elements are positive (ABC-PO with AEC in a frozen tissue, hematoxylin counterstain). *Figure 5–59.*

SLIDE 52
Focal and segmental sclerosis. This figure shows deposits of C3 in sclerotic segments of a glomerulus. The nonsclerotic portion is clearly visible (IMPAS for C3, hematoxylin counterstain). *Figure 6–4.*

SLIDE 53
Poststreptococcal glomerulonephritis. Epimembranous and mesangial deposits of C3 are visible (IMPAS for C3, hematoxylin counterstain). *Figure 6–9.*

SLIDE 54
Membranous glomerulonephritis. The generalized deposits of C3 (arrows) are clearly localized in the epimembranous area (IMPAS for C3). *Figure 6–11.*

SLIDE 55
Membranoproliferative glomerulonephritis. Subendothelial (double arrows) and epimembranous deposits (single arrow) of C3 are visible (IMPAS for C3). *Figure 6–18.*

SLIDE 56
Diffuse lupus glomerulonephritis. Slides 56 and 57 are from the same case. Subendothelial dense deposits of C3 (arrows) and prominent mesangial deposits are visible (IMPAS for C3, hematoxylin counterstain). *Figure 6–20.*

SLIDE 57
Diffuse lupus glomerulonephritis. Electron micrograph shows prominent subendothelial dense deposits (lead citrate and uranyl acetate). *Figure 6–21.*

SLIDE 58
Diffuse lupus glomerulonephritis. Slides 58 and 59 are from the same case. Prominent intraluminal/subendothelial deposits of C3 (arrows) are visible. Adjacent capillary loops also exhibit subendothelial deposits of C3 (IMPAS for C3, hematoxylin counterstain). *Figure 6–22.*

SLIDE 59
Diffuse lupus glomerulonephritis. Electron micrograph shows prominent intraluminal, subendothelial, and mesangial deposits (lead citrate and uranyl acetate). *Figure 6–23.*

SLIDE 60
Anti–glomerular basement membrane disease. Linear deposits of IgG are visible in the peripheral glomerular basement membrane (IMP for IgG). *Figure 6–24.*

SLIDE 61
Anti–glomerular basement membrane disease. Linear deposits of IgG (brown) are visible in the glomerular basement membrane (IMPAS for IgG, hematoxylin counterstain). *Figure 6–25.*

SLIDE 62
κ light chain deposition disease. Slides 62 through 64 are from the same case. Diffuse deposits of κ immunoglobulin light chains in glomeruli, vessels, and tubular basement membranes are visible (IMP for κ immunoglobulin light chains). *Figure 6–27.*

SLIDE 63
κ light chain nephropathy. Diffuse deposits of κ immunoglobulin light chains are visible in a glomerulus and adjacent tubular basement membranes (IMPAS for κ immunoglobulin light chains, hematoxylin counterstain). *Figure 6–28.*

SLIDE 64
κ light chain nephropathy. Electron micrograph shows continuous, finely granular, dense deposits concentrated in the internal aspect of the glomerular basement membrane (lead citrate and uranyl acetate). *Figure 6–30.*

SLIDE 65
Renal amyloidosis. Slides 65 and 66 are from the same case. Generalized granular to homogeneous glomerular deposits of IgM are visible (IMPAS for IgM, hematoxylin counterstain). *Figure 6–31.*

SLIDE 66
Renal amyloidosis. Generalized glomerular staining for κ immunoglobulin light chains (IMP for κ immunoglobulin light chains, no counterstain). *Figure 6–32.*

SLIDE 67
Lupus nephritis. Prominent tubular deposits of C3 are visible. Glomerular deposits of C3 (arrows) are also present in this photograph (IMP for C3, no counterstain). *Figure 6–36.*

SLIDE 68
Lupus nephritis. Deposits of C3 in tubular basement membranes. Interstitial cellular infiltrates are also present (IMPAS for C3, hematoxylin counterstain). *Figure 6–37.*

SLIDE 69
Lupus nephritis. Vascular deposits (arrows) and mesangial and peripheral glomerular basement membrane deposits of IgG in severe diffuse lupus nephritis (IMPAS for IgG, hematoxylin counterstain). *Figure 6–38.*

SLIDE 70
Acute cellular rejection. The majority of mononuclear (lymphocytic) interstitial infiltrates are positive for T11 (arrows), a pan-T-cell marker (IMP, hematoxylin counterstain). *Figure 6–40.*

SLIDE 71
Lupus pneumonitis. Prominent vascular deposits of C3 (arrows) are visible. (IMPAS for C3, hematoxylin counterstain). *Figure 7–2.*

SLIDE 72
Pulmonary vasculitis/Wegener's granulomatosis. $T8^+$ cells (cytotoxic/suppressor subset of T-cells) are visible in the vascular infiltrate (ABC-PO with AEC, hematoxylin counterstain). *Figure 7–4.*

SLIDE 73
Immunoblastic sarcoma, primary in the lung. The majority of cells exhibit the LN2 antigen, indicating B-lymphocytic origin of the cytologically malignant cells (ABC-PO with AEC in a paraffin section of Hollende's-fixed tissue, hematoxylin counterstain). *Figure 7–19.*

SLIDE 74
Small cell undifferentiated carcinoma of the lung. Slides 74 and 75 are from the same case. In this slide, CEA is expressed in scattered cells (ABC-PO with AEC, hematoxylin counterstain). *Figure 7–22.*

SLIDE 75
Small cell undifferentiated carcinoma of the lung. Lymphocytes adjacent to the undifferentiated small cell carcinoma (left) are positive for common leukocyte antigen, whereas the carcinoma (center and right) is negative for this antigen (ABC-PO with AEC, hematoxylin counterstain). *Figure 7–23.*

SLIDE 76
Carcinoid tumor of the lung. Cells are positive for ACTH. This patient had Cushing's syndrome, which was cured following resection of the tumor (ABC-PO with AEC, hematoxylin counterstain). *Figure 7–25.*

SLIDE 77
Malignant mesothelioma diffusely involving the pleura. Slides 77 and 78 are from the same case. This section shows negative staining for CEA (ABC-PO with AEC, hematoxylin counterstain). *Figure 7–27.*

SLIDE 78
Malignant mesothelioma diffusely involving the pleura. Cytokeratins (detected with AE1/3) are present in a majority of neoplastic cells (ABC-PO with AEC in a pronase-digested paraffin section, hematoxylin counterstain). *Figure 7–29.*

SLIDE 79
Metastatic adenocarcinoma involving the pleura. CEA is present in most of the cells. The majority of neoplastic cells were also positive when stained for cytokeratins with AE1/3, an antibody to low molecular weight cytokeratins (ABC-PO with AEC for CEA, hematoxylin counterstain). *Figure 7–31.*

SLIDE 80
Desquamative interstitial pneumonia with prominent alveolar macrophages. Slides 80 and 81 are from the same case. In this slide, muramidase activity in alveolar macrophages is visible (ABC-PO with AEC in a paraffin section, hematoxylin counterstain). *Figure 7–33.*

SLIDE 81
Desquamative interstitial pneumonia with prominent alveolar macrophages. Epithelial membrane antigen is limited to alveolar lining cells. Alveolar macrophages are negative (ABC-PO with AEC, hematoxylin counterstain). *Figure 7–35.*

SLIDE 82
Endodermal sinus tumor of the testis immunostained for α-fetoprotein (ABC-PO with AEC, hematoxylin counterstain). *Figure 8–1.*

SLIDE 83
Mixed germ cell tumor of the testis immunostained for the β subunit of human chorionic gonadotropin (β-HCG; ABC-PO with AEC, hematoxylin counterstain). *Figure 8–2.*

SLIDE 84
Paget's disease of the vulva. This view shows neoplastic cells containing cytokeratins defined by AE1/3 (ABC-PO with AEC, hematoxylin counterstain). *Figure 8–8.*

SLIDE 85
Metastatic carcinoma in bone marrow from a patient without elevation of serum prostatic acid phosphatase. Prostate-specific antigen is expressed by metastatic carcinoma in bone marrow (ABC-PO with AEC, hematoxylin counterstain). *Figure 8–16.*

SLIDE 86
Poorly differentiated invasive malignant neoplasm in the prostate gland. Despite the absence of architectural differentiation, phenotypic expression of prostate-specific antigen is documented (ABC-PO with AEC, hematoxylin counterstain). *Figure 8–18.*

SLIDE 87
Stage 0 transitional cell carcinoma of the urinary bladder. The neoplastic urothelium expresses H substance in concert with the patient's blood type. Note the positive red blood cells and endothelium (ABC-PO with AEC, biotinylated antibody modification [biotinylated anti-*Ulex*], hematoxylin counterstain). *Figure 8–23.*

SLIDE 88
Stage 0 transitional cell carcinoma of the urinary bladder immunostained for monoclonal antibody to blood group O (H substance). This case shows deletion of H substance. The endothelium and red blood cells remain positive (red), an internal positive control (ABC-PO with AEC, biotinylated antibody modification [biotinylated anti-*Ulex*], hematoxylin counterstain). *Figure 8–24.*

SLIDE 89
Rhabdomyosarcoma immunostained for myoglobin. Occasional tumor cells are positive (ABC-PO with AEC, hematoxylin counterstain). *Figure 9–3.*

SLIDE 90
Metastatic spindle cell and epithelioid amelanotic melanoma presenting as idiopathic lymphadenopathy immunostained for S-100 protein. A small portion of noneffaced lymph node is present in the upper right (ABC-PO with AEC, hematoxylin counterstain). *Figure 9–5.*

SLIDE 91
Spindle cell dermal and subcutaneous neoplasm suggestive of spindle cell squamous carcinoma. This view shows positive staining of tumor cells for cytokeratins (ABC-PO with AEC, hematoxylin counterstain). *Figure 9–7.*

SLIDE 92
Gastrinoma of the duodenal wall immunostained for gastrin (red) from a patient with Zollinger-Ellison syndrome (ABC-PO with AEC, hematoxylin counterstain). *Figure 10–1.*

SLIDE 93
Chronic hepatitis. Slides 93 and 94 are from the same case. Diffuse cytoplasmic immunostaining in hepatocytes for HBsAg is present in this slide. Focal membrane-associated immunostaining is also demonstrated (ABC-PO with AEC, hematoxylin counterstain). *Figure 10–10.*

SLIDE 94
Chronic hepatitis. Many nuclei illustrated are positive for immunoreactive HBcAg. Note the color distinction between true-red positive nuclei and negative blue nuclei (ABC-PO with AEC, hematoxylin counterstain). *Figure 10–11.*

SLIDE 95
Hepatocellular carcinoma immunostained for carcinoembryonic antigen (CEA). Note the striking canalicular positivity (ABC-PO with AEC, hematoxylin counterstain). Figure courtesy of Thomas Bauer, MD, PhD. *Figure 10–12.*

SLIDE 96
Adenocarcinoma metastatic to liver. In contrast to Slide 95, this tumor shows cytoplasmic rather than canalicular CEA within the tumor cells (ABC-PO with AEC, hematoxylin counterstain). *Figure 10–13.*

SLIDE 97
Metastatic amelanotic malignant melanoma in the brain. The tumor cells contain S-100 protein (ABC-PO with AEC, hematoxylin counterstain). *Figure 11–2.*

SLIDE 98
Undifferentiated malignant neoplasm presenting as a large neck mass. Slides 98 and 99 are from the same case. While large tumor cells do not express common leukocyte antigen, the latter is identified in small contiguous lymphocytes (ABC-PO with AEC, hematoxylin counterstain). *Figure 12–1.*

SLIDE 99
Undifferentiated malignant neoplasm presenting as a large neck mass. Cytokeratins (AE1/3) are expressed by large tumor cells. Lymphocytes are negative for AE1/3 (ABC-PO with AEC, hematoxylin counterstain). *Figure 12–2.*

SLIDE 100
Undifferentiated large cell carcinoma, lung aspiration specimen. A Papanicolaou cytologic preparation overstained with antibody to epithelial membrane antigen shows positive staining in nucleolated tumor cells (ABC-PO with AEC, Papanicolaou counterstain). Preparation courtesy of Steven Becker, MD. *Figure 12–6.*

SLIDE 101
Cytomegalovirus adrenalitis. In situ hybridization. Viral DNA is identified in the obvious nuclear inclusion, in cytoplasmic inclusions (arrows), and in a nucleus without an obvious inclusion (double arrow; ABC-PO, biotinylated primary modification, with AEC, hematoxylin counterstain). *Figure 12–11.*

Bibliography

Chapter 1: Principles and Practice

GENERAL REVIEW ARTICLES

Battifora H: Recent progress in the immunohistochemistry of solid tumors. *Semin Diagn Pathol* 1984;1:251–271.

Erlandson RA: Diagnostic immunohistochemistry of human tumors. *Am J Surg Pathol* 1984;8:615–624.

Falini B, Taylor CR: New developments in immunoperoxidase techniques and their application. *Arch Pathol Lab Med* 1983;107:105–117.

Farr AG, Nikane PK: Immunohistochemistry with enzyme-labeled antibodies: A brief review. *J Immunol Methods* 1981;47:129–144.

Gatter KC, Cordell JL, Falini B, et al: Monoclonal antibodies in diagnostic pathology: Techniques and applications. *J Biol Response Mod* 1983;2:369–395.

Heyderman E: Immunoperoxidase technique in histopathology: Applications, methods, and controls. *J Clin Pathol* 1979;32:971–978.

Sheibani K, Tubbs RR: Enzyme immunohistochemistry: Technical aspects. *Semin Diagn Pathol* 1984;1:235–250.

Tubbs RR, Sheibani K, Deodhar SD, et al: Enzyme immunohistochemistry: Review of technical aspects and diagnostic applications. *Cleve Clin Q* 1981;48:245–282.

TEXTBOOKS

DeLellis RA (ed): *Diagnostic Immunohistochemistry.* New York, Masson Publishing USA Inc, 1981, pp 61–74.

Mukai K, Rosai J: Application of immunoperoxidase techniques in surgical pathology, in Fenoglio CM, Wolff M (eds): *Progress in Surgical Pathology.* New York, Masson Publishing USA Inc, 1980, vol 1.

Sternberger LA: *Immunocytochemistry,* ed 2. New York, John Wiley & Sons Inc, 1978.

Chapter 2: Immunohistologic Methods

TECHNIQUES

Celio MR, Lutz H, Binz H, et al: Protein A in immunoperoxidase techniques. *J Histochem Cytochem* 1979;27:691–693.

Guesdon JL, Ternynck T, Avrameas S: The use of avidin-biotin interaction in immunoenzymatic techniques. *J Histochem Cytochem* 1979;27:1131–1139.

Holgate CS, Jackson P, Cowen PN, et al: Immunogold-silver staining: New method of immunostaining with enhanced sensitivity. *J Histochem Cytochem* 1983;31:938–944.

Hsu SM, Raine L, Fanger H: A comparative study of the PAP method and avidin-biotin-complex method for studying polypeptide hormones with radioimmunoassay antibodies. *Am J Clin Pathol* 1981;75:734–738.

Lloyd RV, Schmidt K, Blaivas L, et al: A rapid immunostaining method utilizing preformed antibody-avidin-biotin-peroxidase complexes. *Am J Clin Path* 1985;83:636–639.

Roth J: Applications of immunocolloids in light microscopy. *J Histochem Cytochem* 1982;30:691–696.

Stein H, Gatter KC, Heryet A, et al: Freeze-dried paraffin-embedded human tissue for antigen labelling with monoclonal antibodies. *Lancet* 1984;II:71–73.

Tubbs RR, Sheibani K, Deodhar SD, et al: Enzyme immunohistochemistry: Review of technical aspects and diagnostic applications. *Cleve Clin Q* 1981;48:245–282.

PEROXIDASE CHROMOGENS

Bioassay of 3-amino-9-ethylcarbazole hydrochloride for possible carcinogenicity. National Cancer Institute Carcinogenesis technical report series, No. 93, 1978, pp 1–180.

Griswold DP, Casey AE, Weisburger EK, et al: The carcinogenicity of multiple intragastric doses of aromatic heterocyclic nitro or amino derivatives in young female Sprague-Dawley rats. *Cancer Res* 1968;28:924–933.

Hanker JS, Yates PE, Metz CB, et al: A new specific sensitive and noncarcinogenic reagent for the demonstration of horseradish peroxidase. *Histochem J* 1977;9:789–792.

Hsu SM, Soban E: Color modification of diaminobenzidine (DAB) precipitation by metallic ions and its application for double immunohistochemistry. *J Histochem Cytochem* 1982;30:1079–1082.

Mesulam MM, Rosene DL: Differential sensitivity between blue and brown reaction products for HRP neurohistochemistry. *Neurosci Lett* 1977;5:7–14.

Mesulam MM, Rosene DL: Sensitivity of horseradish peroxidase neurohistochemistry: A comparative and quantitative study of nine methods. *J Histochem Cytochem* 1979;27:763–767.

Occupational Safety and Health Administration Standards, part 1910–1010, title 29, Code of Federal Regulations. *Federal Register,* 1979, pp 3825–3845.

Reiner A, Gamin P: On noncarcinogenic chromogens for horseradish peroxidase histochemistry. *J Histochem Cytochem* 1980;28:187–188.

Sonlag JM: Carcinogenicity of substituted benzenediamines (phenylenediamines) in rats and mice. *J Natl Cancer Inst* 1981;66:591–602.

Sternberger LA, Joseph SA: The unlabeled antibody method: Contrasting color staining of paired pituitary hormones without antibody removal. *J Histochem Cytochem* 1979;27:1424–1429.

Tubbs RR, Sheibani K: Chromogens for immunohistochemistry. *J Histochem Cytochem* 1981;29:684.

ALTERNATIVE ENZYMES FOR LABELING

Bondi A, Chieregatti G, Eusebi V, et al: The use of β-galactosidase as a tracer in immunocytochemistry. *Histochemistry* 1982;76:153–158.

Clark CA, Downs EC, Primus FJ: An unlabeled antibody method using glucose oxidase-antiglucose oxidase complexes (GAC): A sensitive alternative to immunoperoxidase for the detection of tissue antigens. *J Histochem Cytochem* 1982;30:27–34.

Cordell JL, Falini B, Erber WN, et al: Immunoenzymatic labeling of monoclonal antibodies using immune complexes of alkaline phosphatase and monoclonal anti-alkaline phosphatase (APAAP) complexes. *J Histochem Cytochem* 1984;32:219–229.

Erber WN, Pinching AJ, Mason DY: Immunocytochemical detection of T and B cell populations in routine blood smears. *Lancet* 1984;I:1042–1045.

Mason DY, Sammons R: Alkaline phosphatase and peroxidase for double immunoenzymatic labelling of cellular constituents. *J Clin Pathol* 1978;31:454–460.

Robb JA: A new enzyme immunoelectron tissue stain. *Diagn Med* 1981;4:87–95.

METALLIC IMMUNOCOLLOIDS

DeWaele M, DeMey D, Moeremans M, et al: The immunogold staining method: An immunocytochemical procedure for leukocyte characterization by monoclonal antibodies, in Knapp W (ed): *Leukemia Markers.* New York, Academic Press Inc, 1981, pp 173–176.

Roth J: Applications of immunocolloids in light microscopy: Preparation of protein-A silver and protein-A gold complexes and their application for localization of single and multiple antigens in paraffin sections. *J Histochem Cytochem* 1982;30:691–696.

Chapter 3: Specimen Processing and Quality Assurance

Hume DA, Gordon S: Mononuclear phagocyte system of the mouse defined by immunohistochemical localization of antigen F4/80. *J Exp Med* 1983;157:1704–1709.

Chapter 4: Endocrine Pathology

PANCREATIC NEUROENDOCRINE TUMORS

Choe B, Pontes E, Rose N, et al: Expression of human prostatic acid phosphatase in a pancreatic islet cell carcinoma. *Invest Urol* 1978;15:312–318.

Cohen C, Bentz M, Budgeon L: Prostatic acid phosphatase in carcinoid and islet cell tumors. *Arch Pathol Lab Med* 1983;107:277.

Creutzfeldt W, Arnold R, Creutzfeldt C, et al: Pathomorphologic, biochemical, and diagnostic aspects of gastrinomas (Zollinger-Ellison syndrome). *Hum Pathol* 1975;6:47–76.

Dayal Y, O'Briain DS: The pathology of the pancreatic endocrine cells, in DeLellis RA (ed): *Diagnostic Immunohistochemistry*. New York, Masson Publishing USA Inc, 1981, pp 111–135.

Falkmer S: Immunocytochemical studies of the evolution of islet hormones. *J Histochem Cytochem* 1979;27:1281–1282.

Hammar S, Sale G: Multiple hormone-producing islet cell carcinomas of the pancreas: A morphologic and biochemical investigation. *Hum Pathol* 1975;6:349–362.

Heitz P, Kasper M, Polak J, et al: Pancreatic endocrine tumors: Immunocytochemical analysis of 125 tumors. *Hum Pathol* 1982;13:263–271.

Kahn C, Rosen S, Weintraub B, et al: Ectopic production of chorionic gonadotropin and its subunits in islet cell tumors: A specific marker for malignancy. *N Engl J Med* 1977;297:565–569.

Klöppel G, Heitz P: *Pancreatic Pathology*. New York, Churchill Livingstone Inc, 1984.

Larsson L: Endocrine pancreatic tumors. *Hum Pathol* 1978;9:401–416.

Mukai K, Greider M, Grotting J, et al: Retrospective study of 77 pancreatic endocrine tumors using the immunoperoxidase method. *Am J Surg Pathol* 1982;6:387–399.

Nieuwenhuijzen Kruseman AC, Knijnenburg G, Erutel de la Riviere G, et al: Morphology and immunohistochemically defined endocrine function of pancreatic islet cell tumors. *Histopathology* 1978;2:389–399.

Öberg K, Wide L, Boström H: HCG-alpha and HCG-beta subunits as tumor markers during therapy in a case with so-called nonfunctioning islet cell tumor. *Acta Med Scand* 1981;210:231–233.

Ordonez N, Manning J, Hanssen G: Alpha-1 antitrypsin in islet cell tumors of the pancreas. *Am J Clin Pathol* 1983;80:277–282.

PITUITARY ADENOMAS

Fukaya T, Kageyama N, Kuwayama A, et al: Morphofunctional study of pituitary adenomas with acromegaly by immunoperoxidase technique and electron microscopy. *Cancer* 1980;45:1598–1603.

Halmi NS, Duello T: Acidophilic pituitary tumors: A reappraisal with differential staining and immunocytochemical techniques. *Arch Pathol Lab Med* 1976;100:346–351.

Heitz P: Multihormonal pituitary adenomas. *Horm Res* 1979;10:1–13.

Lloyd R, Gikas P, Chandler W: Prolactin in growth hormone-producing pituitary adenomas: An immunohistochemical and ultrastructural study. *Am J Surg Pathol* 1983;7:251–260.

Mukai K: Pituitary adenomas: Immunocytochemical study of 150 tumors with clinicopathologic correlation. *Cancer* 1983;52:648–653.

THYROID TUMORS

Alvores-Saavedra J, Nadji M, Civantos F, et al: Thyroglobulin in carcinoma of the thyroid: An immunohistochemical study. *Hum Pathol* 1983;14:62–66.

Bigner S, Cox E, Mendelsohn G, et al: Medullary carcinoma of the thyroid in multiple endocrine neoplasia type II-A syndrome. *Am J Surg Pathol* 1981;5:459–472.

Böcker W, Dralle H, Dorn G: Thyroglobulin: An

immunohistochemical marker in thyroid disease, in DeLellis RA (ed): *Diagnostic Immunohistochemistry*. New York, Masson Publishing USA Inc, 1981, pp 37–61.

Böcker W, Dralle H, Husselmann H, et al: Immunohistochemical analysis of thyroglobulin synthesis in thyroid carcinomas. *Virchows Arch [Pathol Anat]* 1980;385:187–200.

Burt A, Goudie RB: Diagnosis of primary thyroid carcinoma by immunohistological demonstration of thyroglobulin. *Histopathology* 1979;3:279–286.

DeLellis RA, Wolfe H: Calcitonin immunohistochemistry, in DeLellis RA (ed): *Diagnostic Immunohistochemistry*. New York, Masson Publishing USA Inc, 1981, pp 61–74.

Graze K, Spiler I, Tashjian A, et al: The natural history of familial medullary thyroid carcinoma: Effect of a program for early diagnosis. *N Engl J Med* 1978;299:280–285.

Kawaoi A, Okano T, Nemoto N, et al: Production of thyroxin (T4) and tri-iodothyronine (T3) in non-toxic thyroid tumors: An immunohistochemical study. *Virchows Arch [Pathol Anat]* 1981;390: 249–257.

Livolsi V: Calcitonin: The hormone, its significance and its progress, in Fenoglio CM, Wolff M (eds): *Progress in Surgical Pathology*. New York, Masson Publishing USA Inc, 1980, pp 71–103.

Livolsi V, Find C: Incidental medullary thyroid carcinoma in sporadic hyperparathyroidism: An expansion of the concept of C cell hyperplasia. *Am J Clin Pathol* 1979;71:595–599.

Mendelsohn G, Baylin S, Bigner S, et al: Anaplastic variants of medullary thyroid carcinoma: A light microscopic immunohistochemical study. *Am J Surg Pathol* 1980;4:333–341.

Mendelsohn G, Wells SA, Baylin SB: Relationship of tissue carcinoembryonic antigen and calcitonin to tumor virulence in medullary thyroid carcinoma. *Cancer* 1984;54:657–662.

Wolfe H, Melvin K, Cervi-Skinner S, et al: C cell hyperplasia preceding medullary thyroid carcinoma. *N Engl J Med* 1973;289:437–441.

Wolfe H, Voelkel E, Tashjian A: Distribution of calcitonin-containing cells in the normal adult human thyroid gland: A correlation of morphology with peptide content. *J Clin Endocrinol Metab* 1974;38:688–694.

OTHER APPLICATIONS

Forman B, Marban E, Kayne R, et al: Ectopic ACTH syndrome due to a pheochromocytoma: Case report and review of the literature. *Yale J Biol Med* 1979;52:181–189.

Kurman RJ, Andrade D, Goebelsmann U, et al: An immunohistological study of steroid localization in Sertoli-Leydig tumors of the ovary and testis. *Cancer* 1978;42:1772–1783.

Sano T, Saito H, Inaba H, et al: Immunoreactive somatostatin in vasoactive intestinal polypeptide in adrenal pheochromocytoma: An immunochemical and ultrastructural study. *Cancer* 1983;52:282–289.

Spark R, Connolly P, Gluckin B, et al: ACTH secretion from a functioning pheochromocytoma. *N Engl J Med* 1979;301:416–418.

Chapter 5: Lymphoproliferative Disorders

GENERAL IMMUNOTYPES OF LYMPHOPROLIFERATIVE DISORDERS

Aisenberg AC, Wilkes BM, Long JC, et al: Cell surface phenotype in lymphoproliferative disease. *Am J Med* 1980;68:206–213.

Garvin AJ, Spicer SS, Parmley RT, et al: Immunohistochemical demonstration of IgG on Reed-Sternberg and other cells in Hodgkin's disease. *J Exp Med* 1974;139:1077–1083.

Gold EJ, Mertelsman RH, Filippa DA, et al: Prognostic significance of receptors for the third component of complement and heavy chain phenotype in diffuse B-cell lymphoma. *Blood* 1983;62:107–111.

Horning SJ, Doggett RS, Warnke RA, et al: Clinical relevance of immunologic phenotype of diffuse large-cell lymphoma. *Blood* 1984;63:1209–1215.

Knowles DM, Halper JP: Human T-cell malignancies: Correlative clinical, histopathologic, immunologic, and cytochemical analysis of 23 cases. *Am J Pathol* 1982;106:187–203.

Levy R, Warnke R, Dorfman RF, et al: The

monoclonality of human B-cell lymphomas. *J Exp Med* 1977;145:1014–1028.

Mann RB, Jaffe ES, Berard CW: Malignant lymphomas: A conceptual understanding of morphologic diversity. *Am J Pathol* 1979;94:105–192.

Pinkus GS, Said JW: Characterization of non-Hodgkin's lymphomas using multiple cell markers: Immunologic, morphologic and cytochemical studies of 72 cases. *Am J Pathol* 1978;94:349–380.

Reinherz EL, Kung PC, Goldstein G, et al: Discrete stages of human intrathymic differentiation: Analysis of normal thymocytes and leukemic lymphoblasts of T-cell lineage. *Proc Natl Acad Sci USA* 1980;77:1588–1592.

Stein H, Bonk A, Tolksdorf G, et al: Immunohistologic analysis of the organization of normal lymphoid tissue and non-Hodgkin's lymphomas. *J Histochem Cytochem* 1980;28:746–760.

Stein H, Gatter KC, Heryet A, et al: Freeze-dried paraffin-embedded human tissue for antigen labelling with monoclonal antibodies. *Lancet* 1984;II:71–73.

Tubbs RR: Immunocytochemistry of lymphomas in frozen tissue sections, in Russo J (ed): *Immunocytochemistry in Tumor Diagnosis*. Boston, Mortimus Nijhoff Publishing Co, 1985, pp 116–140.

Tubbs RR, Fishleder A, Weiss RA, et al: Immunohistologic cellular phenotypes of lymphoproliferative disorders: Comprehensive evaluation of 564 cases including 257 non-Hodgkin's lymphomas classified by the International Working Formulation. *Am J Pathol* 1983;113:207–221.

Tubbs RR, Sheibani K: Immunohistology of lymphoproliferative disorders. *Semin Diagn Pathol* 1984;I:272–284.

Warnke RA: Alteration of immunoglobulin-bearing lymphoma cells by fixation. *J Histochem Cytochem* 1979;27:1195–1196.

LEUKEMIA IMMUNOTYPES

Erber WN, Pinching AJ, Mason DY: Immunocytochemical detection of T & B cell populations in routine blood smears. *Lancet* 1984;I:1042–1045.

Fishleder A, Tubbs RR, Savage RA, et al: Immunophenotypic characterization of acute leukemia by immunocytology. *Am J Clin Pathol* 1984;81:611–617.

Foon KA, Schroff RW, Gale RP: Surface markers on leukemia and lymphoma cells: Recent advances. *Blood* 1982;60:1–19.

Salmon M, Bacon PA, Johnson GD, et al: The use of cytocentrifuge preparations for the demonstration of T-cell surface antigens. *J Immunol Methods* 1984;66:327–330.

Sandhaus LM, Gajl-Peczalska KJ, Brunning RD: Immunophenotyping of leukemia: An immunoperoxidase method using air-dried smears. *Br J Haematol* 1984;56:131–138.

THYMOMA IMMUNOHISTOLOGY

Chilosi M, Menestrina F, Iannucci AM, et al: Immunohistochemical analysis of thymoma: Evidence for medullary origin of epithelial cells. *Am J Surg Pathol* 1984;8:309–318.

Cossman J, Deegan MJ, Schnitzer B: Thymoma: An immunologic and electron microscopic study. *Cancer* 1978;41:2183–2191.

Mokhtar N, Hsu S-M, Lad RP, et al: Thymoma: Lymphoid and epithelial components mirror the phenotype of normal thymus. *Hum Pathol* 1984;15:378–384.

Woda BA, Bain K, Vander Salm T: The phenotype of lymphocytes in a thymoma as studied with monoclonal antibodies. *Clin Immunol Immunopathol* 1984;30:197–201.

Chapter 6: Nephropathology

METHODOLOGY

Choi YJ, Reiner L: Immunofluorescence of renal lesions in paraffin-embedded and fresh-frozen sections. *Am J Clin Pathol* 1980;73:116–119.

Curran RC, Gegory J: The unmasking of antigens in paraffin sections of tissue by trypsin. *Experientia* 1977;33:1400–1401.

Davey FR, Busch GJ: Immunohistochemistry of glomerulonephritis using horseradish peroxidase and fluorescein-labeled antibody: A comparison of two technics. *Am J Clin Pathol* 1970;53:531–536.

Denk H, Syre G, Weirich E: Immunomorphologic methods in routine pathology: Application of immunofluorescence and the unlabeled antibody-enzyme (peroxidase-antiperoxidase) technique to formalin-fixed paraffin-embedded kidney biopsies. *Beitr Pathol* 1977;160:187–194.

Elias JM, Miller F: A comparison of the unlabeled enzyme method with immunofluorescence for the evaluation of human immunologic renal disease. *Am J Clin Pathol* 1975;64:464–471.

MacIver AG, Giddings J, Mepham BL: Demonstration of extracellular immunoproteins in formalin-fixed renal biopsy specimens. *Kidney Int* 1979;16:632–636.

Qualman SJ, Keren DF: Immunofluorescence of deparaffinized trypsin-treated renal tissues. Preservation of antigens as an adjunct to diagnosis of disease. *Lab Invest* 1979;41:483–489.

Sheibani K, Tubbs RR, Gephardt GN, et al: Comparison of alternative chromogens for renal immunohistochemistry. *Human Pathol* 1981;12: 349–354.

Tubbs RR, Gephardt GN, Valenzuela R, et al: An approach to immunomicroscopy of renal disease with immunoperoxidase and periodic acid–Schiff counterstain (IMPAS stain). *Am J Clin Pathol* 1980;73:240–244.

Turner DR, Wilson D, Cameron JS: Peroxidase-labelled IgG and complement in plastic-embedded human renal tissue, in Feldmann G, Druet P, Bignon J, et al (eds): *First International Symposium on Immunoenzymatic Techniques*, INSERM Symposium No. 2. Amsterdam, North-Holland Publishing Co, 1976, pp 105–108.

INTERPRETATION OF RENAL IMMUNOPEROXIDASE PREPARATIONS

Tubbs RR, Gephardt GN: Use and interpretation of immunoperoxidase procedures in renal disease, in Seymour R (ed): *Contemporary Issues in Surgical Pathology: Glomerular Disease*. New York, Churchill Livingstone Inc, 1983, pp 11–34.

Turner DR, Wilson DM, Lake A, et al: An evaluation of the immunoperoxidase technique in renal biopsy diagnosis. *Clin Nephrol* 1979;11:13–17.

Chapter 7: Diseases of the Lung and Pleura

AUTOIMMUNE LUNG DISEASE

Bateman E, Turner-Warwick M, Haslam PL, et al: Cryptogenic fibrosing alveolitis: Prediction of fibrinogenic activity from immunohistochemical studies of collagen types in lung biopsy specimens. *Thorax* 1983;38:93–101.

Churg A, Franklin W, Chan KL, et al: Pulmonary hemorrhage and immune-complex deposition in the lung: Complications in a patient with systemic lupus erythematosus. *Arch Pathol Lab Med* 1980;104:388–391.

Eagen JW, Memoli VA, Roberts JL, et al: Pulmonary hemorrhage in systemic lupus erythematosus. *Medicine* 1978;57:545–560.

Inoue T, Kanayama Y, Ohe A: Immunopathologic studies of pneumonitis in systemic lupus erythematosus. *Ann Intern Med* 1979;91:30–34.

CELLULAR ANTIGENS AND NEOPLASIA

Battifora H: Recent progress in the immunohistochemistry of solid tumors. *Semin Diagn Pathol* 1984;1:251–271.

Corson JM, Pinkus GS: Mesothelioma: Profile of keratin proteins and carcinoembryonic antigen: An immunoperoxidase study of 20 cases and comparison with pulmonary adenocarcinomas. *Am J Pathol* 1982;108:80–87.

Epstein AL, Marder RJ, Winter JN, et al: Two new monoclonal antibodies (LN-1, LN-2) reactive in B5 formalin-fixed, paraffin-embedded tissues with follicular center and mantle zone human B lymphocytes and derived tumors. *J Immunol* 1984;133:1028–1036.

Goslin RH, O'Brien MJ, Skarin AT, et al: Immunocytochemical staining for CEA in small-cell carcinoma of lung predicts clinical usefulness of the plasma assay. *Cancer* 1983;52:301–306.

Holden J, Churg A: Immunohistochemical staining for keratin and carcinoembryonic antigen in the diagnosis of malignant mesothelioma. *Am J Surg Pathol* 1984;8:277–279.

LaRocca PJ, Rheinwald JG: Coexpression of simple

epithelial keratins and vimentin by human mesothelium and mesothelioma *in vivo* and in culture. *Cancer Res* 1984;44:2991–2999.

Marshall RJ, Herbert A, Braye SG, et al: Use of antibodies to carcinoembryonic antigen and human milk fat globule to distinguish carcinoma, mesothelioma, and reactive mesothelium. *J Clin Pathol* 1984;37:1215–1221.

Primus FJ, Wang RH, Sharkey RM, et al: Detection of carcinoembryonic antigen in tissue sections by immunoperoxidase. *J Immunol Methods* 1975;8:267–276.

Said JW, Nash G, Banks-Schlegel S, et al: Keratin in human lung tumors: Patterns of localization of different-molecular-weight keratin proteins. *Am J Pathol* 1983;113:27–32.

Schlegel R, Banks-Schlegel S, Pinkus GS: Immunohistochemical localization of keratin in normal human tissues. *Lab Invest* 1980;42:91–96.

Tubbs RR, Fishleder A, Weiss RA, et al: Immunohistologic cellular phenotypes of lymphoproliferative disorders: Comprehensive evaluation of 564 cases including 257 non-Hodgkin's lymphomas classified by the International Working Formulation. *Am J Pathol* 1983;113:207–221.

Walts AE, Said JW, Shintaku IP, et al: Keratins of different molecular weight in exfoliated mesothelial and adenocarcinoma cells: An aid to cell identification. *Am J Clin Pathol* 1984;81:442–446.

Wang NS, Huang SN, Gold P: Absence of carcinoembryonic antigen-like material in mesothelioma: An immunohistochemical differentiation from other lung cancers. *Cancer* 1979;44:937–943.

Warnke RA, Gatter KC, Falini B, et al: Diagnosis of human lymphoma with monoclonal antileukocyte antibodies. *N Engl J Med* 1983;309:1275–1281.

Whitaker D, Shilkin KB: CEA in tissue diagnosis of malignant mesothelioma. *Lancet* 1981;1:1369.

PULMONARY VASCULITIS

Gephardt GN, Ahmad M, Tubbs RR: Pulmonary vasculitis (Wegener's granulomatosis): Immunohistochemical study of T- and B-cell markers. *Am J Med* 1983;74:700–704.

Chapter 8: Genitourinary Pathology

PROSTATE

Jobsis AC, DeVries GP, Anholt RR, et al: Demonstration of the prostatic origin of metastases: An immunohistochemical method for formalin-fixed embedded tissue. *Cancer* 1978;41:1788–1793.

Nadji M, Tabei SZ, Castro A, et al: Prostatic origin of tumors: An immunohistochemical study. *Am J Clin Pathol* 1980;73:735–739.

GERM CELL AND GENITOURINARY EPITHELIAL TUMORS

Cohen C, Shulman G, Budgeon LR: Immunohistochemical ferritin in testicular seminoma. *Cancer* 1984;54:2190–2194.

Hattori M, Fukase M, Yoshimi H, et al: Ectopic production of human chorionic gonadotropin in malignant tumors. *Cancer* 1978;42:2328–2333.

Heald J, Buckley CH, Fox H: An immunohistochemical study of the distribution of carcinoembryonic antigen in epithelial tumors of the ovary. *J Clin Pathol* 1979;32:918–926.

Javadpour N, McIntire KR, Waldemann TA: Human chorionic gonadotropin (HCG) and alpha-fetoprotein (AFP) in sera and tumor cells of patients with testicular seminoma: A prospective study. *Cancer* 1978;42:2768–2772.

Kurman RJ, Scardino PT, McIntire KR, et al: Cellular localization of alpha-fetoprotein and human chorionic gonadotropin in germ cell tumors of the testis using an indirect immunoperoxidase technique: A new approach to classification utilizing tumor markers. *Cancer* 1977;40:2136–2151.

Kurman RJ, Young RH, Norris HJ, et al: Immunocytochemical localization of placental lactogen and chorionic gonadotropin in the normal placenta and trophoblastic tumors, with emphasis on intermediate trophoblast and the placental site trophoblastic tumor. *Int J Gynecol Pathol* 1984;3:101–121.

Rutanen EM, Lindgren J, Sipponen P, et al: Carcinoembryonic antigen in malignant and nonmalignant gynecologic tumors. *Cancer* 1978;42:581–590.

Stachura I, Mendelow H: Endodermal sinus tumor originating in the region of the pineal gland: Ultrastructural and immunohistochemical study. *Cancer* 1980;45:2131–2137.

Van Nagell JR, Donaldson ES, Gay EC, et al: Carcinoembryonic antigen in ovarian epithelial cystadenocarcinomas: The prognostic value of tumor and serial plasma determinations. *Cancer* 1978;41:2335–2340.

URINARY BLADDER

Cummings KB: Carcinoma of the bladder: Predictors. *Cancer* 1980;45:1849–1855.

Johnson JD, Lamm DL: Prediction of bladder tumor invasion with the mixed-cell agglutination test. *J Urol* 1980;123:25–28.

Limas C, Lange P, Fraley EE, et al: A, B, H antigens in transitional cell tumors of the urinary bladder: Correlation with the clinical course. *Cancer* 1979;44:2099–2107.

Weinstein RS, Alroy J, Farrow GM, et al: Blood group isoantigen deletion in carcinoma *in situ* of the urinary bladder. *Cancer* 1979;43:661–668.

KIDNEY TUMORS

Cordon-Cardo C, Bander NH, Fradet Y, et al: Immunoanatomic dissection of the human urinary tract by monoclonal antibodies. *J Histochem Cytochem* 1984;32:1035–1040.

Ueda R, Ogata SI, Morrissey DM, et al: Cell surface antigens of human renal cancer defined by mouse monoclonal antibodies: Identification of tissue-specific kidney glycoproteins. *Proc Natl Acad Sci USA* 1981;78:5122–5126.

Chapter 9: Soft Tissue Tumors

GENERAL

Erlandson RA: Diagnostic immunohistochemistry of human tumors: An interim evaluation. *Am J Surg Pathol* 1984;8:615–625.

Stern R: Current concepts in the diagnosis of human soft tissue sarcomas. *Hum Pathol* 1981;12:777–781.

MYOGLOBIN

Brooks JJ: Immunohistochemistry of soft tissue tumors: Myoglobin as a tumor marker for rhabdomyosarcoma. *Cancer* 1982;50:1757–1763.

Corson JM, Pinkus GS: Intracellular myoglobin: A specific marker for skeletal muscle differentiation in soft tissue sarcomas: An immunoperoxidase study. *Am J Pathol* 1981;103:384–389.

DeJong ASH, Van Raamsdonk W, Van Vark M, et al: Myosin and myoglobin as tumor markers in the diagnosis of rhabdomyosarcoma: A comparative study. *Am J Surg Pathol* 1984; 8:521–528.

Eusebi V, Bondi A, Rosai J: Immunohistochemical localization of myoglobin in nonmuscular cells. *Am J Surg Pathol* 1984;8:51–55.

Mukai K, Rosai J, Halloway BE: Localization of myoglobin in normal and neoplastic human skeletal muscle cells using an immunoperoxidase method. *Am J Surg Pathol* 1979;3:373–376.

Tsokos M, Howard R, Costa J: Immunohistochemical study of alveolar and embryonal rhabdomyosarcoma. *Lab Invest* 1983;48:148–155.

KERATIN AND OTHER INTERMEDIATE FILAMENTS

Corson JM, Weiss LM, Banks-Schlegel SP, et al: Keratin proteins and carcinoembryonic antigen: An immunohistochemical study of 24 cases. *Hum Pathol* 1984;15:615–621.

Denk H, Krepler R, Artlieb U, et al: Proteins of intermediate filaments: An immunohistochemical and biochemical classification of soft tissue tumors. *Am J Pathol* 1983;110:193–208.

Miettinen M, Virtanen I: Synovial sarcoma: A misnomer. *Am J Pathol* 1984;117:18–25.

S-100 PROTEIN

Armin A, Connelly EM, Rowden G: An immunoperoxidase investigation of S-100 protein in granular cell myoblastomas: Evidence for Schwann cell derivation. *Am J Clin Pathol* 1983;79:37–44.

Cochran AJ, Wen D-R, Herschman HR, et al: Detection of S-100 protein as an aid to the identification of melanocytic tumors. *Int J Cancer* 1982;30:295–297.

Kahn HJ, Marks A, Thom H, et al: Role of antibody

to S-100 protein in diagnostic pathology. *Am J Clin Pathol* 1983;79:341–347.

Mukai M: Immunohistochemical localization of S-100 protein and peripheral nerve myelin proteins (P2 protein, PO protein) in granular cell tumors. *Am J Pathol* 1983;112:139–146.

Nakajima T, Kameya T, Watanabe S, et al: An immunoperoxidase study of S-100 protein distribution in normal and neoplastic tissues. *Am J Surg Pathol* 1982;6:715–727.

Nakajima T, Watanabe S, Sato Y, et al: Immunohistochemical demonstration of S-100 protein in malignant melanoma and pigmented nevus, and its diagnostic application. *Cancer* 1982;50:912–918.

Nakajima T, Watanabe S, Sato Y, et al: S-100 protein in Langerhans cells, interdigitating reticulum cells and histiocytosis X cells. *Gann* 1982;73:429–432.

Nakamura Y, Becker LE, Marks A: S-100 protein in tumors of cartilage and bone: An immunohistochemical study. *Cancer* 1983;52:1820–1824.

Nakazato Y, Ishizeki J, Takahashi K, et al: Immunohistochemical localization of S-100 protein in granular cell myoblastoma. *Cancer* 1982;49: 1624–1628.

Stefansson K, Wollmann RL: S-100 protein in granular cell tumors (granular-cell myoblastomas). *Cancer* 1982;49:1834–1838.

Weiss SW, Langloss JM, Enzinger FM: Value of S-100 protein in the diagnosis of soft-tissue tumors with particular reference to benign and malignant Schwann cell tumors. *Lab Invest* 1983;49:299–308.

ENOLASE

Rode J, Dhillon AP, Papadaki L: Immunohistochemical staining of granular-cell tumour for neurone-specific enolase: Evidence in support of a neural origin. *Diagn Histopathol* 1982;5:205–211.

FACTOR VIII–RELATED ANTIGEN

Mukai K, Rosai J, Burgdorf WHC: Localization of factor VIII-related antigen in vascular endothelial cells using an immunoperoxidase method. *Am J Surg Pathol* 1980;4:273–276.

Nadji M, Morales AR, Ziegles-Weissman J, et al: Kaposi's sarcoma: Immunohistologic evidence for an endothelial origin. *Arch Pathol Lab Med* 1981;105:274–275.

Sehested M, Hou-Jensen K: Factor VIII-related antigen as an endothelial cell marker in benign and malignant diseases. *Virchows Arch [Pathol Anat]* 1981;391:217–225.

ULEX

Holthöfer H, Virtanen I, Kariniemi A-L, et al: *Ulex europaeus* I lectin as a marker for vascular endothelium in human tissues. *Lab Invest* 1982;47:60–66.

Miettinen M, Holthöfer H, Lehto V-P, et al: *Ulex europaeus* I lectin as a marker for tumors derived from endothelial cells. *Am J Clin Pathol* 1983;79: 32–36.

FIBRONECTIN

Irish PS, Hasty DL: Immunocytochemical localization of fibronectin in human fibroblast cultures using a cell surface replica technique. *J Histochem Cytochem* 1983;31:69–77.

Kindblom L-G, Jacobsen GK, Jacobsen M: Immunohistochemical investigations of tumors of supposed fibroblastic-histiocytic origin. *Hum Pathol* 1982;13:834–840.

MURAMIDASE, α-1-ANTITRYPSIN, α-1-CHYMOTRYPSIN, AND PHAGOCYTOSIS

DuBoulay CEH: Demonstration of alpha-1-antitrypsin and alpha-1-antichymotrypsin in fibrous histiocytomas using the immunoperoxidase technique. *Am J Surg Pathol* 1982;6:559–564.

Iwasaki H, Kikuchi M, Takii M, et al: Benign and malignant fibrous histiocytomas of the soft tissues: Functional characterization of the cultured cells. *Cancer* 1982;50:520–530.

Meister P, Nathrath M: Immunohistochemical characterization of histiocytic tumours. *Diagn Histopathol* 1981;4:79–87.

MONOCLONAL ANTIBODIES

Brooks JJ: Immunohistochemistry of soft-tissue tumors: Progress and prospects. *Hum Pathol* 1982;13:969–974.

Brown JM: Detection of a human sarcoma-associated

antigen with monoclonal antibodies. *Cancer Res* 1983;43:2113–2120.

Ghandour S, Langley K, Gombos G, et al: A surface marker for murine vascular endothelial cells defined by monoclonal antibody. *J Histochem Cytochem* 1982;30:165–170.

Chapter 10: Gastrointestinal and Hepatic Pathology

GASTROINTESTINAL NEUROENDOCRINE CELLS AND NEOPLASMS

Alumets J, Alm P, Falkmer S, et al: Immunohistochemical evidence of peptide hormones in endocrine tumors of the rectum. *Cancer* 1981;48:2409–2415.

Lewin K, Elashoff J, Yang K, et al: Primary gastrin cell hyperplasia. *Am J Surg Pathol* 1984;8:821–832.

Mukai K, Rosai J: Application of immunoperoxidase techniques in surgical pathology, in Fenoglio CM, Wolff M (eds): *Progress in Surgical Pathology*. New York, Masson Publishing USA Inc, 1980, pp 15–49.

O'Briain D, Dayal Y: The pathology of the gastrointestinal endocrine cells, in DeLellis RA (ed): *Diagnostic Immunohistochemistry*. New York, Masson Publishing USA Inc, 1980, pp 75–109.

O'Briain D, Tischler A, Dayal Y, et al: Rectal carcinoids as tumors of hindgut endocrine cells: A morphological and immunohistochemical analysis. *Am J Surg Pathol* 1982;6:131–142.

Yang K, Ulich T, Cheng L, et al: The neuroendocrine products of intestinal carcinoids: An immunoperoxidase study of 35 carcinoid tumors stained for serotonin and eight polypeptide hormones. *Cancer* 1983;51:1918–1926.

GASTROINTESTINAL LYMPHOPROLIFERATIVE DISORDERS

Brooks J, Enterline H: Primary gastric lymphomas: A clinical pathologic study of 58 cases with long-term follow-up and literature review. *Cancer* 1983;51:701–711.

Foucar K, Foucar E, Mitros F, et al: Epitheliotropic lymphoma of the small bowel. *Cancer* 1984;54:54–60.

Grody W, Magidson J, Weiss L, et al: Gastrointestinal lymphomas: Immunohistochemical studies on the cell of origin. *Am J Surg Pathol* 1985;9:328-337.

Isaacson P, Wright D: Malignant lymphoma of mucosa associated lymphoid tissue: A distinctive type of B-cell lymphoma. *Cancer* 1983;52:1410–1416.

Isaacson P, Wright D, Judd M, et al: Primary gastrointestinal lymphomas: A classification of 66 cases. *Cancer* 1979;43:1805–1819.

Knowles D, Halper J, Jakobiec F: The immunologic characterization of 40 extranodal lymphoid infiltrates: Usefulness in distinguishing between benign pseudolymphoma and malignant lymphoma. *Cancer* 1982;49:2321–2335.

Saraga P, Hurlimann J, Ozzello L: Lymphomas and pseudolymphomas of the alimentary tract: An immunohistochemical study with clinical pathologic correlations. *Hum Pathol* 1981;12:713–723.

Vanden Heule B, Taylor C, Terry R, et al: Presentation of malignant lymphoma in the rectum. *Cancer* 1982;49:2602–2607.

Vimadalal S, Said J, Voyles H: Gastric lymphoreticular neoplasms: An immunologic study of 36 cases. *Am J Clin Pathol* 1983;80:792–799.

Wolf J, Spjut H: Focal lymphoid hyperplasia of the stomach preceding gastric lymphoma: Case report and review of the literature. *Cancer* 1981;48:2518–2523.

LIVER

Bianchi L, Zimmerly-Ning M, Gudat F: Viral hepatitis, in MacSween RNM, Anthony PP, Scheuer PJ (eds): *Pathology of the Liver*. New York, Churchill Livingstone Inc, 1979, pp 164–191.

Burns J: Immunoperoxidase localization of hepatitis B antigen (HB) in formalin-paraffin processed liver tissue. *Histochemistry* 1975;44:133–135.

Gordon H, Dickson J, Rogers J, et al: Alpha-1-antitrypsin accumulation and livers of emphysematous patients with alpha-1-antitrypsin deficiency. *Hum Pathol* 1972;3:361–370.

Millward-Sadler G, Czaykowski A, Wright R: Diagnosis of alpha-1-antitrypsin deficiency. *Lancet* 1975;2:1050.

Omata M, Liew CT, Ashcavai M, et al: Nonimmunologic binding of horseradish peroxidase to hepatitis B surface antigen: A possible source of error in immunohistochemistry. *Am J Clin Pathol* 1980;73:626–632.

Sumithran E: Methods for detection of hepatitis B surface antigen in paraffin sections of liver: A guideline for their use. *J Clin Pathol* 1976;30:460–463.

Tapp E, Jones M: HBsAg and HBcAg in the livers of asymptomatic hepatitis B antigen carriers. *J Clin Pathol* 1977;30:671–677.

Theodoropoulos G, Nakapoulou L, Repanti M, et al: Detection of hepatitis B surface antigen in fixed tissues of patients with cirrhosis and hepatoma. *Virchows Arch* [*Pathol Anat*] 1979;382:293–300.

Ulich T, Thorne C, Cheng L, et al: Chronic active hepatitis of hepatitis B and non-A, non-B etiology: Immunoperoxidase staining of hepatitis B surface antigen in a series of 66 needle biopsies. *Am J Surg Pathol* 1982;6:33–39.

Wu PC, Lam KC: Cytoplasmic hepatitis B surface antigen and the ground-glass appearance in hepatocellular carcinoma. *Am J Clin Pathol* 1979;71:229–234.

Additional references pertaining to S-100 protein and pan-reactive leukocyte and epithelial antigens are given in Chapters 5, 9, and 12.

Chapter 11: Other Applications

Clark HB: Immunohistochemistry of nervous system antigens: Diagnostic applications in surgical neuropathology. *Semin Diagn Pathol* 1984;1:309–316.

Eng LF, Bigbee JW: Immunohistochemistry of nervous system antigens, in Agranoff BW, Aprison MH (eds): *Advances in Neurochemistry*. New York, Plenum Publishing Corp, 1978, vol 3, pp 43–98.

Roessmann U, Velasco ME, Gambetti P, et al: Neuronal and astrocytic differentiation in human neuroepithelial neoplasms: An immunohistochemical study. *J Neuropathol Exp Neurol* 1983;42:113–121.

Tascos NA, Parr J, Gontas NK: Immunocytochemical study of the glial fibrillary acidic protein in human neoplasms of the central nervous system. *Hum Pathol* 1982;13:454–458.

Velasco ME, Dahl D, Roessmann U, et al: Immunohistochemical localization of glial fibrillary acidic protein in human glial neoplasms. *Cancer* 1980;45:484–494.

Chapter 12: Future Directions

INTERMEDIATE FILAMENTS

Altmannsberger M, Osborn M, Weber K, et al: Expression of intermediate filaments in different human epithelial and mesenchymal tumors. *Pathol Res Pract* 1982;175:227–237.

Barsky SH, Siegal GP, Jannotta F, et al: Loss of basement membrane components by invasive tumors but not by their benign counterparts. *Lab Invest* 1983;49:140–147.

Battifora H: Recent progress in the immunohistochemistry of solid tumors. *Semin Diagn Pathol* 1984;1:251–271.

Bussolati G, Alfani V, Weber K, et al: Immunocytochemical detection of actin on fixed and embedded tissues: Its potential use in routine pathology. *J Histochem Cytochem* 1980;28:169–173.

Denk H, Krepler R, Artlieb U, et al: Proteins of intermediate filaments: An immunohistochemical and biochemical approach to the classification of soft-tissue tumors. *Am J Pathol* 1983;110:193–208.

Erlandson RA: Diagnostic immunohistochemistry of human tumors: An interim evaluation. *Am J Surg Pathol* 1984;8:615–624.

Evans DJ, Lampert IA, Jacobs M: Intermediate filaments in smooth-muscle tumours. *J Clin Pathol* 1983;36:57–61.

Gabbiani G, Kapanci Y, Barazzone P, et al: Immunochemical identification of intermediate-sized filaments in human neoplastic cells: A diagnostic aid for the surgical pathologist. *Am J Pathol* 1981;104:206–216.

Huszar M, Halkin H, Herczeg E, et al: Use of antibodies to intermediate filaments in the diagnosis of metastatic amelanotic malignant melanoma. *Hum Pathol* 1983;14:1006–1008.

Macartney JC, Trebithick MA, Kricka L, et al: Identification of myosin in human epithelial cancers with immunofluorescence. *Lab Invest* 1979;41:437–445.

Miettinen M, Foidart J-M, Ekblom P: Immunohistochemical demonstration of laminin, the major glycoprotein of basement membranes, as an aid in the diagnosis of soft tissue tumors. *Am J Clin Pathol* 1983;79:306–311.

Miettinen M, Lehto V-P, Badley RA, et al: Expression of intermediate filaments in soft tissue sarcomas. *Int J Cancer* 1982;30:541–546.

Mukai K, Schollmeyer JV, Rosai J: Immunohistochemical localization of actin: Applications in surgical pathology. *Am J Surg Pathol* 1981;5:91–97.

Osborn M, Weber K: Biology of disease: Tumor diagnosis by intermediate filament typing: A novel tool for surgical pathology. *Lab Invest* 1983;48:327–394.

TISSUE MONOSPECIFIC AND OLIGOSPECIFIC ANTIGENS

Bender RA, Weintraub BD, Rosen SW: Prospective evaluation of two tumor-associated proteins in pancreatic adenocarcinoma. *Cancer* 1979;43:591–595.

Cordon-Cardo C, Bander NH, Fradet Y, et al: Immunoanatomic dissection of the human urinary tract by monoclonal antibodies. *J Histochem Cytochem* 1984;32:1035–1040.

Dippold WG, Lloyd KO, Li LTC, et al: Cell surface antigens of human malignant melanoma: Definition of six antigenic systems with mouse monoclonal antibodies. *Proc Natl Acad Sci USA* 1980;77:6114–6118.

Houghton AN, Eisenger A, Albino AP, et al: Surface antigens of melanocytes and melanomas: Markers of melanocyte differentiation and melanoma subsets. *J Exp Med* 1982;156:1755–1766.

Loor R, Kuriyama M, Bodziak MLM, et al: Simultaneous evaluation of a pancreas-specific antigen and a pancreatic-cancer associated antigen in pancreatic carcinoma. *Cancer Res* 1984;44:3604–3607.

Marko O, Houghton AN, Eisinger M: Purification of human melanocytes by monoclonal antibody combined with Percoll gradients. *Exp Cell Res* 1982;142:309–315.

Pukel CS, Lloyd KO, Travassos LR, et al: GD_3, a prominent ganglioside of human melanoma: Detection and characterization by monoclonal antibody. *J Exp Med* 1982;155:1133–1147.

Sloane JP, Ormerod MG: Distribution of epithelial membrane antigen in normal and neoplastic tissues and its value in diagnostic tumor pathology. *Cancer* 1981;47:1786–1795.

Ueda R, Ogata SI, Morrissey DM, et al: Cell surface antigens of human renal cancer defined by mouse monoclonal antibodies: Identification of tissue-specific kidney glycoproteins. *Proc Natl Acad Sci USA* 1981;78:5122–5126.

Warnke RA, Gatter KC, Falini B, et al: Diagnosis of human lymphoma with monoclonal anti-leukocyte antibodies. *N Engl J Med* 1983;309:1275–1281.

DIAGNOSTIC EFFICIENCY ASSESSMENTS

Galen RS: Application of the predictive-value model in the analysis of test effectiveness. *Clin Lab Med* 1982;2:685–699.

Sedmak DD, Tubbs RR, Galen RS: The diagnostic utility of monoclonal antibodies to tumor-associated antigens in surgical pathology. *Am J Clin Pathol* 1985;83:260.

IN SITU HYBRIDIZATION APPLICATIONS

Myerson D, Hackman RC, Nelson JA, et al: Widespread presence of histologically occult cytomegalovirus. *Hum Pathol* 1984;15:430–439.

HORMONE RECEPTORS

King WJ, Greene GL: Monoclonal antibodies localize receptors in the nuclei of target cells. *Nature* 1984;I:745–748.

McCarty KS, McCarty KS: Histochemical approaches to steroid receptor analyses. *Semin Diagn Pathol* 1984;2:297–308.

ONCOGENE PRODUCTS

Thor A, Hand PH, Wunderlich D, et al: Monoclonal antibodies define differential *ras* gene expression in malignant and benign colonic diseases. *Nature* 1984;311:562–565.

Glossary of Abbreviations

ABC avidin-biotin complex
ABC-AP avidin-biotinylated alkaline phosphatase complex
ABC-GO avidin-biotinylated glucose oxidase complex
ABC-PO avidin-biotinylated peroxidase complex
ACTH adrenocorticotropic hormone
AEC aminoethylcarbazole, or 3-amino-9-ethylcarbazole
APAAP alkaline phosphatase–anti-alkaline phosphatase
CALLA common acute lymphocytic leukemia antigen
CEA carcinoembryonic antigen
4CN 4-chloro-1-naphthol
CLA common leukocyte antigen
DAB 3,3′-diaminobenzidine
EM electron micrograph
FSH follicle-stimulating hormone
GFAP glial fibrillary acidic protein
GH growth hormone
HBcAg hepatitis-B core antigen
HBsAg hepatitis-B surface antigen
HCG human chorionic gonadotropin
β-HCG beta subunit of HCG
H & E hematoxylin and eosin
HPO horseradish peroxidase
HYR Hanker-Yates reagent (*p*-phenylenediamine and pyrocatechol)
Ig immunoglobulin
IMP immunoperoxidase
IMPAS immunoperoxidase with periodic acid–Schiff counterstain
κ κ immunoglobulin light chain
λ λ immunoglobulin light chain
LH luteinizing hormone
MPD *m*-phenylenediamine
MW molecular weight
OPD *o*-phenylenediamine
PAP peroxidase-antiperoxidase
PAS periodic acid–Schiff
PBS phosphate-buffered saline
SLE systemic lupus erythematosus
TMB tetramethylbenzidine
TSH thyroid-stimulating hormone
VIP vasoactive intestinal polypeptide

Index

Pages on which color illustrations appear are indicated in **bold.** Pages on which tables appear are indicated in *italics*. Slide numbers refer to the slides in the optional slide set.